.

Diseases of Companion Animals

Diseases of Companion Animals

Edited by Isabela Burton

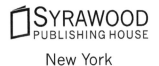
SYRAWOOD
PUBLISHING HOUSE

New York

Published by Syrawood Publishing House,
750 Third Avenue, 9th Floor,
New York, NY 10017, USA
www.syrawoodpublishinghouse.com

Diseases of Companion Animals
Edited by Isabela Burton

International Standard Book Number: 978-1-64740-375-1 (Hardback)

Trademark Notice: Registered trademark of products or corporate names are used only for explanation and identification without intent to infringe.

Cataloging-in-publication Data

Diseases of companion animals / edited by Isabela Burton.
    p. cm.
Includes bibliographical references and index.
ISBN 978-1-64740-375-1
1. Pets--Diseases. 2. Domestic animals--Diseases. 3. Pets. I. Burton, Isabela.
SF981 .D57 2023
636.089--dc23

TABLE OF CONTENTS

Preface...IX

Chapter 1   **Evaluation of Electrolyte Concentration and Pro-Inflammatory and Oxidative Status in Dogs with Advanced Chronic Kidney Disease under Dietary Treatment**.......................1
Doris Pereira Halfen, Douglas Segalla Caragelasco,
Juliana Paschoalin de Souza Nogueira, Juliana Toloi Jeremias, Vivian Pedrinelli,
Patrícia Massae Oba, Bruna Ruberti, Cristiana Fonseca Ferreira Pontieri,
Marcia Mery Kogika and Marcio Antonio Brunetto

Chapter 2   **Feline Infectious Peritonitis as a Systemic Inflammatory Disease: Contribution of Liver and Heart to the Pathogenesis**.......................12
Alexandra J Malbon, Sonja Fonfara, Marina L Meli, Shelley Hahn,
Herman Egberink and Anja Kipar

Chapter 3   **Prevalence of the Mutations Responsible for Glanzmann Thrombasthenia in Horses**.......................28
Raíssa O. Leite, Júlia F. Ferreira, César E. T. Araújo, Diego J. Z. Delfiol,
Regina K. Takahira, Alexandre S. Borges and Jose P. Oliveira-Filho

Chapter 4   **Deleterious *AGXT* Missense Variant Associated with Type 1 Primary Hyperoxaluria (PH1) in Zwartbles Sheep**.......................32
Anna Letko, Reinie Dijkman, Ben Strugnell, Irene M. Häfliger, Julia M. Paris,
Katrina Henderson, Tim Geraghty, Hannah Orr,
Sandra Scholes and Cord Drögemüller

Chapter 5   **A Deletion in *GDF7* is Associated with a Heritable Forebrain Commissural Malformation Concurrent with Ventriculomegaly and Interhemispheric Cysts in Cats**.......................41
Yoshihiko Yu, Erica K. Creighton, Reuben M. Buckley and Leslie A. Lyons

Chapter 6   ***LAMB3* Missense Variant in Australian Shepherd Dogs with Junctional Epidermolysis Bullosa**.......................56
Sarah Kiener, Aurore Laprais, Elizabeth A. Mauldin, Vidhya Jagannathan,
Thierry Olivry and Tosso Leeb

Chapter 7   ***NSDHL* Frameshift Deletion in a Mixed Breed Dog with Progressive Epidermal Nevi**.......................66
Matthias Christen, Michaela Austel, Frane Banovic,
Vidhya Jagannathan and Tosso Leeb

Chapter 8   **A *CNTNAP1* Missense Variant is Associated with Canine Laryngeal Paralysis and Polyneuropathy**.......................74
Anna Letko, Katie M. Minor, Steven G. Friedenberg, G. Diane Shelton,
Jill Pesayco Salvador, Paul J. J. Mandigers, Peter A. J. Leegwater, Paige A.Winkler,
Simon M. Petersen-Jones, Bryden J. Stanley, Kari J. Ekenstedt, Gary S. Johnson,
Liz Hansen, Vidhya Jagannathan, James R. Mickelson and Cord Drögemüller

Chapter 9   **A Missense Variant Affecting the C-Terminal Tail of UNC93B1 in Dogs with Exfoliative Cutaneous Lupus Erythematosus (ECLE)**............................88
Tosso Leeb, Fabienne Leuthard, Vidhya Jagannathan, Sarah Kiener, Anna Letko,
Petra Roosje, Monika M. Welle, Katherine L. Gailbreath, Andrea Cannon,
Monika Linek, Frane Banovic, Thierry Olivry, Stephen D. White, Kevin Batcher,
Danika Bannasch, Katie M. Minor, James R. Mickelson, Marjo K. Hytönen,
Hannes Lohi, Elizabeth A. Mauldin and Margret L. Casal

Chapter 10   **Deletion in the Bardet–Biedl Syndrome Gene *TTC8* Results in a Syndromic Retinal Degeneration in Dogs**............................98
Suvi Mäkeläinen, Minas Hellsand, Anna Darlene van der Heiden, Elina Andersson,
Elina Thorsson, Bodil S. Holst, Jens Häggström, Ingrid Ljungvall, Cathryn Mellersh,
Finn Hallböök, Göran Andersson, Björn Ekesten and Tomas F. Bergström

Chapter 11   **Mapping of Diabetes Susceptibility Loci in a Domestic Cat Breed with an Unusually High Incidence of Diabetes Mellitus**............................125
Lois Balmer, Caroline Ann O'Leary, Marilyn Menotti-Raymond, Victor David,
Stephen O'Brien, Belinda Penglis, Sher Hendrickson, Mia Reeves-Johnson,
Susan Gottlieb, Linda Fleeman, Dianne Vankan, Jacquie Rand and Grant Morahan

Chapter 12   **Whole Genome Sequencing Indicates Heterogeneity of Hyperostotic Disorders in Dogs**............................136
Anna Letko, Fabienne Leuthard, Vidhya Jagannathan, Daniele Corlazzoli,
Kaspar Matiasek, Daniela Schweizer, Marjo K. Hytönen, Hannes Lohi,
Tosso Leeb and Cord Drögemüller

Chapter 13   **Mitochondrial PCK2 Missense Variant in Shetland Sheepdogs with Paroxysmal Exercise-Induced Dyskinesia (PED)**............................147
Jasmin Nessler, Petra Hug, Paul J. J. Mandigers, Peter A. J. Leegwater,
Vidhya Jagannathan, Anibh M. Das, Marco Rosati, Kaspar Matiasek,
Adrian C. Sewell, Marion Kornberg, Marina Hoffmann, Petra Wolf,
Andrea Fischer, Andrea Tipold and Tosso Leeb

Chapter 14   ***SLC19A3* Loss-of-Function Variant in Yorkshire Terriers with Leigh-Like Subacute Necrotizing Encephalopathy**............................161
Michaela Drögemüller, Anna Letko, Kaspar Matiasek, Vidhya Jagannathan,
Daniele Corlazzoli, Marco Rosati, Konrad Jurina, Susanne Medl, Thomas Gödde,
Stefan Rupp, Andrea Fischer, Alejandro Luján Feliu-Pascual and Cord Drögemüller

Chapter 15   ***ATP2A2* SINE Insertion in an Irish Terrier with Darier Disease and Associated Infundibular Cyst Formation**............................169
Monika Linek, Maren Doelle, Tosso Leeb, Anina Bauer, Fabienne Leuthard,
Jan Henkel, Danika Bannasch, Vidhya Jagannathan and Monika M. Welle

Chapter 16   **The Genetic Basis of Obesity and Related Metabolic Diseases in Humans and Companion Animals**............................180
Natalie Wallis and Eleanor Raffan

Chapter 17   **A Missense Variant in *ALDH5A1* Associated with Canine Succinic Semialdehyde Dehydrogenase Deficiency (SSADHD) in the Saluki Dog**............................209
Karen M. Vernau, Eduard Struys, Anna Letko, Kevin D. Woolard, Miriam Aguilar,
Emily A. Brown, Derek D. Cissell, Peter J. Dickinson, G. Diane Shelton,
Michael R. Broome, K. Michael Gibson, Phillip L. Pearl, Florian König,
Thomas J. Van Winkle, Dennis O'Brien, B. Roos, Kaspar Matiasek,
Vidhya Jagannathan, Cord Drögemüller, Tamer A. Mansour,
C. Titus Brown and Danika L. Bannasch

Chapter 18   **X-Linked Duchenne-Type Muscular Dystrophy in Jack Russell Terrier Associated with a Partial Deletion of the Canine *DMD* Gene**...229
Barbara Brunetti, Luisa V. Muscatello, Anna Letko, Valentina Papa,
Giovanna Cenacchi, Marco Grillini, Leonardo Murgiano,
Vidhya Jagannathan and Cord Drögemüller

Permissions

List of Contributors

Index

PREFACE

Companion animals are the animals which are domesticated primarily for providing companionship or amusement rather than being used as a working animal, a laboratory animal, or livestock. Cats, birds, rabbits, guinea pigs, dogs, horses, ferrets, small fishes and certain reptiles are kept as companion animals. This excludes all types of wild animals and poultry. Various diseases affect the companion animals such as Canine influenza, Canine parvovirus, External parasites, cryptococcosis, rabies, Salmonellosis, Cryptosporidiosis, Giardiasis, anthrax, black quarter, foot-and-mouth disease, mastitis, equine infectious anemia virus, west nile virus, streptococcus equi, and tetanus. There are a number of diseases that can spread from animals to humans, and are called zoonotic diseases. Some of the diseases of companion animals include leptospirosis, campylobacteriosis, salmonellosis, rabies, influenza, brucellosis, and plague. This book unravels the recent studies on the diseases which affect companion animals. It will prove to be immensely beneficial to students and researchers in the field of veterinary science.

This book is the end result of constructive efforts and intensive research done by experts in this field. The aim of this book is to enlighten the readers with recent information in this area of research. The information provided in this profound book would serve as a valuable reference to students and researchers in this field.

At the end, I would like to thank all the authors for devoting their precious time and providing their valuable contribution to this book. I would also like to express my gratitude to my fellow colleagues who encouraged me throughout the process.

Editor

Evaluation of Electrolyte Concentration and Pro-Inflammatory and Oxidative Status in Dogs with Advanced Chronic Kidney Disease under Dietary Treatment

Doris Pereira Halfen [1], Douglas Segalla Caragelasco [1], Juliana Paschoalin de Souza Nogueira [2], Juliana Toloi Jeremias [3], Vivian Pedrinelli [1], Patrícia Massae Oba [2], Bruna Ruberti [1], Cristiana Fonseca Ferreira Pontieri [3], Marcia Mery Kogika [1,*] and Marcio Antonio Brunetto [1]

[1] School of Veterinary Medicine and Animal Science, University of São Paulo, Av. Prof. Dr. Orlando Marques de Paiva, 87, Cidade Universitária, São Paulo, SP 05508-270, Brazil; dorisph2@yahoo.com.br (D.P.H.); mv.douglas@yahoo.com.br (D.S.C.); vivian.pedrinelli@gmail.com (V.P.); brunaruberti@usp.br (B.R.); mabrunetto@usp.br (M.A.B.)

[2] Animal Sciences Department, College of Agricultural, Consumer & Environmental Sciences, University of Illinois at Urbana-Champaign, Champaign, IL 217-333-3131, USA; juliana_nog@hotmail.com (J.P.d.S.N.); obapm@illinois.edu (P.M.O.)

[3] Nutrition Development Center, Grand Food Industria e Comercio Ltda (Premier Pet), Dourado, SP 13590-000, Brazil; jjeremias@premierpet.com.br (J.T.J.); cristiana@premierpet.com.br (C.F.F.P.)

* Correspondence: mmkogika@usp.br

Abstract: An integrated study on the effect of renal diet on mineral metabolism, fibroblast growth factor 23 (FGF-23), total antioxidant capacity, and inflammatory markers has not been performed previously. In this study, we evaluated the effects of renal diet on mineral metabolism, oxidative stress and inflammation in dogs with stage 3 or 4 of chronic kidney disease (CKD). Body condition score (BCS), muscle condition score (MCS), serum biochemical profile, ionized calcium (i-Ca), total calcium (t-Ca), phosphorus (P), urea, creatinine, parathyroid hormone (PTH), FGF-23, interleukin 6 (IL-6), interleukin 10 (IL-10), tumor necrosis factor alpha (TNF-α) and total antioxidant capacity (TAC) were measured at baseline (T0) and after 6 months of dietary treatment (T6). Serum urea, P, t-Ca, i-Ca, PTH, FGF-23, IL-6, IL-10, TNF-α and TAC measurements did not differ between T0 and T6. Serum creatinine (SCr) was increased at T6 and serum PTH concentrations were positively correlated with serum SCr and urea. i-Ca was negatively correlated with urea and serum phosphorus was positively correlated with FGF-23. Urea and creatinine were positively correlated. The combination of renal diet and support treatment over 6 months in dogs with CKD stage 3 or 4 was effective in controlling uremia, acid–base balance, blood pressure, total antioxidant capacity, and inflammatory cytokine levels and in maintaining BCS and MCS.

Keywords: secondary renal hyperparathyroidism; oxidative stress; inflammation; canine

Key Contribution: This is the first study to our knowledge to analyze the FGF-23 concentrations in dogs with advanced chronic kidney disease under dietary treatment.

1. Introduction

Chronic kidney disease (CKD) is considered the most common renal disease in dogs [1]. Throughout the progression of this disease, several changes occur in the organism, such as disorders of calcium and phosphorus metabolism, development of secondary renal hyperparathyroidism (SRHP), and increases in serum fibroblast growth factor 23 (FGF-23), oxidative stress and inflammation [2–12]. There is consensus that use of renal diets is essential for decreasing the progression rate of CKD and improving the survival of affected animals [13–20]. In addition to the restriction of protein and phosphorus, ω-3 polyunsaturated fatty acids (PUFAs) can attenuate the inflammatory process of CKD, and antioxidants may attenuate oxidative stress [7,21–23]. FGF-23 is a phosphatonin that is involved in the pathogenesis of mineral metabolism in CKD [24]. However, few studies in animals have been conducted to study the effects of dietary modulation of FGF-23 [25–28]. SRHP is one of the consequences of CKD, and parathyroid hormone (PTH) is considered a major uremic toxin [3,5]. Reactive oxygen species (ROS) are usually formed at a low rate in renal tissue; however, in CKD, the remaining nephrons are hyperfunctioning, increasing oxidative phosphorylation and ROS production [29]. Oxidative stress generates tissue injury and inflammation, directly contributing to the progression of CKD [11,30,31] as inflammatory cytokines increase protein catabolism and inhibit appetite, exacerbating cachexia [11,32,33]. In addition, scientific evidence indicates that patients with CKD have antioxidant and ω-3 PUFAs deficiencies and that those nutrients are capable of reducing inflammation [6,7,23,34]. Although studies have reported associations among oxidative stress, inflammation, and mineral metabolism, few have investigated dietary interactions with these parameters in dogs. The present study aimed to evaluate the effects of a renal diet in dogs with CKD stage 3 or 4, on mineral metabolism, blood pressure, acid–base balance, body condition score (BCS), muscle condition score (MCS), inflammatory cytokine levels, and total antioxidant capacity (TAC).

2. Results

2.1. Animals

Ten client-owned dogs were enrolled with a mean ± SD body weight of 16.33 ±14.64 kg, a mean age of 8.89 ± 4.46 years, various breeds and seven out of 10 were females and three of them were sterilized. Diagnosis of CKD was based on persistent azotemia over 3 months as well as imaging (ultrasound) findings of chronic kidney abnormalities. CKD classification was according to IRIS and 80% of CKD dogs were in stage 3 at T0 [35]. All animals had good acceptance of the diet, though one animal experienced an episode of diarrhea during the diet change. Three animals needed treatment with 1–2 mg/kg BW H_2 blockers (ranitidine) every 8 or 12 h and sodium bicarbonate according to blood gas results. Two animals required 0.5–1 mg/kg BW appetite stimulants (cyproheptadine hydrochloride) every 12 h, and five animals were treated with 30–60 mg/kg BW/day phosphorus binder (aluminum hydroxide). One animal had an episode of acute decompensation of CKD and received medical treatment. Dogs were also closely monitored to detect dehydration and no parenteral fluid administration was needed, excepted for that dog that had acute renal dysfunction. Free access of tap water was assured.

2.2. Body Weight, BCS and MCS

A reduction in body weight was observed between T0 (16.34 ± 14.64 kg) and T6 (14.78 ± 13.32 kg; $p = 0.045$). However, BCS (T0: 5.70 ± 0.67 versus T6: 5.30 ± 1.05) and MCS (T0: 2.20 ± 0.42 versus T6: 2.40 ± 0.51) showed no significant differences ($p = 0.375$ and $p = 0.625$, respectively) between T0 and T6.

2.3. Urine Profile

Urinary pH remained within the reference range during the experiment, without a difference between T0 and T6 ($p = 0.687$). No differences in urine specific gravity (USG) were found between the two time points, showing isosthenuria at both times ($p = 0.384$) (Table 1). Proteinuria by semi quantitative method was not found by urine dipstick analysis along the period of observation.

Table 1. Urine pH, urine specific gravity, systolic blood pressure, blood pH and blood bicarbonate concentration parameters during the 6-month follow-up compared to the initial value.

Variables	T0 (n = 10)	T6 (n = 10)	p Value
Urine pH	6.50 ± 1.08	6.40 ± 0.96	0.687
Urine specific gravity	1.014 ± 0.006	1.016 ± 0.004	0.384
Systolic blood pressure (mmHg)	138.8 ± 8.3	138.4 ± 5.49	0.853
Blood pH	7.33 ± 0.04	7.32 ± 0.07	0.704
Blood bicarbonate (mEq/L)	21.36 ± 1.96	19.64 ± 2.67	0.072

T0, baseline; T6, 6-month time point. Data are presented as the mean ± SD.

2.4. Blood Pressure

Systolic blood pressure was within the reference range [36] and showed no difference ($p = 0.853$) between T0 and T6 (138.4 ± 5.49 mmHg) (Table 1).

2.5. Acid–Base Balance

Blood pH ($p = 0.704$) and blood bicarbonate concentration ($p = 0.072$) showed no differences between the two time points and were within the reference range (Table 1).

2.6. Biochemical Profile

Serum triglycerides (T0: 47.70 mg/dL versus T6: 41.29 mg/dL; RI, 20–112) and serum cholesterol were slightly elevated at T0 and T6 (T0: 294 ± 80.20 mg/dL versus T6: 274.40 ± 100.14 mg/dL, RI 125–270 mg/dL), but only cholesterol was significantly different between assessment periods ($p = 0.0350$). Sodium (T0: 146.36 mEq/L versus T6: 148.54 mEq/L; RI, 143–148 mEq/L), potassium (T0: 4.53 mmol/L versus T6: 4.66 mmol/L; RI, 4.37–5.65 mmol/L), alanine aminotransferase (ALT) (T0: 54.45 UI/L versus T6: 35.29 UI/L; RI, 10–88 UI/L) and alkaline phosphatase (ALP) (T0: 40.87 UI/L versus T6: 27.59 UI/L; RI, 20–150 UI/L) were within the reference ranges at both time points. Moreover, serum total protein (T0: 6.12 ± 0.45 g/dL versus T6: 6.17 ± 0.63 g/dL; RI 5.3–7.6 g/dL) and albumin (T0: 3.23 ± 0.16 g/dL versus T6: 3.18 ± 0.42 g/dL; RI 2.3–3.8 g/dL) did not differ between T0 and T6 ($p = 0.777$ and $p = 1.000$, respectively). The packed cell volume (PCV) showed a decrease between T0 (35.3 ± 6.83%) and T6 (31.2 ± 6.74%; $p = 0.032$) and was below reference values at both points (RI 37–55%). Notably, serum creatinine (SCr) was increased at T6 ($p = 0.0022$; Table 2). Serum urea, phosphorus, total calcium (t-Ca) and ionized calcium (i-Ca) showed no difference between time points ($p = 0.187$, 0.630, 0.312, and 0.232, respectively; Table 2).

Table 2. Serum urea, creatinine, phosphorus, total calcium, ionic calcium, PTH and fibroblast growth factor 23 (FGF-23) concentrations and number of dogs who had increased or decreased parameters during the 6-month follow-up compared to the initial value.

Variables	T0 (n = 10)	T6 (n = 10)	p Value
Creatinine (mg/dL)	3.11 ± 1.06	4.30 ± 1.71	0.002
Urea (mg/dL)	206.07 ± 44.69	235.34 ± 74.24	0.187
Phosphorus (mg/dL)	5.15 ± 1.46	5.36 ± 1.05	0.630
Total calcium (mg/dL)	11.33 ± 1.11	11.94 ± 1.85	0.312
Ionized calcium (mmol/L)	1.41 ± 0.08	1.38 ± 0.11	0.232
PTH (pg/mL)	145.81 ± 190.69	336.48 ± 392.48	0.125
FGF-23 (pg/mL)	5645.67 ± 4720.67	5788.56 ± 5655.2	0.858

T0, baseline; T6, 6-month time point; PTH, parathyroid hormone; FGF-23, fibroblast growth factor 23. Data are presented as the mean ± SD.

2.7. PTH and FGF-23

Serum PTH and FGF-23 showed no difference between T0 and T6 ($p = 0.125$ and 0.858, respectively; Table 2).

2.8. Correlation between PTH, Total Calcium, Ionized Calcium, Phosphorus, FGF-23, Creatinine and Urea

PTH concentration was positively correlated with creatinine ($r = 0.45$; $p < 0.05$) and urea ($r = 0.67$; $p < 0.01$), and i-Ca had a negative correlation with urea ($r = -0.59$; $p < 0.01$). Urea and SCr were positively correlated ($r = 0.45$; $p < 0.05$), and FGF-23 was positively correlated with phosphorus ($r = 0.51$; $p < 0.05$).

2.9. Cytokines and TAC

The serum cytokines interleukin 6 (IL-6), interleukin 10 (IL-10), and tumor necrosis factor alpha (TNF-α) and TAC showed no difference between T0 and T6 ($p = 0.148$, 0.627, 0.289, and 0.6758, respectively; Table 3).

Table 3. Serum concentrations of the IL-6, IL-10 and TNF-α cytokines and the number of animals that had increased or decreased cytokine levels at the 6-month follow-up.

Variables	T0 (n = 10)	T6 (n = 10)	p Value
IL-6 (pg/mL)	52.67 ± 116.28	97.26 ± 138.13	0.148
IL-10 (pg/mL)	6.93 ± 10.11	9.04 ± 11.16	0.627
TNF-α (pg/mL)	9.34 ± 20.14	15.87 ± 23.65	0.289
TAC (µmol) [3]	50.64 ± 46.74	62.71 ± 62.63	0.675

T0, baseline; T6, 6-month time point; IL-6, interleukin 6; IL-10, interleukin 10; TNF-α, tumor necrosis factor alpha; TAC, total antioxidant capacity. Data are presented as the mean ± SD.

3. Discussion

Few studies have evaluated the role of the renal diet in CKD at different stages of the disease [14,15,20]. In the present study, the effects of a renal diet on advanced CKD in dogs were evaluated, and most of the parameters assessed were stable after feeding with renal diet and therapeutic support. Although some animals lost weight, the dietary intake was able to maintain an ideal BCS [37] and prevent the loss of MCS in the majority of animals. The maintenance of a BCS over a 3/9 score has been associated with a lower mortality rate and is an indicator of better prognosis in CKD patients [38,39].

The severity of anemia is proportional to the loss of kidney function [1], and in this study, PCV decreased between T0 and T6. Almost all dogs were able to maintain acid–base balance. Since there is an increased glomerular filtration rate (GFR) per nephron, the excretion of fixed buffers is also increased, and consequently, the excretion rate of acid titratable by the kidneys remains stable until the advanced stages of CKD [40]. Additionally, dogs with stage 3 CKD had higher bicarbonate resorption in the proximal and distal tubules compared to dogs in stage 1, showing renal adaptation, even in advanced CKD stages [41].

Feeding a renal diet did not prevent the increase in SCr; thus, the progression of renal disease was not avoided. Although the renal diet cannot itself prevent the progression of the disease, it may help to increase longevity and improve quality of life [14]. Serum phosphorus stability during the trial suggests that the combination of coadjuvant diet and therapeutic treatment was effective in maintaining a constant concentration, even with advanced CKD. Dietary restriction of phosphorus contributes to slowing the disease progression rate, as it helps to maintain phosphorus concentrations [1].

Accumulation of phosphate, caused by renal impairment, favors ionized hypocalcemia [1,42]. Both serum i-Ca and t-Ca levels remained constant during the trial, which may be positive since hypocalcemia is frequent in CKD patients, especially in the advanced stages [3,5,43]. In previous studies, the prediction of serum calcium concentration by t-Ca measurement in dogs with CKD had a 55% diagnostic discordance [42], and the correlation between t-Ca and i-Ca indicated that only 25% of the variation in t-Ca could be explained by i-Ca variation [43].

Serum PTH did not differ between T0 and T6. High levels of PTH were already expected, and one objective of this study was to maintain the stability of PTH since there is evidence that the development of SRHP occurs in the early stages of CKD and reaches up to 100% in stage 4 [3,5]. There was considerable variation in the results at T0 and T6, which may be explained by the small number of animals. Notably, high variance in PTH results was also reported in another study [44]. The main regulatory factor of PTH secretion is serum calcium, which varies inversely with its concentration, and small i-Ca oscillations cause large variations in PTH secretion [40]. In a previous study on dogs with CKD, the renal diet was unable to prevent the increase in PTH, although the animals had fewer uremic crises and increased survival time compared to the group fed a maintenance diet [15]. In the present study, serum PTH showed a positive correlation with creatinine and urea, but the correlation with phosphorus was not significant, although other studies have identified a positive correlation between PTH and phosphorus [3,5,44,45]. Similar to the present study, a previous report did not find a relationship between PTH and phosphorus and suggested that other variables in addition to phosphorus and calcium may be involved in the regulation of PTH. The positive correlation with creatinine and urea was expected because, with the deterioration of renal function, PTH concentrations tend to increase as a compensatory mechanism to maintain phosphate concentrations [4].

The increase in FGF-23 has been shown to occur prior to changes in calcium, phosphorus or PTH concentrations, which is why this metabolite has been considered one of the first biomarkers of CKD [12,25,27,46,47]. Therefore, high concentrations of FGF-23 were already expected in animals in advanced stages of the disease. Mean FGF-23 values were higher in dogs with CKD fed a renal diet than in healthy animals [26]. In the present study, the mean FGF-23 concentrations remained stable after consuming the renal diet for six months, which may have occurred because the concentrations of phosphorus, PTH, i-Ca, and t-Ca remained stable as well. In a study on cats diagnosed with CKD, feeding a renal diet for 12 months was able to reduce serum FGF-23, phosphate and PTH in hyperphosphatemic cats [28]. In the present study, a positive correlation between phosphorus and FGF-23 was found, which was expected since FGF-23 is a phosphatonin and the small number of animals could have made it difficult to find other correlations between these parameters.

The maintenance of values of TNF-α, IL-6, and IL-10 may be considered a positive result since they are usually increased in humans with CKD [48,49] due to decreased renal clearance and increased production of proinflammatory cytokines [10]. IL-10 is mainly eliminated by the kidneys, and thus, its plasma half-life may be increased in renal failure [11,50,51]. Furthermore, diets are known to influence the reduction in inflammation through the action of ω-3 PUFAs [7,21,52–54]. Higher ω-3 concentrations can modulate the production of eicosanoids, which is less potent in inducing vasoconstriction and aggregation [7,21,52]. Therefore, higher concentrations of ω-3 PUFAs, as used in the present study, may be required to control the immune response in advanced CKD stages.

No difference in TAC was found in the literature between CKD and healthy cats and dogs, corroborating the results found in this study and suggesting that systemic antioxidant defense systems might not be exhausted in CKD [8,55,56]. Evidence indicates that CKD is a pro-oxidative state [57–61] and that malnutrition status in advanced CKD patients usually culminates in a reduction in antioxidant vitamins [6,7]. This study cannot ensure that the diet was fundamental to the stabilization of TAC because all animals consumed the same diet enriched with antioxidants, but dietary supplementation with antioxidants is known to benefit CKD animals, reducing oxidative stress [22,23].

The limitations of the present study were the small size of the sample, no control group, and no urine protein:creatinine ratio (UPC) analysis, as well as different treatments that had to be initiated to control clinical and laboratory alterations. The best delineation would be the inclusion of a group of animals with CKD fed with a maintenance diet. However, the use of a maintenance diet in this situation may reduce the life expectancy of the dogs included in the control group. In advanced stages of CKD, finding animals with stable renal function and no appetite changes is difficult.

4. Conclusions

In conclusion, feeding dogs with advanced CKD with a renal diet for 6 months in combination with support treatment was effective in controlling uremia, acid–base balance, blood pressure, antioxidant capacity, and production of inflammatory cytokines, as well as in the maintenance of BCS and MCS. Further studies are needed to better explore how a renal diet can improve the quality of life in CKD dogs.

5. Materials and Methods

5.1. Animals and Study Design

This study was conducted at the Veterinary Hospital of the School of Veterinary Medicine and Animal Science of the University of São Paulo (FMVZ/USP), São Paulo—SP, Brazil and approved by the Ethics Committee of the Veterinary Medicine and Animal Science School of the University of São Paulo (FMVZ/USP) on 4 September 2013, protocol number 3138/2013. The research was a prospective, 6-month longitudinal dietary trial utilizing a before (T0) and after (T6) design. Ten client-owned dogs with CKD at stage 3 or 4 [35] were included. The dogs had a stable renal function, without symptoms such as anorexia or impairment of appetite, nausea/vomiting or associated conditions, and had not consumed a renal diet previously.

5.2. Diet and Feeding Protocol

Nutritional contents of the diet were balanced and met all requirements for the maintenance of adult dogs [62,63]; however, the diet had a baseline concentration of protein and phosphorus and the addition of ω-3 PUFAs and vitamin E, as described in Table 4. Owners received the recommendation that no other food should be provided. Adherence to the balanced diet was assessed through a questionnaire applied monthly when the dogs returned to the hospital for recheck. There was a 4 day adaptation period to the new diet when prior food and the experimental diet were mixed (Appendix A—a). The amount of food to be fed daily was calculated using the equation: 95 kcal × (body weight) 0.75/day [62]. The result was divided by the metabolizable energy of the diet to calculate daily food intake.

Table 4. Diet composition * as fed and per 1000 kcal and ingredients according to the manufacturer.

	Nutrients	
	Per 100 g of diet	Per 1000 kcal
Dry matter (g)	90.00	–
Protein (g)	14.50	35.60
Fat (g)	18.00	44.20
Ash (g)	5.50	13.50
Crude fiber (g)	3.50	8.60
Minimum calcium (g)	0.40	0.98
Maximum calcium (g)	0.90	2.21
Phosphorus (g/kg)	0.30	0.74
Potassium (g/kg)	0.60	1.47
Omega 6 (g)	2.00	4.91
Omega 3 (g)	0.52	1.27
EPA + DHA ** (g)	0.35	0.86
Food base excess (mEq)	11.30	27.75
Metabolizable energy (Kcal/g)	4.072 ***	

* Premier Nutrição Clínica Renal Cães. ** Eicosapentaenoic and Docosahexaenoic *** Metabolizable energy of the diet, previously calculated in a metabolism assay at the Premier Pet Center for Nutritional Development. * Ingredients: poultry meal, soy protein isolate, dried egg spray, broken rice, ground whole corn, barley, beet pulp, poultry fat, stabilized animal fat, fish oil, hydrolyzed poultry, antioxidants Buthylated Hydroxyanisole, potassium citrate, potassium chloride, dried brewer's yeast, vitamin and mineral premix.

5.3. Determination of Blood Pressure, BCS and MCS

Systolic blood pressure was measured indirectly with ultrasonic Doppler (Parks Medical® Model 811-B, Oregon, United States). Blood pressure was evaluated before any clinical examination or sample collection was performed. Six measurements were performed at each time point, and the mean value was recorded. The BCS was determined according to a nine-point scale [37], and MCS was determined using a four-point scale [64]. The same trained veterinarian determined the BCS and MCS at all times to reduce possible differences in the evaluation due to subjectivity.

5.4. Blood, Urine Sampling and Laboratory Evaluation

The periods of blood and urine collection were labeled as times, with T0 before animals received the diet, followed by subsequent times T1 (30 days after T0), T2 (60 days after T0), T3 (90 days after T0), T4 (120 days after T0), T5 (150 days after T0) and T6 (6 months after T0). After a 12 h fasting period, blood samples were obtained from all dogs for a complete blood count (CBC) and serum biochemistry [urea, SCr, albumin, total protein, globulins, glucose, triglycerides, cholesterol, ALP, ALT, sodium, potassium, i-Ca, t-Ca, and phosphorus]. For analysis of PTH, FGF-23, cytokines and TAC, blood samples were collected and immediately placed on ice and centrifuged at 4 °C later. Serum aliquots of 1 mL were stored at −80 °C. Urine samples were obtained by cystocentesis for urinalysis (urine dipstick analysis), USG (by refractometry method), urine culture and sediment microscopic examination. Blood pH and bicarbonate measurements were performed using a blood gas analyzer (Appendix A—b); blood was collected in syringes coated with lithium heparin (Blood Gas Monovette, Sarstedt, Nümbrecht, Germany) (Appendix A—b).

5.5. Additional Laboratory Evaluations

For PTH, serum samples stored at −80 °C were shipped to a reference laboratory (Appendix A—c), and the concentration was determined by radioimmunoassay. Samples used to assess TNF-α, IL-6 and IL-10 cytokines were sent to a commercial laboratory (Appendix A—d) and quantified by a cytokine panel (Appendix A—e) validated for dogs; TAC samples were sent to a commercial laboratory and measured using a commercial kit (Appendix A—f). TAC was measured by quantitative colorimetric assay. In this method, Cu^{2+} is reduced to Cu^+, and the resulting Cu^+ forms colorful complexes. The color intensity at 570 nm is proportional to the amount of TAC in the sample, and the antioxidant concentrations were expressed in μm Trolox equivalents. FGF-23 was analyzed with a human-specific FGF-23 ELISA (Appendix A—g) validated for dogs [26] according to the manufacturer's protocol, including dilution with the zero standard supplied in the assay kit.

5.6. Statistical Analysis

Statistical analyses were performed using statistical software—Statistical Analysis System (SAS) (Appendix A—h) (Statistical Analysis System 8.2, SAS Institute Inc., Cary, NC, USA). Data were assessed for normality by the Shapiro–Wilk test and tested for homogeneity by the F test. The results were arranged in 2 groups: CKD T0 (CKD dogs at baseline) and CKD T6 (CKD dogs after 6 months). The data were analyzed by a paired T-test (CKD T0 vs. CKD T6). If, after transformations, the results still had not reached normality and/or homogeneity, the data were analyzed by nonparametric statistics (SAS PROC NPAR1WAY) by the Wilcoxon test, corresponding to a paired T-test. The correlations between variables were analyzed by nonparametric statistics (Spearman correlation). Significance was set at $p \leq 0.05$. Although some variables were assessed throughout the study (every 30 days), the values at T0 and T6 were used for the statistical analyses. The data are expressed as the mean ± SD.

Author Contributions: Funding acquisition, M.M.K. and M.A.B.; Investigation, D.P.H., D.S.C., J.P.d.S.N., M.M.K. and M.A.B.; Methodology, D.P.H., D.S.C., J.P.d.S.N., J.T.J., C.F.F.P., M.M.K. and M.A.B.; Resources, J.T.J. and C.F.F.P.; Writing—original draft, D.P.H., C.F.F.P., M.M.K. and M.A.B.; Writing—review and editing, V.P., P.M.O. and B.R. All authors have read and agreed to the published version of the manuscript.

Acknowledgments: The authors are grateful to CAPES for the Ph.D. studentship awarded to the first author and to Premier Pet for financial support. The authors wish to thank all owners and their pets for participating in the study.

Appendix A

[a] The daily food requirement was calculated according to the NRC- National Research Council (NRC). *Nutrient Requirements of Dogs and Cats* (2006) adult dogs energy requirements for adult dogs, equation: 95 × (BW) 0.75 = Kcal/day divided by diet metabolizable energy;

[b] OMNI C, COBAS B 121—Roche®;

[c] Diagnostic Center for Population and Animal Health (DCPAH, Michigan State University, East Lansing, Michigan, USA);

[d] Specialized Laboratory in Scientific Analysis—LEAC, São Paulo—SP;

[e] Milliplex™ MAP kit CCYTO-90K-03 (MILLIPORE, Billerica, Massachusetts, USA);

[f] Quantichrom™ Antioxidant Assay (DTAC-100, Bioassay Systems, California, USA);

[g] Kainos, Tokyo, Japan;

[h] Statistical Analysis System 8.2, SAS Institute Inc., Cary, NC, USA.

References

1. Polzin, D.J. Chronic kidney disease. In *Nephrology and Urology of Small Animals*; Bartges, J., Polzin, D.J., Eds.; Blackwell Publishing: Ames, IA, USA, 2011; pp. 433–471.
2. Schenck, P.A.; Chew, D.J. Determination of calcium fractionation in dogs with chronic renal failure. *Am. J. Vet. Res.* **2003**, *64*, 1181–1184. [CrossRef]
3. Cortadellas, O.; Fernández del Palacio, M.J.; Talavera, J.; Bayón, A. Calcium and phosphorus homeostasis in dogs with spontaneous chronic kidney disease at different stages of severity. *J. Vet. Intern. Med.* **2010**, *24*, 73–79. [CrossRef] [PubMed]
4. Finch, N.C.; Syme, H.M.; Elliott, J. Parathyroid hormone concentration in geriatric cats with various degrees of renal function. *J. Am. Vet. Med. Assoc.* **2012**, *241*, 1326–1335. [CrossRef] [PubMed]
5. Barber, P.J.; Elliott, J. Feline chronic renal failure: Calcium homeostasis in 80 cases diagnosed between 1992 and 1995. *J. Small Anim. Pract.* **1998**, *39*, 108–116. [CrossRef] [PubMed]
6. Locatelli, F.; Canaud, B.; Eckardt, K.U.; Stenvinkel, P.; Wanner, C.; Zoccali, C. Oxidative stress in end-stage renal disease: An emerging treat to patient outcome. *Nephrol. Dial. Transplant.* **2003**, *18*, 1272–1280. [CrossRef] [PubMed]
7. Brown, S.A. Oxidative Stress and Chronic Kidney Disease. *Vet. Clin. North Am. Small Anim. Pract.* **2008**, *38*, 157–166. [CrossRef] [PubMed]
8. Krofič Žel, M.; Tozon, N.; Nemec Svete, A. Plasma and Erythrocyte Glutathione Peroxidase Activity, Serum Selenium Concentration, and Plasma Total Antioxidant Capacity in Cats with IRIS Stages I–IV Chronic Kidney Disease. *J. Vet. Intern. Med.* **2014**, *28*, 130–136. [CrossRef]
9. Keegan, R.; Webb, C. Oxidative stress and neutrophil function in cats with chronic renal failure. *J. Vet. Intern. Med.* **2010**, *24*, 514–519. [CrossRef]
10. Cheung, W.W.; Paik, K.H.; Mak, R.H. Inflammation and cachexia in chronic kidney disease. *Pediatr. Nephrol.* **2010**, *25*, 711–724. [CrossRef]
11. Stenvinkel, P.; Ketteler, M.; Johnson, R.J.; Lindholm, B.; Pecoits-Filho, R.; Riella, M.; Heimbürger, O.; Cederholm, T.; Girndt, M. IL-10, IL-6, and TNF-α: Central factors in the altered cytokine network of uremia—The good, the bad, and the ugly. *Kidney Int.* **2005**, *67*, 1216–1233. [CrossRef]
12. Hardcastle, M.R.; Dittmer, K.E. Fibroblast Growth Factor 23: A New Dimension to Diseases of Calcium-Phosphorus Metabolism. *Vet. Pathol.* **2015**, *52*, 770–784. [CrossRef] [PubMed]
13. Plantinga, E.; Everts, H.; Kastelein, A.; Beynen, A. Retrospective study of the survival of cats with acquired chronic renal insufficiency offered different commercial diets. *Vet. Rec.* **2005**, *157*, 185–187. [CrossRef] [PubMed]
14. Ross, S.J.; Osborne, C.A.; Kirk, C.A.; Lowry, S.R.; Koehler, L.A.; Polzin, D.J. Clinical evaluation of dietary modification for treatment of spontaneous chronic kidney disease in cats. *J. Am. Vet. Med. Assoc.* **2006**, *229*, 949–957. [CrossRef] [PubMed]
15. Jacob, F.; Polzin, D.J.; Osborne, C.A.; Allen, T.A.; Kirk, C.A.; Neaton, J.D.; Lekcharoensuk, C.; Swanson, L.L. Clinical evaluation of dietary modification for treatment of spontaneous chronic renal failure in dogs. *J. Am. Vet. Med. Assoc.* **2002**, *220*, 1163–1170. [CrossRef]

16. Polzin, D.; Osborne, C.; Hayden, D.; Stevens, J. Influence of reduced protein diets on morbidity, mortality, and renal function in dogs with induced chronic renal failure. *Am. J. Vet. Res.* **1984**, *45*, 506–517.

17. Burkholder, W.; Lees, G.; LeBlanc, A.; Slater, M.; Bauer, J.; Kashtan, C.; McCracken, B.; Hannah, S. Diet Modulates Proteinuria in Heterozygous Female Dogs with X-Linked Hereditary Nephropathy. *J. Vet. Intern. Med.* **2004**, *18*, 165–175. [CrossRef]

18. Elliott, J.; Rawlings, J.M.; Markwell, P.J.; Barber, P.J. Survival of cats with naturally occurring chronic renal failure: Effect of dietary management. *J. Small Anim. Pract.* **2000**, *41*, 235–242. [CrossRef]

19. Leibetseder, J.L.; Neufeld, K.W. Effects of Medium Protein Diets in Dogs with Chronic Renal Failure. *J. Nutr.* **1991**, *121*, S145–S149. [CrossRef]

20. Hall, J.A.; Fritsch, D.A.; Yerramilli, M.; Obare, E.; Yerramilli, M.; Jewell, D.E. A longitudinal study on the acceptance and effects of a therapeutic renal food in pet dogs with IRIS-Stage 1 chronic kidney disease. *J. Anim. Physiol. Anim. Nutr.* **2018**, *102*, 297–307. [CrossRef]

21. Brown, S.A.; Brown, C.A.; Crowell, W.A.; Barsanti, J.A.; Allen, T.; Cowell, C.; Finco, D.R. Beneficial effects of chronic administration of dietary ω-3 polyunsaturated fatty acids in dogs with renal insufficiency. *J. Lab. Clin. Med.* **1998**, *131*, 447–455. [CrossRef]

22. Yu, S.; Gross, K.; Allen, T. A renal food supplemented with vitamins E, C and beta-carotene reduces oxidative stress and improves kidney function in client-owned dogs with stages 2 or 3 kidney disease. *J. Vet. Intern. Med.* **2006**, *20*, 1537.

23. Yu, S.; Paetau-Robinson, I. Dietary supplements of vitamins E and C and β-carotene reduce oxidative stress in cats with renal insufficiency. *Vet. Res. Commun.* **2006**, *30*, 403–413. [CrossRef] [PubMed]

24. Moe, S.; Drüeke, T.; Cunningham, J.; Goodman, W.; Martin, K.; Olgaard, K.; Ott, S.; Sprague, S.; Lameire, N.; Eknoyan, G. Definition, evaluation, and classification of renal osteodystrophy: A position statement from Kidney Disease: Improving Global Outcomes (KDIGO). *Kidney Int.* **2006**, *69*, 1945–1953. [CrossRef] [PubMed]

25. Geddes, R.; Finch, N.; Elliott, J.; Syme, H. Fibroblast growth factor 23 in feline chronic kidney disease. *J. Vet. Intern. Med.* **2013**, *27*, 1407–1519. [CrossRef] [PubMed]

26. Harjes, L.M.; Parker, V.J.; Dembek, K.; Young, G.S.; Giovaninni, L.H.; Kogika, M.M.; Chew, D.J.; Toribio, R.E. Fibroblast Growth Factor-23 Concentration in Dogs with Chronic Kidney Disease. *J. Vet. Intern. Med.* **2017**, *31*, 784–790. [CrossRef]

27. Finch, N.; Geddes, R.; Syme, H.; Elliott, J. Fibroblast growth factor 23 (FGF-23) concentrations in cats with early nonazotemic chronic kidney disease (CKD) and in healthy geriatric cats. *J. Vet. Intern. Med.* **2013**, *27*, 227–233. [CrossRef]

28. Geddes, R.; Elliott, J.; Syme, H. The Effect of Feeding a Renal Diet on Plasma Fibroblast Growth Factor 23 Concentrations in Cats with Stable Azotemic Chronic Kidney Disease. *J. Vet. Intern. Med.* **2013**, *27*, 1354–1361. [CrossRef]

29. Galle, J. Oxidative stress in chronic renal failure. *Nephrol. Dial. Transpl.* **2001**, *16*, 2135–2137. [CrossRef]

30. Pecoits-Filho, R.; Sylvestre, L.C.; Stenvinkel, P. Chronic kidney disease and inflammation in pediatric patients: From bench to playground. *Pediatr. Nephrol.* **2005**, *20*, 714–720. [CrossRef]

31. Vianna, H.R.; Soares, C.M.B.M.; Tavares, M.S.; Teixeira, M.M.; Silva, A.C.S.E. Inflammation in chronic kidney disease: The role of cytokines. *Braz. J. Nephrol.* **2011**, *33*, 351–364. [CrossRef]

32. Garibotto Giacomo, G.; Sofia, A.; Saffioti, S.; Bonanni, A.; Mannucci, I.; Verzola, D. Amino acid and protein metabolism in the human kidney and in patients with chronic kidney disease. *Clin. Nutr.* **2010**, *29*, 424–433. [CrossRef] [PubMed]

33. Stenvinkel, P.; Barany, P.; Heimbürger, O.; Pecoits-Filho, R.; Lindholm, B. Mortality, malnutrition, and atherosclerosis in ESRD: What is the role of interleukin-6? *Kidney Int. Suppl.* **2002**, *61*, 103–108. [CrossRef] [PubMed]

34. Madsen, T.; Christensen, J.H.; Svensson, M.; Witt, P.M.; Toft, E.; Schmidt, E.B. Marine n-3 Polyunsaturated Fatty Acids in Patients With End-stage Renal Failure and in Subjects Without Kidney Disease: A Comparative Study. *J. Ren. Nutr.* **2011**, *21*, 169–175. [CrossRef] [PubMed]

35. IRIS Staging of CKD. Available online: http://www.iris-kidney.com/guidelines/ (accessed on 26 November 2019).

36. Brown, S.; Atkins, C.; Bagley, R.; Carr, A.; Cowgill, L.; Davidson, M.; Egner, B.; Elliott, J.; Henik, R.; Labato, M.; et al. Guidelines for the Identification, Evaluation, and Management of Systemic Hypertension in Dogs and Cats. *J. Vet. Intern. Med.* **2007**, *21*, 542–558. [CrossRef] [PubMed]

37. Laflamme, D. Development and Validation of a Body Condition Score System for Dogs. *Canine Pract.* **1997**, *22*, 10–15.

38. Parker, V.J.; Freeman, L.M. Association between body condition and survival in dogs with acquired chronic kidney disease. *J. Vet. Intern. Med.* **2011**, *25*, 1306–1311. [CrossRef]

39. Nobre, M.C.; Santos, M.C.S.; Vieira, A.B.; Salomão, M.C.; Gershony, L.C.; Soares, A.M.B.; Ferreira, A.M.R. Escore de condição corporal como indicador do prognóstico de gatos com doença renal crônica. *Cienc. Rural* **2010**, *40*, 365–370.

40. Zatz, R. *Bases Fisiológicas da Nefrologia*; Atheneu: São Paulo, Brasil, 2011.

41. Wong, N.L.M.; Quamme, G.A.; Dirks, J.H. Tubular handling of bicarbonate in dogs with experimental renal failure. *Kidney Int.* **1984**, *25*, 912–918. [CrossRef]

42. Schenck, P.A.; Chew, D.J. Prediction of serum ionized calcium concentration by use of serum total calcium concentration in dogs. *Am. J. Vet. Res.* **2005**, *66*, 1330–1336. [CrossRef]

43. Kogika, M.M.; Lustoza, M.D.; Notomi, M.K.; Wirthl, V.A.B.F.; Mirandola, R.M.S.; Hagiwara, M.K. Serum ionized calcium in dogs with chronic renal failure and metabolic acidosis. *Vet. Clin. Pathol.* **2006**, *35*, 441–445. [CrossRef]

44. Lazaretti, P.; Kogika, M.M.; Hagiwara, M.K.; Lustoza, M.D.; Mirandola, R.M.S. Serum concentration of intact parathormone in dogs with chronic renal failure. *Arq. Bras. Med. Vet. Zootec.* **2006**, *58*, 489–494. [CrossRef]

45. Giovaninni, L.H.; Kogika, M.M.; Lustoza, M.D.; Reche Junior, A.; Wirthl, V.A.B.F.; Simões, D.M.N.; Coelho, B.M. Serum intact parathyroid hormone levels in cats with chronic kidney disease. *Pesqui. Vet. Bras.* **2013**, *33*, 229–235. [CrossRef]

46. Isakova, T.; Wahl, P.; Vargas, G.S.; Gutiérrez, O.M.; Scialla, J.; Xie, H.; Appleby, D.; Nessel, L.; Bellovich, K.; Chen, J.; et al. Fibroblast growth factor 23 is elevated before parathyroid hormone and phosphate in chronic kidney disease. *Kidney Int.* **2011**, *79*, 1370–1378. [CrossRef] [PubMed]

47. Gutierrez, O.; Isakova, T.; Rhee, E.; Shah, A.; Holmes, J.; Collerone, G.; Jüppner, H.; Wolf, M. Fibroblast growth factor-23 mitigates hyperphosphatemia but accentuates calcitriol deficiency in chronic kidney disease. *J. Am. Soc. Nephrol.* **2005**, *16*, 2205–2215. [CrossRef] [PubMed]

48. Lee, B.T.; Ahmed, F.A.; Hamm, L.L.; Teran, F.J.; Chen, C.-S.; Liu, Y.; Shah, K.; Rifai, N.; Batuman, V.; Simon, E.E.; et al. Association of C-reactive protein, tumor necrosis factor-alpha, and interleukin-6 with chronic kidney disease. *BMC Nephrol.* **2011**. [CrossRef]

49. Yilmaz, M.I.; Solak, Y.; Saglam, M.; Cayci, T.; Acikel, C.; Unal, H.U.; Eyileten, T.; Oguz, Y.; Sari, S.; Carrero, J.J.; et al. The Relationship between IL-10 Levels and Cardiovascular Events in Patients with CKD. *Clin. J. Am. Soc. Nephrol.* **2014**, *9*, 1207–1216. [CrossRef]

50. Morita, Y.; Yamamura, M.; Kashihara, N.; Makino, H. Increased production of interleukin-10 and inflammatory cytokines in blood monocytes of hemodialysis patients. *Res. Commun. Mol. Pathol. Pharmacol.* **1997**, *98*, 19–33.

51. Brunet, P.; Capo, C.; Dellacasagrande, J.; Thirion, X.; Mege, J.L.; Berland, Y. IL-10 synthesis and secretion by peripheral blood mononuclear cells in haemodialysis patients. *Nephrol. Dial. Transplant.* **1998**, *13*, 1745–1751. [CrossRef]

52. Allen, T.; Forrester, D.; Adams, L. Chronic Kidney Disease. In *Small Animal Clinical Nutrition*; Hand, M., Thatcher, C., Remillard, R., Roudebusch, P., Eds.; Mark Morris Institute: Topeka, KS, USA, 2010; pp. 765–812.

53. Himmelfarb, J.; Phinney, S.; Ikizler, T.A.; Kane, J.; McMonagle, E.; Miller, G. Gamma-Tocopherol and Docosahexaenoic Acid Decrease Inflammation in Dialysis Patients. *J. Ren. Nutr.* **2007**, *17*, 296–304. [CrossRef]

54. Guebre-Egziabher, F.; Debard, C.; Drai, J.; Denis, L.; Pesenti, S.; Bienvenu, J.; Vidal, H.; Laville, M.; Fouque, D. Differential dose effect of fish oil on inflammation and adipose tissue gene expression in chronic kidney disease patients. *Nutrition* **2013**, *29*, 730–736. [CrossRef]

55. Silva, A.C.R.A.; de Almeida, B.F.M.; Soeiro, C.S.; Ferreira, W.L.; de Lima, V.M.F.; Ciarlini, P.C. Oxidative stress, superoxide production, and apoptosis of neutrophils in dogs with chronic kidney disease. *Can. J. Vet. Res.* **2013**, *77*, 136–141. [PubMed]

56. Galvão, A.L.B. Estresse Oxidativo em Cães com Doença Renal Crônica. PH.D. Thesis, Universidade Estadual Paulista (UNESP), São Paulo, Brasil, 2014.

57. Nguyen-Khoa, T.; Massy, Z.A.; De Bandt, J.P.; Kebede, M.; Salama, L.; Lambrey, G.; Witko-Sarsat, V.; Drüeke, T.B.; Lacour, B.; Thévenin, M. Oxidative stress and haemodialysis: Role of inflammation and duration of dialysis treatment. *Nephrol. Dial. Transplant.* **2001**, *16*, 335–340. [CrossRef] [PubMed]

58. Witko-Sarsat, V.; Friedlander, M.; Capeillère-Blandin, C.; Nguyen-Khoa, T.; Nguyen, A.T.; Zingraff, J.; Jungers, P.; Descamps-Latscha, B. Advanced oxidation protein products as a novel marker of oxidative stress in uremia. *Kidney Int.* **1996**, *49*, 1304–1313. [CrossRef] [PubMed]

59. Oberg, B.P.; McMenamin, E.; Lucas, F.L.; McMonagle, E.; Morrow, J.; Ikizler, T.A.; Himmelfarb, J. Increased prevalence of oxidant stress and inflammation in patients with moderate to severe chronic kidney disease. *Kidney Int.* **2004**, *65*, 1009–1016. [CrossRef]

60. Massy, Z.A.; Stenvinkel, P.; Drueke, T.B. The role of oxidative stress in chronic kidney disease. *Semin. Dial.* **2009**, *22*, 405–408. [CrossRef]

61. Dounousi, E.; Papavasiliou, E.; Makedou, A.; Ioannou, K.; Katopodis, K.P.; Tselepis, A.; Siamopoulos, K.C.; Tsakiris, D. Oxidative Stress Is Progressively Enhanced With Advancing Stages of CKD. *Am. J. Kidney Dis.* **2006**, *48*, 752–760. [CrossRef]

62. National Research Council (NRC). *Nutrient Requirements of Dogs and Cats*; The National Academies Press: Washington, DC, USA, 2006.

63. FEDIAF. *FEDIAF's Nutritional Guidelines 2019*; FEDIAF: Brussels, Belgium, 2019.

64. Michel, K.E.; Anderson, W.; Cupp, C.; Laflamme, D.P. Correlation of a feline muscle mass score with body composition determined by dual-energy X-ray absorptiometry. *Br. J. Nutr.* **2011**, *106*, S57–S59. [CrossRef]

Feline Infectious Peritonitis as a Systemic Inflammatory Disease: Contribution of Liver and Heart to the Pathogenesis

Alexandra J Malbon [1,2,*,†], **Sonja Fonfara** [3,4,5], **Marina L Meli** [2,6]🔟, **Shelley Hahn** [5,‡], **Herman Egberink** [7]🔟 and **Anja Kipar** [1,2,5]

1   Institute of Veterinary Pathology, Vetsuisse Faculty, University of Zurich, 8057 Zurich, Switzerland; anja.kipar@uzh.ch

2   Center for Clinical Studies, Vetsuisse Faculty, University of Zurich, 8057 Zurich, Switzerland; mmeli@vetclinics.uzh.ch

3   Department of Clinical Studies, Ontario Veterinary College, University of Guelph, Guelph, ON N1G 2W1, Canada; sfonfara@uoguelph.ca

4   Small Animal Hospital, Faculty of Veterinary Medicine, University of Helsinki, 00014 Helsinki, Finland

5   Department of Basic Veterinary Sciences, Faculty of Veterinary Medicine, University of Helsinki, 00014 Helsinki, Finland; shelley.hahn@tufts.edu

6   Clinical Laboratory, Vetsuisse Faculty, University of Zurich, 8057 Zurich, Switzerland

7   Virology Division, Department of Infectious Diseases and Immunology, Faculty of Veterinary Medicine, Utrecht University, 3584 CL Utrecht, The Netherlands; h.f.egberink@uu.nl

*   Correspondence: alexandra.malbon@uzh.ch

†   Current addresses: The Royal (Dick) School of Veterinary Studies, Easter Bush Campus, University of Edinburgh, Edinburgh EH25 9RG, UK.

‡   Current addresses: Cummings School of Veterinary Medicine, Tufts University, N. Grafton, MA 01536, USA.

Abstract: Feline infectious peritonitis (FIP) is a fatal immune-mediated disease of cats, induced by feline coronavirus (FCoV). A combination of as yet poorly understood host and viral factors combine to cause a minority of FCoV-infected cats to develop FIP. Clinicopathological features include fever, vasculitis, and serositis, with or without effusions; all of which indicate a pro-inflammatory state with cytokine release. As a result, primary immune organs, as well as circulating leukocytes, have thus far been of most interest in previous studies to determine the likely sources of these cytokines. Results have suggested that these tissues alone may not be sufficient to induce the observed inflammation. The current study therefore focussed on the liver and heart, organs with a demonstrated ability to produce cytokines and therefore with huge potential to exacerbate inflammatory processes. The IL-12:IL-10 ratio, a marker of the immune system's inflammatory balance, was skewed towards the pro-inflammatory IL-12 in the liver of cats with FIP. Both organs were found to upregulate mRNA expression of the inflammatory triad of cytokines IL-1β, IL-6, and TNF-α in FIP. This amplifying step may be one of the missing links in the pathogenesis of this enigmatic disease.

Keywords: feline infectious peritonitis; feline coronavirus; hepatocytes; cardiomyocytes; inflammatory cytokines; pathogenesis; systemic inflammatory response

---

1. Introduction

Feline infectious peritonitis (FIP) is a coronavirus-induced fatal immune-mediated disease in cats, characterised by serofibrinous and granulomatous serositis, often with protein-rich effusions into body cavities, granulomatous phlebitis and periphlebitis, and granulomatous inflammatory lesions in several organs [1–4]. The disease presents clinically with recurrent fever and signs reflecting the distribution of organ lesions. The development of FIP lesions is triggered by activated, virus infected monocytes. In the presence of a generalised activation of venous endothelial cells, these monocytes induce the granulomatous phlebitis that is considered to be the first and hallmark lesion and can occur in a range of organs [4]. Endothelial cell activation, together with other systemic changes such as fever, indicates excessive systemic cytokine release though the precise sources remain unclear [4–6].

Pro-inflammatory cytokines are the main mediators of the innate immune response, allowing communication between and priming of the various components of the innate immune system, e.g., activation of leukocytes and endothelial cells (reviewed by [6,7]). In cats, interleukin (IL)-1β, IL-6, and tumour necrosis factor (TNF)-α are the main mediators of the acute phase inflammatory response [8] and cats with FIP exhibit clear clinical and histological evidence of overt inflammatory processes. Despite this, there are conflicting results on the presence and systemic levels of these cytokines in FIP. Early studies found high IL-1 and IL-6 activity in sera, ascitic fluid, and the supernatant of cultured peritoneal exudate cells of cats with FIP [9,10]. However, IL-6 mRNA levels in peripheral blood mononuclear cells (PBMC) were found to be unaltered, only mildly increased, or variable in FIP [11–13], whilst IL-10 and IL-12 transcription was markedly depressed [11].

In vitro transcriptome studies have also not shown these classical inflammatory mediators to be significantly altered between feline infectious peritonitis virus (FIPV) infected and uninfected cells; however, these have focussed on cell culture experiments using CRFK cells, so may not reflect the complex immune interactions in vivo [14,15]. Additionally, CRFK cells are not primary immune cells so are unlikely to exhibit the same response. In vitro studies using peritoneal macrophages, a system that is closer to the disease scenario, provided evidence of the importance of TNF-α. FIPV induced TNF-α production in infected cells; as TNF-α can itself upregulate the type II FCoV receptor aminopeptidase N, cells may thus enhance their own infection rate [16,17]. In turn TNF-α functions as a possible contributor to the lymphocyte apoptosis observed in FIP [18,19]. Despite this, in natural disease, end stage FIP is associated with only a low increase or in some cases even a decrease in TNF-α transcription in the lymphatic tissues themselves [20,21]. In conjunction, IL-1β and IL-6 transcription showed no to low increases in the lymphatic tissues in FIP whilst IL-10 and IL-12 decreased or remained unchanged [20,21].

These previous results suggest that lymphatic tissues are not by themselves mass producing inflammatory cytokines at the levels required in order to contribute to and potentiate a systemic activation of endothelial cells and monocytes, and that other organ systems may play a role. We therefore first hypothesised a role for hepatocytes in cytokine production, as these have already been shown to be active in the disease. In cats with FIP, hepatocyte produced acute phase proteins such as haptoglobin, serum amyloid A, and in particular alpha1-acid glycoprotein (AGP) have been shown to be elevated; to the extent that they are considered key elements of the diagnostic process [22–24]. Although not thus far studied in felines, human and murine hepatocytes have also been shown capable of producing cytokines, including IL-1, IL-6, IL-10, IL-12, and TNF-α [25–30]. Additionally, our group has previously identified constitutive pro-inflammatory cytokine expression by feline cardiomyocytes, which increases in systemic inflammatory disease [31]. This led to the second hypothesis that the heart is an additional source of cytokines and thereby contributes to the systemic inflammatory status that allows FIP lesions to develop.

To evaluate these hypotheses, we measured relative mRNA levels of IL-1β, IL-6, and TNF-α in liver and heart by quantitative reverse transcriptase polymerase chain reaction (RT-qPCR). We then used a palette of methods on selected cases to confirm translation and identify the cell source of the cytokines. In light of both our previous findings in lymphatic tissues [20,21] and the importance of these cytokines in determining the balance of the immune response (Th1 vs. Th2/pro- vs. anti-inflammatory [32,33]), we also evaluated the hepatic IL-10 and IL-12p40 mRNA levels in an attempt to assess whether this ratio correlated with the clinical picture.

We demonstrated that both hepatocytes and cardiomyocytes are sources of inflammatory cytokines in FIP, and that the hepatic IL-12:IL-10 balance is skewed towards IL-12 in diseased animals.

2. Materials and Methods

2.1. Animals and Tissue Processing

2.1.1. Liver Study (Groups 1.1–1.3)

This study was undertaken on three groups of cats. Group 1.1 comprised 16 cats with FIP, further subdivided into natural infection (12 pet cats; age: 5 months to 2 years; Group 1.1a) and experimental infection (four female specific pathogen free (SPF) cats; age: 14–16 weeks; Group 1.1b), see Table 1. All 1.1a cats were submitted for diagnostic post mortem examination with full owner consent. The 1.1b cats had been euthanased with FIP after experimental intra-peritoneal infection with the serotype I FCoV strain FIPV-UCD at the University of Utrecht, The Netherlands. Approval for this experiment was obtained from the Ethical Committee of Utrecht University (approval number: 0502.0802). All Group 1.1b cats showed clinical signs of FIP which necessitated euthanasia of two cats at 3.5 and 4 weeks post infection (p.i.) whilst the remaining two were euthanased at the end of the experiment (11 weeks p.i.).

The diagnosis of FIP was confirmed in all cases by gross, histological, and immunohistological examination [3]. Six of the 16 cats with FIP had effusions, including three of the four experimental cases (data was unavailable for three animals).

Group 1.2 consisted of 14 clinically healthy, male SPF cats that had been per-orally infected at an age of 8.5 to 27 weeks with previously isolated serotype I FCoV field strains of enteric pathotype (FCoVZu1, 2, 3, and 5 -feline enteric coronavirus; FECV) and had been euthanased between 2 and 12 weeks p.i. [34]. This experiment was performed under the Swiss regional legislation (project license number TVB 66/2000). All cats had tested positive for FCoV shedding and those euthanased more than 2 weeks p.i. seroconverted. All were confirmed to be systemically FCoV infected by the presence of a FCoV viraemia [34]. These cats were used as a comparison group to provide relatively uniform baseline cytokine level as pet cats without FIP would be subject to wide variations in terms of pathogen exposure, FCoV infection status, and concurrent disease. This also allowed evaluation of the effect of FIP on the animal rather than FCoV infection per se.

All group 1.1 and 1.2 animals were necropsied within 1 h of death. Liver samples from grossly normal regions (i.e., without FIP lesions) were collected and immediately frozen at −80 °C for RNA extraction, whilst normal and lesion samples were fixed in 10% buffered formalin for 24–48 h and routinely paraffin wax embedded for histological and immunohistological examination.

The third group (Group 1.3) comprised six healthy untreated SPF cats, aged 36–38 months, that had been euthanased at the University of Glasgow, UK as part of a study performed under UK Home Office Project Licence PPL 60/3735. From these cats, formalin fixed, paraffin embedded liver samples were kindly provided by Prof M Hosie.

Table 1. Signalment and lesion distribution of cats in Group 1 (naturally and experimentally infected cats with feline infectious peritonitis (FIP) used for the liver study).

Cat	Group	Signalment	Lesion Distribution	Presence of Effusions
1	1.1a	6 m, MN, DSH	Peritoneum	Y
2	1.1a	6 m, FE, DSH	Peritoneum	Y
3	1.1a	1.5 y, FN, DLH	Kidney, lung	Y
4	1.1a	5 m, ME, DSH	Kidney, eye, brain	N
5	1.1a	Juvenile, FE, BSH	Kidneys, liver, spleen, lung, CNS	N
6	1.1a	Juvenile, MN, DSH	Liver, spleen, lungs, peritoneum, pleura	N
7	1.1a	8 m, MN, Burmese	Lung, kidney, brain, eye	N
8	1.1a	1 y, FN, DSH	Lung, brain	N
9	1.1a	2 y, MN, DSH	Lung, kidney, liver, peritoneum	N
10	1.1a	2 y, FE, DSH	NR	NR

Table 1. *Cont.*

Cat	Group	Signalment	Lesion Distribution	Presence of Effusions
11	1.1a	3 y, FN, DLH	NR	NR
12	1.1a	4 y, MN, DSH	NR	NR
13	1.1b	14–16 w, FE, DSH	Heart, lungs, spleen	N
14	1.1b	14–16 w, FE, DSH	Peritoneum, liver, kidney, omentum, spleen	Y
15	1.1b	14–16 w, FE, DSH	Peritoneum, liver, kidney, omentum, spleen	Y
16	1.1b	14–16 w, FE, DSH	Peritoneum, liver, omentum, spleen	Y

m: months; y: years; ME: male entire; MN: male neutered; FE: female entire; CNS: brain and spinal cord; N: no effusions; Y: effusions present; blank: data not available; NR: not recorded.

2.1.2. Heart Study (Groups 2.1–2.3)

This study was undertaken on three additional groups of cats. Group 2.1 comprised 18 pet cats (age: 2 months to 3 years; mean age: 14 months) that had died or were euthanased with FIP; the diagnosis was confirmed as described above. See Table 2.

Group 2.2 comprised 10 cats that had been euthanased due to non-inflammatory diseases not expected to have any systemic impact (24 months to 19 years; mean age: 9 years) which were further grouped by age (Group 2.2a (*n* = 4), (two each); Group 2.2b (*n* = 6), aged 9–19 years, mean age: 13.4 years) to acknowledge the fact that age has an effect on constitutive cytokine expression in the myocardium [35]. See Table 2.

Group 2.3 comprised three cats with systemic inflammatory diseases other than FIP. See Table 2.

Table 2. Signalment and lesion distribution of cats in Group 2.

Cat	Group	Signalment	Lesion Distribution */Disease [†]	Presence of Effusions
1	2.1	4 m, ME, Birman	Pleuritis, peritonitis, med ln	Y
2	2.1	7 m, ME, Devon Rex	Peritoneum, mes ln	Y
3	2.1	7 m, MN, BSH	Peritoneum, lung, liver, kidney, mes ln	Y
4	2.1	9 m, FN, DSH	Peritoneum, liver, mes ln, kidney	Y
5	2.1	1 y, MN, BSH	Pleura, liver, kidney, lung, mes ln	Y
6	2.1	11 m, ME, Birman	Pleura, peritoneum, liver, mes ln	Y
7	2.1	11 m, FN, Ragdoll	Peritoneum, intestinal wall, mes ln	Y
8	2.1	1 y, FN, DSH	Pleura, peritoneum, leptomeninx, lung, liver, kidneys	Y
9	2.1	1 y, MN, DLH	Peritoneum, liver, spleen, mes ln	Y
10	2.1	1 y, MN, Birman	Kidney, colon (BALT), liver, ln	Y
11	2.1	2 y, MN, DSH	Peritoneum, mes ln	Y
12	2.1	2 y, ME, British Blue	Widespread visceral lesions	Y
13	2.1	3 y, MN, Siamese	Pleuritis, peritoneum	Y
14	2.1	3 y, ME, Birman	Pleura	Y
15	2.1	4 m, ME, DSH	Liver, kidney, mes ln	N
16	2.1	8 m, MN, Ragdoll	Kidney, liver	N
17	2.1	9 m, ME, Birman	Brain	N
18	2.1	1 y, FN, DLH	NR	NR
19	2.2a	2 y, FN, DSH	Nasal polyp	
20	2.2a	2 y, FN, DSH	Oesophageal stricture	
21	2.2a	3 y, FN, DSH	Vertebral disc prolapse	
22	2.2a	3 y, MN, DLH	Lymphocytic cholangiohepatitis	
23	2.2b	9 y, FN, DSH	Unknown, no lesions	
24	2.2b	10 y, FN, DLH	Behavioural	
25	2.2b	10 y, FN, DSH	Behavioural	
26	2.2b	14 y, ME, DSH	Age-related	
27	2.2b	14 y, FN, DSH	Nasal osteosarcoma	
28	2.2b	19 y, FN, DSH	Gastrointestinal stromal tumour	
29	2.3	5 y, FN, Oriental Shorthair	Chlamydial infection	
30	2.3	5 y, MN, Oriental Shorthair	Chlamydial infection	
31	2.3	11 y, FN, DLH	Septic peritonitis	

* in the case of FIP; [†] in all non FIP cats; m: months; y: years; ME: male entire; MN: male neutered; FE: female entire; mes: mesenteric; med: mediastinal; ln: lymph node.

All cats had been euthanased and submitted for diagnostic post mortem examination with full owner consent. They were necropsied within 1 h of death. Pleuritis involving the outer pericardium was observed in one of the FIP cats, however, neither this cat nor any of the others exhibited any gross changes in the heart. 14 of the 18 cats with FIP had effusions (data was unavailable for one animal). Hearts were removed and samples collected from both atria, both ventricular free walls, and the interventricular septum into RNA*later*™ Stabilization Solution (Thermo Fisher Scientific, Ilkirch Cedex, France) and stored at −80 °C until RNA extraction. The remaining heart was fixed in 10% buffered formalin for 24–48 h, trimmed, routinely paraffin wax embedded and subjected to a histological examination. This did not reveal pathological changes in the myocardium of any of the cats.

2.2. Assessment of Cytokine Transcription

2.2.1. Reverse Transcription and Quantitative Polymerase Chain Reaction (RT-qPCR) for Feline Cytokines

From each frozen liver and heart sample, approximately 50–100 mg was taken for RNA extraction and subsequent cDNA synthesis, following published protocols [21,34]. For the liver, RT-qPCR for feline IL-1β, IL-6, IL-10, IL-12p40, and TNF-α was carried out on the cDNA samples, using previously published assays [21,36,37]. For the heart, IL-1β, IL-6, and TNF-α transcription was assessed. The mRNA levels of the housekeeping gene feline glyceraldehyde-3-phosphate dehydrogenase (GAPDH) served as internal controls. All reactions were run in duplicate, using previously published amplification conditions and assay compositions [21,35,37]. Briefly, the thermal profile was as follows: 50 °C for 2 min, 95 °C for 10 min, and 45 cycles of 95 °C for 10 s, and 60 °C for 1 min. Data collection occurred during the extension phase (60 °C).

2.2.2. Laser Capture Microdissection (LCM)

This was performed as proof of principle on a single FIP cat heart (Group 2.1) to confirm that cardiomyocytes are themselves responsible for the detected mRNA transcription, and was therefore not subject to any statistical analysis.

Frozen RNA*later*™ samples were embedded in Tissue-Tek® O.C.T. Compound (Sakura® Finetek USA Inc., Alphen aan den Rijn, The Netherlands) in a cryostat at −20 °C before sectioning at 8–10 μm onto PEN Membrane Glass Slides (Applied Biosystems™, Waltham, MA, USA) and staining according to published protocols ([38]). The slides were completely air dried before LCM to allow for proper excision performance.

The ArcturusXT™ Laser Capture Microdissection System (Thermo Fisher Scientific) and Arcturus® CapSure® Macro LCM Caps (Thermo Fisher Scientific) were used for the LCM process itself. Areas of myocardium with highly enriched populations of cardiomyocytes (i.e., avoiding all small to large vessels and adipocytes) were identified and isolated. The isolation of cells of interest was verified by microscopic examination of the LCM cap as well as of the excised region after microdissection.

The Qiagen RNeasy Microkit (Qiagen, Hilden, Germany) was used for RNA extraction as per the manufacturer's protocol; briefly, the LCM cap was placed on a 500 μL Eppendorf tube containing extraction buffer and incubated inverted at 42 °C for 30 min before proceeding to the next steps. From the final elute of 12 μL of RNA, 8 μL was used for cDNA synthesis using the SuperScript IV VILO Master Mix kit (Thermo Fisher Scientific) with an integrated DNase step to remove traces of genomic DNA. This was followed by target specific pre-amplification using the primers described above and the TaqMan® PreAmp Master Mix (2 ×) (Applied Biosystems™) to produce sufficient cDNA for qPCR analysis. The pre-amplification was performed according to the manufacturer's protocol using 20 PCR cycles. The resulting product was then diluted 1:20 and used for all RT-qPCR reactions as described above.

2.2.3. Relative Quantification of Cytokine Transcripts and Statistical Analysis

Relative quantification of cytokine signals was done by the comparative threshold cycle (C_T) method [39] using fGAPDH as the internal reference gene. This serves to normalise for differences in the amount of total nucleic acid added to each reaction and the efficiency of the reverse transcriptase step [21,37]. The programme IBM SPSS® was used for statistical comparisons; a two-tailed Mann–Whitney test was applied at the 95% confidence level on the premise that cytokine levels in the two groups were different.

In the liver study (1), first the natural FIP cases (Group 1.1a) were compared with the experimental FIP cases (Group 1.1b) to determine if they could be classed as one group. As no statistically significant difference was found between these subgroups, all of Group 1.1 was compared to Group 1.2. Both Group 1.1a and 1.1b were also compared separately to Group 1.2. Within Group 1.1, cytokine mRNA levels from cats with and without effusions were compared. Each disease form subgroup of FIP cats was then compared with control cats. Where clinical information regarding the presence of effusions was lacking, the individuals were excluded from these comparisons. The IL-12p40:IL-10 mRNA ratio was evaluated using the Independent Samples Median Test.

In the heart study (2), cats with FIP (Group 2.1) were compared to control cats (Group 2.2) and cats with systemic inflammatory disease (Group 2.3). To take a potential age influence into account, FIP cats and cats with systemic diseases were subsequently each compared to young (Group 2.2a) and old (Group 2.2b) control cats. Within Group 2.1, FIP cases were split into those with and without effusions. These were first compared to each other and then separately to control cats, age subgroups of the control cats, and cats with systemic inflammatory diseases.

2.3. Assessment of Cytokine Protein Expression

2.3.1. Antibodies Specific for Feline Cytokines

Since antibodies reacting with the feline cytokines of our interest were not available, a panel of rabbit anti-peptide antibodies, specific for feline IL-1β, IL-6, IL-10, IL-12p40, and TNF-α was commercially produced (Genosphere Biotechnologies, Paris, France). Antibodies were raised against the C-terminus of the proteins by using 14 amino acid long synthetic peptides with an additional cysteine residue at the N-terminus coupled to keyhole limpet hemocyanin (KLH) carrier (see supplemental Table S1). All antisera had been determined by the supplier by ELISA to have a titre greater than 1:10,000 when tested against the peptide antigen. Antibody specificity was confirmed by ELISA and dot blot, using recombinant cytokines where available (human IL-1β and TNF-α (Peprotech, London, UK); feline IL-6 (Serotec (now Bio-Rad, Oxford, UK)); feline IL-1β, IL-10, TNF-α, IL-12 (R&D Systems, Zug, Switzerland), and following routine protocols. Immunoblotting was also performed following routine protocols on a homogenised liver sample from an experimental FIP cat to confirm reaction with the 'native' protein. The antibodies were subsequently used in immunohistology. As IL-6 specificity could not be confirmed in the Western blot system, a mouse monoclonal antibody directed against feline IL-6 (MAB23051, R&D Systems) that became commercially available following completion of the initial liver study was tested on a small set of liver samples. This antibody has been previously published [40] and served here to further confirm IL-6 protein expression in the myocardium.

2.3.2. Immunohistology for Feline Cytokines

Staining protocols for the anti-peptide antibodies were optimised using FIP lesions from a diagnostic case, in which a mixed inflammatory cell population was present. The staining was then applied to a selection of cases (five cats from Group 1.1a, all four cats from Group 1.1b, all cats from Group 1.3) from the liver study (1). Briefly, formalin-fixed, paraffin embedded liver sections (3–5 μm) were subjected to immunohistological staining following the previously published peroxidase anti-peroxidase (PAP) method [3], with diaminobenzidine as the chromogen and Papanicolaou's haematoxylin counterstaining. Sections incubated with rabbit pre-immune serum and/or PBS instead of the primary antibody, and sections incubated with antibodies blocked by the respective peptide served as negative controls. These did not yield any reaction. Stained liver sections were assessed independently by two pathologists (AJM and AK) and staining was graded in a semi-quantitative manner as negative, weak, moderate or strong, based on the number of positive hepatocytes and average staining intensity.

For the heart study (2), formalin-fixed, paraffin embedded sections from the left and right ventricular free wall and atrium and from the interventricular septum were stained for IL-6, using the commercial IL-6 antibody (see above; the custom-made antibodies were no longer available at this time). Briefly, protocols were as follows: pre-treatment with citrate buffer followed by 15 min serum block, incubation with primary antibody (diluted 1:500 in dilution buffer (Dako, Basel, Switzerland; S2022) at room temperature for 1 h, use of the EnVision Mouse (Dako Cytomation) detection system. Chromogen, counterstaining methods, and controls were as described above.

3. Results

3.1. Inflammatory Cytokine Transcription in the Liver

Hepatic transcription of all tested cytokines was detectable in all groups, and in the majority of animals (81–100%, cytokine dependent; Table S2).

Relative transcription levels of all cytokines were significantly higher ($p < 0.05$) in cats with FIP. Variation between animals was observed in all groups, this being greater in the FIP group (Figure 1). In the latter, the within group variation for each cytokine was lower in the experimentally infected group (1.1b) than in natural infection (Group 1.1a), and so were the transcription levels overall (though not significantly so) (Table S2). When comparing naturally and experimentally infected cats with FIP separately with the FECV-infected healthy cats, a significant difference was observed for the experimentally infected animals with FIP only for IL-6 which was transcribed at a higher level in cats with FIP (Figure 1; Table 3).

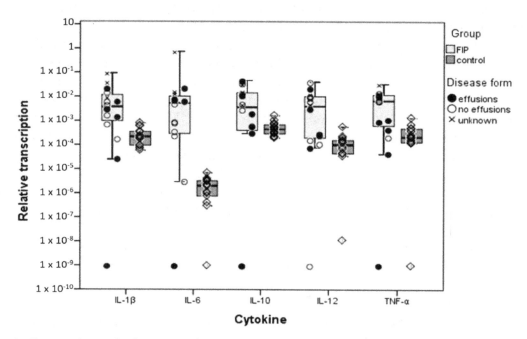

Figure 1. Comparison of relative cytokine transcription levels in the liver between cats with feline infectious peritonitis (FIP) and healthy, feline coronavirus (FCoV)-infected cats; box and whisker plots together with illustration of individual cat values and presence or absence of effusions in the case of FIP. 'FIP' includes Group 1.1a–natural FIP cases in the left-hand column of the box, and 1.1b–experimentally infected cats with FIP at the right-hand side; 'control' cats are Group 1.2–FCoV-infected cats without FIP. Boxes indicate the median value and the interquartile range, whilst whiskers indicate the spread of values with the exception of outliers (calculated by SPSS as >1.5 box lengths).

The IL-12p40:IL-10 mRNA ratio was assessed as an accepted indicator of the inflammatory balance of the immune system [32,33]. This was overall significantly higher in cats with FIP ($p = 0.047$), indicating the balance is tipped towards a pro-inflammatory state. In fact, IL-10 levels were higher than IL-12 levels in each individual control cat, whereas in half of the naturally infected FIP cats IL-10 levels were lower than IL-12 levels. Experimental FIP cats were again in between the groups, with slightly higher IL-10 than IL-12 levels in all animals.

Il-6 showed the largest quantitative difference in medians between cats with and without FIP, with mRNA levels nearly 1000 fold higher in disease. Interestingly, this was owing to lower relative transcription levels for IL-6 in healthy cats than of the other cytokines (though the difference was not statistically significant), whereas in cats with FIP, IL-6 levels were on a par with those of other cytokines. IL-6 was also the only cytokine that varied depending on the presence or absence of effusions; its transcription was significantly higher ($p = 0.04$) in cats with effusions than in those without (Table 3). For IL-12 and TNF-α, a close to 100 fold increase in relative transcription was seen between cats with and without disease, whilst the smallest quantitative difference was found for IL-1β and IL-10; for both cytokines, mRNA levels were only ~10 fold higher in FIP.

Table 3. Results of statistical comparisons (p values of a two-tailed Mann–Whitney) between cytokine mRNA transcription in the livers of naturally and experimentally infected cats with FIP and of experimentally FCoV-infected, healthy cats (FCoV-infected cats without FIP).

Group Comparison	p Values for Each Cytokine; * = Significant at 95% CI				
	IL-1β	IL-6	IL-10	IL-12p40	TNF-α
1.1a vs. 1.1b	0.103	0.770	0.170	0.133	0.078
1.1 vs. 1.2	0.002 *	0.001 *	0.034 *	0.001 *	0.017 *
1.1a vs. 1.2	0.000 *	0.003 *	0.031 *	0.002 *	0.004 *
1.1b vs.1. 2	0.721	0.012 *	0.382	0.061	0.878
1.1 eff vs. 1.1 no eff	0.628	0.035 *	1.000	0.836	0.234
1.1 eff vs. 1.2	0.274	0.020 *	0.312	0.009 *	0.494
1.1 no eff vs. 1.2	0.003 *	0.025 *	0.224	0.067	0.046 *

In all cases where the difference is significant, the first of the pair is higher. 1.1a: natural FIP cases; 1.1b: experimental FIP cases; 1.2: controls cats; 1.1 eff: FIP cats with effusions; 1.1 no eff: FIP cats without effusions.

3.2. Hepatocytes Are a Source of Inflammatory Cytokines in FIP

Immunohistology was then used to identify the cell sources of the cytokines. The SPF cat livers were histologically unaltered and served to assess FCoV-independent constitutive protein expression. Cytokine expression was mainly evident in the bile duct epithelium which exhibited variable expression of all cytokines (Figure 2). There was also occasional evidence (i.e., in one or two animals for each cytokine) of very low level expression by hepatocytes, represented by a weak, finely granular cytoplasmic staining (Figure 2G,I). Furthermore, Kupffer cells in all SPF cats occasionally expressed IL-1β and in two and one cat respectively also IL-6 and IL-12 (Figure 2G).

The livers of FCoV-infected cats without FIP often exhibited mild portal lymphocyte infiltration as well as occasional small clusters of lymphocytes and scattered individual neutrophils within the sinusoids. The cytokine expression pattern and intensity were similar to that seen in SPF cats; hepatocytes largely exhibited either no or very weak staining.

In cats with FIP, the majority of livers exhibited typical lesions, i.e., fibrinosuppurative perihepatitis and/or focal to multifocal granulomatous-necrotising inflammation. Cytokine expression by inflammatory cells was generally weak, but all cytokines were found to be expressed by macrophages and neutrophils as well as low numbers of Kupffer cells (Figure 2H). Hepatocytes were shown to express all cytokines. This was seen either as a diffuse staining of all hepatocytes (Figure 2F,H,J) or appeared to vary in its intensity between individual cells (Figure 2B,D). A direct correlation between protein expression and mRNA levels was not observed by semi-quantitative assessment of cytokine expression.

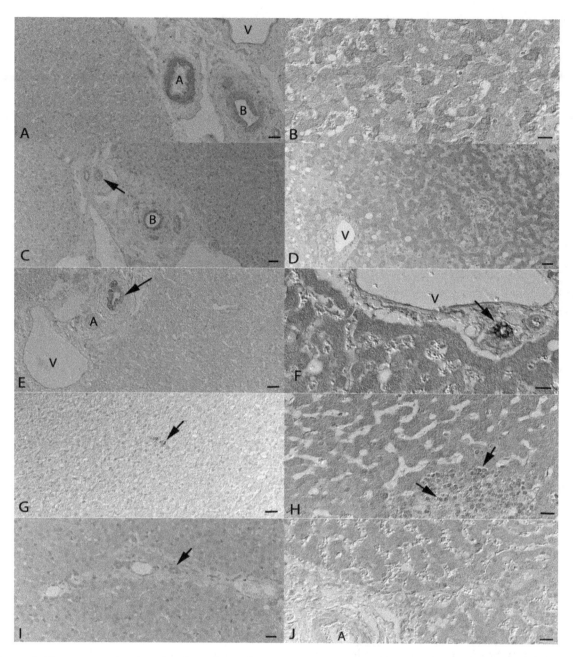

Figure 2. Representative immunohistological staining for the expression of cytokines in the liver. Left column: specific pathogen free (SPF) cats; right column: cats with FIP. (**A,B**): Expression of IL-1β. (**A**): In SPF cats, expression is restricted to bile duct (B) epithelial cells and the media of small arteries (A). V: vein in portal area. (**B**): In a FIP cat, hepatocytes exhibit variably intense expression. (**C,D**): Expression of IL-6. (**C**): In SPF cats, expression is restricted to a weak staining in bile duct (B) epithelial cells and the media of small arteries (arrow). (**D**): In a FIP cat, a large proportion of hepatocytes exhibit variably intense expression. V: vein in portal area. (**E,F**): Expression of IL-10. (**E**): In SPF cats, expression is restricted to bile duct epithelial cells (arrow). A: artery, V: vein in portal area. (**F**): In a FIP cat, hepatocytes exhibit a diffuse strong expression. The staining in bile duct epithelial cells (arrow) is even stronger. V: vein in portal area. (**G,H**): Expression of IL-12p40. (**G**): In a SPF cat, weak expression is seen within hepatocytes. Occasional positive Kupffer cells (arrow) are also seen. (**H**): In a FIP cat, hepatocytes exhibit a diffuse weak to moderate expression. In a granulomatous infiltrate, there are some weakly positive macrophages (arrows). (**I,J**): Expression of TNF-α. (**I**): In a SPF cat, very weak expression is seen within hepatocytes and bile duct epithelial cells (arrow). (**J**): In a cat with FIP, hepatocytes exhibit a diffuse weak staining. Bars represent 50 μm (A, C, D, E, and G) or 20 μm (B, D, H, I, and J) Peroxidase anti-peroxidase method, Papanicolaou's haematoxylin counterstain.

3.3. Inflammatory Cytokine Transcription in the Heart

IL-1β, IL-6, and TNF-α were all constitutively transcribed in the heart.

Cats with FIP exhibited significantly higher myocardial IL-1β ($p = 0.008$), IL-6, and TNF-α (both $p < 0.001$) transcription than control cats. When control cats were split by age, older cats retained the significant differences for all three cytokines ($p < 0.001$) whereas only TNF-α was significantly lower in the young control cats than in cats with FIP (Table 4). There were no significant differences between cats with systemic inflammatory diseases and FIP or between cats with FIP with and without effusions., These FIP subgroups (with and without effusions) were compared in turn to the other groups, with results almost identical to those obtained using the combined FIP group. The exception was in comparing FIP cats without effusions to controls, which were not significantly different despite the combined FIP group and FIP cats with effusions showing significantly higher transcription levels than controls (displayed graphically in Figure 3). Data distribution is summarised in Table S3.

Table 4. Results of statistical comparisons (p values of a two-tailed Mann–Whitney) between cytokine mRNA transcription in the hearts of naturally infected cats with FIP, cats with non-inflammatory conditions, and of cats with other systemic inflammatory diseases.

Group Comparison	p Values for Each Cytokine; * = Significant at 95% CI		
	IL-1β	IL-6	TNF-α
2.1 vs. 2.2	0.008 *	0.000 *	0.000 *
2.1 vs. 2.2a	0.165	0.122	0.000 *
2.1 vs. 2.2b	0.000 *	0.000 *	0.000 *
2.1 vs. 2.3	0.474	0.355	0.614
2.1 eff vs. 2.1 no eff	0.256	0.885	0.155
2.1 eff vs. 2.2	0.001 *	0.000 *	0.000 *
2.1 eff vs. 2.2a	0.410	0.093	0.000 *
2.1 eff vs. 2.2b	0.000 *	0.000 *	0.000 *
2.1 eff vs. 2.3	0.886	0.255	0.437
2.1 no eff vs. 2.2	0.331	0.018 *	0.001 *
2.1 no eff vs. 2.2a	0.159	0.332	0.025 *
2.1 no eff vs. 2.2b	0.013 *	0.002 *	0.000 *
2.1 no eff vs. 2.3	0.217	0.529	0.894

In all cases where the difference is significant, the first of the pair is higher. 2.1: cats with FIP; 2.2: control cats; 2.2a: control cats up to 3 years old; 2.2b: control cats greater than 9 years old; 2.3: cats with systemic inflammatory disease other than FIP; 2.1 eff: FIP cats with effusions; 2.1 no eff: FIP cats without effusions.

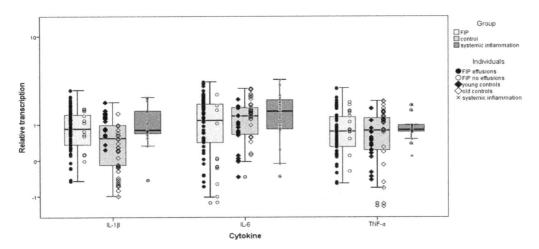

Figure 3. Comparison of relative cytokine transcription levels in the heart between cats with feline infectious peritonitis (FIP), control cats, and cats with systemic inflammatory disease other than FIP; box and whisker plots together with illustration of individual cat values. Group 2.1, FIP cases; 2.2, control cats (young ≤3 years old; old ≥9 years old); 2.3, systemic inflammatory disease. Boxes indicate the median value and the interquartile range, whilst whiskers indicate the spread of values with the exception of outliers (calculated by SPSS as >1.5 box lengths).

3.4. Cardiomyocytes Themselves Contribute to Cytokine Expression

Laser capture microdissection samples of myocardium demonstrated mRNA expression of IL-1β, IL-6, and TNF-α in cardiomyocytes.

Staining of a representative selection of heart samples from cats with FIP for IL-6 confirmed IL-6 production predominantly by cardiomyocytes. Endothelial cells and smooth muscle cells of the tunica media were also positive in some sections and mesothelial cells showed irregular staining.

4. Discussion

Here we present the first functional studies of their kind to focus on the potential contribution of non-immune organs, i.e., the liver and heart, to cytokine production in cats affected by FIP and, more generally, by systemic inflammatory disease per se. The specific panel of cytokines, IL-1, IL-6 and TNF-α as well as IL-10 and IL-12p40, was chosen based on their known effects and to assess their potential role in disease manifestation, as FIP is driven by activated monocytes and characterised by vascular inflammatory lesions and fever.

Using a combination of methods to demonstrate cytokine transcription and in situ protein expression as well, we could show that both organs produce the entire panel of pro-inflammatory and immunomodulatory cytokines, and confirmed the parenchymal cells, hepatocytes and cardiomyocytes, as a source of these.

The varying origins of the different groups of cats reflects the availability of tissue samples. The study aimed to maximise the information gleaned from previous unrelated experimental infections and case collections by utilising these tissues to tackle the hypotheses. Results obtained from the liver study provided a springboard to studying the heart, for which retrospective samples were available. They are presented together here as it was felt that, combined, the results add more to our knowledge of potential pathogenesis. This of course comes with the limitation of inter-group matching, hence we have drawn broad rather than highly specific conclusions and the groups have not been compared between organs.

In the liver, there was a low level of expression observed in healthy FCoV-infected cats, whilst the transcription of IL-1β, IL-6, IL-10, IL-12, and TNF-α was significantly upregulated in FIP. Interestingly, when comparing natural and experimental FIP, the range of cytokine transcription extended higher in the natural cases. It is possible that the prior SPF status of the experimentally infected cats accounts for this as they would not have had previous exposure to FCoVs and/or other common infectious pathogens. They would also be at a more regulated stage of disease and received identical virus and dosage, likely explaining the lower variability of the results. This difference between groups, with higher levels in many of the natural cases, also supports the role of these organs in systemic inflammation generally rather than as a FCoV specific response.

In cats with FIP, not only hepatocytes but also inflammatory cells within the typical macrophage dominated lesions were found, unsurprisingly, to express the examined cytokines. However, the inflammatory cells likely played a minor role in the overall hepatic transcription, since we extracted RNA from tissue specimens without grossly visible FIP lesions and generally found immunohistological evidence of more consistent cytokine expression by hepatocytes than by inflammatory cells. The different antibodies showed variation in their staining patterns, being either relatively diffuse or showing more varying intensity between hepatocytes. The precise cause of this is unknown but may reflect variations in cytokine expression and release beyond the scope of this study.

The heart was not affected by FIP lesions in any case, which is consistent with the known lesion distribution [41]. Despite this, the pyrogenic cytokines IL-6 and TNF-α were upregulated in FIP; this was also seen in other systemic inflammatory diseases, these likely affected the heart in a similar way. Cardiomyocytes were confirmed to be a source of both cytokine mRNA and protein.

These findings suggest that 'bystander' cells such as cardiomyocytes and hepatocytes are likely to play a significant role in amplifying systemic inflammation by responding non-specifically to inflammatory processes. Immunohistological staining results did not allow an accurate quantification of translation, nor could we identify a direct correlation between mRNA and protein levels. This has a number of possible explanations—the different regions sampled, the different sensitivities of the two methods, the time lapse between transcription and translation (with our samples all taken at a single time point), and the manifold levels of pre- and post-translational regulation to which cytokines are exposed. Taking TNF-α alone, there is regulation of mRNA at export, post-transcription, and translation, with multiple mechanisms at each stage [42]. However, our objective was to confirm rather than quantify parenchymal cytokine expression and, together with what is known of cytokine function, our results provide strong evidence that hepatocytes and cardiomyocytes may indeed play a role in systemic inflammatory disease and hence the pathogenesis of FIP. This is supported by data from a mouse study showing that hepatocytes can produce at least as much IL-6 per cell as macrophages [28]. Traditionally thought to have more of a reactive or even bystander role in disease, the parenchymal cells may in fact provide a large amplifying step in a cascade of cytokine release. This role is, however, secondary and rather unspecific, as systemic inflammatory diseases were found to be associated with myocardial transcription of IL-1β, IL-6, and TNF-α at levels similar to those seen in cats with FIP. Whether other organs such as the lung (in which resident macrophages such as pulmonary intravascular macrophages may be targets for FCoV [43]) also have a role to play remains to be investigated.

IL-1β, IL-6, and TNF-α are the major inflammatory cytokines in cats; in FIP, they can be linked to both lesion induction and clinical signs such as fever. IL-1β and TNF-α may also contribute to the hypoalbuminaemia and weight loss seen in FIP via decreased albumin production and increased muscle breakdown respectively [8,44]. Adhesion molecule expression and chemokine production by endothelial cells (EC) is induced by TNF-α and IL-1β, leading to leukocyte binding [45]. In line with this, upregulation of β2-integrins was seen on leukocytes from cats with FIP [4,46]. The cytokines can then be expected to contribute to the destruction of the vascular basal lamina seen in FIP phlebitis [1,3,4,47], as they upregulate matrix metalloproteinase secretion from monocytes [48,49].

IL-6, known to be particularly stimulated by IL-1β and TNF-α [50], showed the greatest hepatic upregulation of the studied cytokines in association with FIP and was the only one to be significantly higher in the effusive form of disease compared to the non-effusive form. In wet FIP, significant IL-6 activity has previously been reported in sera and peritoneal exudate cells [9]. The wet, dry, and mixed forms of FIP indicate overlapping disease states with a variable degree of vascular permeability [51,52]. IL-6 can induce vascular endothelial growth factor (VEGF) production and pulmonary vascular permeability [53–55], and the degree of ascites was found to be correlated with serum VEGF levels in cats with FIP [51]. This could explain, via VEGF upregulation, the particularly high hepatic IL-6 transcription levels seen in FIP cats with effusions in our study. Hepatic IL-6 release could also contribute to the progressive plasma cell infiltration seen in older FIP lesions [3,41], as IL-6 induces the final maturation of B cells into plasma cells [56]. It might also influence myocardial cytokine transcription, which showed a lower increase in FIP when compared to control cats than the liver samples and might therefore suggest a later, reactive involvement of the myocardium in the disease process. Showing a reactive response might also be the reason that no difference in myocardial transcription was observed between the effusive and non-effusive forms of FIP. However, further investigations into the time course of FIPV infection are needed.

Interestingly, IL-1β has been shown experimentally to more than double the half-life of IL-6 mRNA, and TNF-α had a similar, but less intense effect [57]. Accordingly, in addition to its direct effects, IL-1β could have two relevant synergistic effects in FIP; stimulating IL-6 transcription and prolonging the lifespan of IL-6 mRNA [50], thereby potentiating its effects. The similar IL-1β and IL-6 mRNA concentrations in the myocardium of young control cats and cats with FIP confirms our previous finding of a generally more reactive/inflammatory myocardium in young cats [35], which might also contribute to the increased susceptibility of young cats to FIP, with TNF-α subsequently further amplifying the inflammatory process.

IL-10 is an anti-inflammatory and immunosuppressive cytokine that inhibits inflammatory cytokine transcription by monocytes, but also complements IL-6 as it can stimulate antibody production [58,59]. The host's attempt to counteract the pro-inflammatory signals in FIP through increased IL-10 expression may therefore have the negative side effect of promoting anti-FCoV antibody production.

We also found IL-12 upregulation in the liver in association with FIP. The pro-inflammatory effects of IL-12 are usually counteracted by IL-10 which attempts to return the immune response to homeostatic base levels [60]. The IL-12:IL-10 ratio has been used as a measure of the balance between pro- and anti-inflammatory states in a number of disease conditions [61]. In our study we found an overall higher hepatic IL-12:IL-10 mRNA ratio in FIP than in healthy FCoV-infected cats. Despite being archetypally pro-inflammatory, at high concentrations IL-12 can inhibit the immune response and the generation of cytotoxic T lymphocytes [62,63]. In contrast to the liver, the mesenteric lymph nodes were previously found to downregulate IL-12 transcription in FIP, with IL-10 levels unaffected [20,21]. It would appear that neither high IL-12 nor high IL-10 are themselves protective and indeed plasmids encoding IL-12 have been found to enhance susceptibility to disease in FIPV vaccination studies, rather than offering protection as had been predicted [64].

5. Conclusions

This study sheds light on the contribution of non-immune organs, specifically the heart and liver, to systemic disease in which they are not directly targeted. This knowledge helps bridge the gap between the accepted understanding of FIP as an immune-mediated inflammatory disease and the seemingly limited contribution of primary immune organs to inflammatory cytokine production. It also provides avenues for further study into the role of these organs in other feline systemic diseases.

Author Contributions: "conceptualization, A.K., S.F.; methodology, A.K., M.L.M., S.F.; validation, A.J.M., M.L.M., S.F.; formal analysis, A.J.M., S.F.; investigation, A.J.M., S.H., S.F.; resources, A.K., H.E., S.F.; writing—original draft preparation, A.J.M., S.F., A.K.; writing—review and editing, all authors; visualization, A.J.M., A.K.; supervision, A.K., S.F.; project administration, A.K.; funding acquisition, A.K."

Acknowledgments: The authors gratefully acknowledge the help of Keith Baptiste, who provided statistical advice. We wish to thank Margaret Hosie and Os Jarrett, University of Glasgow, Centre for Virus Research, for providing the SPF cat tissue samples and are also most grateful to A. Barth and the technicians in the Histology Laboratory, School of Veterinary Science, University of Liverpool, for excellent technical support. The laboratory work was partly performed using the logistics of the Centre for Clinical Studies at the Vetsuisse Faculty, University of Zurich. This work is dedicated to the memory of Anne Vaughan-Thomas who contributed significantly to the project.

References

1.   Hayashi, T.; Goto, N.; Takahashi, R.; Fujiwara, K. Systemic vascular lesions in feline infectious peritonitis. *Jpn. J. Vet. Sci.* **1977**, *39*, 365–377. [CrossRef] [PubMed]

2.   Weiss, R.C.; Scott, F.W. Pathogenesis of feline infectious peritonitis: Pathologic changes and immunofluorescence. *Am. J. Vet. Res.* **1981**, *42*, 2036–2048. [PubMed]

3.   Kipar, A.; Bellmann, S.; Kremendahl, J.; Köhler, K.; Reinacher, M. Cellular composition, coronavirus antigen expression and production of specific antibodies in lesions in feline infectious peritonitis. *Vet. Immunol. Immunopathol.* **1998**, *65*, 243–257. [CrossRef]

4.   Kipar, A.; May, H.; Menger, S.; Weber, M.; Leukert, W.; Reinacher, M. Morphologic features and development of granulomatous vasculitis in feline infectious peritonitis. *Vet. Pathol.* **2005**, *42*, 321–330. [CrossRef] [PubMed]

5.   Acar, D.D.; Olyslaegers, D.A.J.; Dedeurwaerder, A.; Roukaerts, I.D.M.; Baetens, W.; Van Bockstael, S.; De Gryse, G.M.A.; Desmarets, L.M.B.; Nauwynck, H.J. Upregulation of endothelial cell adhesion molecules characterizes veins close to granulomatous infiltrates in the renal cortex of cats with feline infectious peritonitis and is indirectly triggered by feline infectious peritonitis virus-infected monocytes. *J. Gen. Virol.* **2016**, *97*, 2633–2642. [CrossRef] [PubMed]

6. Dinarello, C.A. Historical Review of Cytokines. *Eur. J. Immunol.* **2007**, *37*, S34–S45. [CrossRef]

7. Akdis, M.; Burgler, S.; Crameri, R.; Eiwegger, T.; Fujita, H.; Gomez, E.; Klunker, S.; Meyer, N.; O'Mahony, L.; Palomares, O.; et al. Interleukins, from 1 to 37, and interferon-γ: Receptors, functions, and roles in diseases. *J. Allergy Clin. Immunol.* **2011**, *127*, 701–721. [CrossRef]

8. Paltrinieri, S. The feline acute phase reaction. *Vet. J.* **2008**, *177*, 26–35. [CrossRef]

9. Goitsuka, R.; Ohashi, T.; Ono, K.; Yasukawa, K.; Koishibara, Y.; Fukui, H.; Ohsugi, Y.; Hasegawa, A. IL-6 activity in feline infectious peritonitis. *J. Immunol.* **1990**, *144*, 2599–2603.

10. Goitsuka, R.; Onda, C.; Hirota, Y.; Hasegawa, A.; Tomoda, I. Feline interleukin 1 production induced by feline infectious peritonitis virus. *Jpn. J. Vet. Sci.* **1988**, *50*, 209–214. [CrossRef]

11. Gunn-Moore, D.A.; Caney, S.M.; Gruffydd-Jones, T.J.; Helps, C.R.; Harbour, D.A. Antibody and cytokine responses in kittens during the development of feline infectious peritonitis (FIP). *Vet. Immunol. Immunopathol.* **1998**, *65*, 221–242. [CrossRef]

12. Kiss, I.; Poland, A.M.; Pedersen, N.C. Disease outcome and cytokine responses in cats immunized with an avirulent feline infectious peritonitis virus (FIPV)-UCD1 and challenge-exposed with virulent FIPV-UCD8. *J. Feline Med. Surg.* **2004**, *6*, 89–97. [CrossRef] [PubMed]

13. Gelain, M.E.; Meli, M.; Paltrinieri, S. Whole blood cytokine profiles in cats infected by feline coronavirus and healthy non-FCoV infected specific pathogen-free cats. *J. Feline Med. Surg.* **2006**, *8*, 389–399. [CrossRef] [PubMed]

14. Mehrbod, P.; Harun, M.S.R.; Shuid, A.N.; Omar, A.R. Transcriptome analysis of feline infectious peritonitis virus infection. *Coronaviruses Methods Protoc. Methods Mol. Biol.* **2015**, *1282*, 241–250.

15. Harun, M.S.R.; Kuan, C.O.; Selvarajah, G.T.; Wei, T.S.; Arshad, S.S.; Hair Bejo, M.; Omar, A.R. Transcriptional profiling of feline infectious peritonitis virus infection in CRFK cells and in PBMCs from FIP diagnosed cats. *Virol. J.* **2013**, *10*, 329. [CrossRef]

16. Takano, T.; Hohdatsu, T.; Toda, A.; Tanabe, M.; Koyama, H. TNF-alpha, produced by feline infectious peritonitis virus (FIPV)-infected macrophages, upregulates expression of type II FIPV receptor feline aminopeptidase N in feline macrophages. *Virology* **2007**, *364*, 64–72. [CrossRef]

17. Takano, T.; Hohdatsu, T.; Hashida, Y.; Kaneko, Y.; Tanabe, M.; Koyama, H. A "possible" involvement of TNF-alpha in apoptosis induction in peripheral blood lymphocytes of cats with feline infectious peritonitis. *Vet. Microbiol.* **2007**, *119*, 121–131. [CrossRef]

18. Haagmans, B.L.; Egberink, H.F.; Horzinek, M.C. Apoptosis and T-cell depletion during feline infectious peritonitis. *J. Virol.* **1996**, *70*, 8977–8983.

19. Kipar, A.; Köhler, K.; Leukert, W.; Reinacher, M. A comparison of lymphatic tissues from cats with spontaneous feline infectious peritonitis (FIP), cats with FIP virus infection but no FIP, and cats with no infection. *J. Comp. Pathol.* **2001**, *125*, 182–191. [CrossRef]

20. Malbon, A.J.; Meli, M.L.; Barker, E.N.; Davidson, A.D.; Tasker, S.; Kipar, A. Inflammatory mediators in the mesenteric lymph nodes, site of a possible intermediate phase in the immune response to feline coronavirus and the pathogenesis of feline infectious peritonitis? *J. Comp. Pathol.* **2019**, *166*, 69–86. [CrossRef]

21. Kipar, A.; Meli, M.L.; Failing, K.; Euler, T.; Gomes-Keller, M.A.; Schwartz, D.; Lutz, H.; Reinacher, M. Natural feline coronavirus infection: Differences in cytokine patterns in association with the outcome of infection. *Vet. Immunol. Immunopathol.* **2006**, *112*, 141–155. [CrossRef] [PubMed]

22. Duthie, S.; Eckersall, P.D.; Addie, D.D.; Lawrence, C.E.; Jarrett, O. Value of alpha 1-acid glycoprotein in the diagnosis of feline infectious peritonitis. *Vet. Rec.* **1997**, *141*, 299–303. [CrossRef] [PubMed]

23. Giordano, A.; Spagnolo, V.; Colombo, A.; Paltrinieri, S. Changes in some acute phase protein and immunoglobulin concentrations in cats affected by feline infectious peritonitis or exposed to feline coronavirus infection. *Vet. J.* **2004**, *167*, 38–44. [CrossRef]

24. Giori, L.; Giordano, A.; Giudice, C.; Grieco, V.; Paltrinieri, S. Performances of different diagnostic tests for feline infectious peritonitis in challenging clinical cases. *J. Small Anim. Pract.* **2011**, *52*, 152–157. [CrossRef] [PubMed]

25. González-Amaro, R.; García-Monzón, C.; García-Buey, L.; Moreno-Otero, R.; Alonso, J.L.; Yagüe, E.; Pivel, J.P.; López-Cabrera, M.; Fernández-Ruiz, E.; Sánchez-Madrid, F. Induction of tumor necrosis factor alpha production by human hepatocytes in chronic viral hepatitis. *J. Exp. Med.* **1994**, *179*, 841–848. [CrossRef] [PubMed]

26. Alfrey, E.J.; Most, D.; Wang, X.; Lee, L.K.; Holm, B.; Krieger, N.R.; Sibley, R.K.; Huie, P.; Dafoe, D.C. Interferon-gamma and interleukin-10 messenger RNA are up-regulated after orthotopic liver transplantation in tolerant rats: Evidence for cytokine-mediated immune dysregulation. *Surgery* **1995**, *118*, 399–405. [CrossRef]

27. Saad, B.; Frei, K.; Scholl, F.A.; Fontana, A.; Maier, P. Hepatocyte-derived interleukin-6 and tumor-necrosis factor alpha mediate the lipopolysaccharide-induced acute-phase response and nitric oxide release by cultured rat hepatocytes. *Eur. J. Biochem.* **1995**, *229*, 349–355. [CrossRef]

28. Panesar, N.; Tolman, K.; Mazuski, J.E. Endotoxin stimulates hepatocyte interleukin-6 production. *J. Surg. Res.* **1999**, *85*, 251–258. [CrossRef]

29. Stonāns, I.; Stonāne, E.; Russwurm, S.; Deigner, H.P.; Böhm, K.J.; Wiederhold, M.; Jäger, L.; Reinhart, K. HepG2 human hepatoma cells express multiple cytokine genes. *Cytokine* **1999**, *11*, 151–156. [CrossRef]

30. Dikopoulos, N.; Wegenka, U.; Kröger, A.; Hauser, H.; Schirmbeck, R.; Reimann, J. Recently Primed CD8+ T Cells Entering the Liver Induce Hepatocytes to Interact with Naïve CD8+ T Cells in the Mouse. *Hepatology* **2004**, *39*, 1256–1266. [CrossRef]

31. Fonfara, S.; Kitz, S.; Hahn, S.; Kipar, A. The influence of age and disease presentation on myocardial transcription in cats with hypertrophic cardiomyopathy. *Res. Vet. Sci.*. in preparation.

32. Levy, J.K.; Ritchey, J.W.; Rottman, J.B.; Davidson, M.G.; Liang, Y.-H.; Jordan, H.L.; Tompkins, W.A.; Tompkins, M.B. Elevated interleukin-10–to–interleukin-12 ratio in feline immunodeficiency virus–infected cats predicts loss of type 1 immunity to Toxoplasma gondii. *J. Infect. Dis.* **1998**, *178*, 503–511. [CrossRef] [PubMed]

33. Van Hemert, S.; Meijerink, M.; Molenaar, D.; Bron, P.A.; De Vos, P.; Kleerebezem, M.; Wells, J.M.; Marco, M.L. Identification of Lactobacillus plantarum genes modulating the cytokine response of human peripheral blood mononuclear cells. *BMC Microbiol.* **2010**, *10*, 293. [CrossRef] [PubMed]

34. Meli, M.L.; Kipar, A.; Müller, C.; Jenal, K.; Gönczi, E.; Borel, N.; Gunn-Moore, D.; Chalmers, S.; Lin, F.; Reinacher, M.; et al. High viral loads despite absence of clinical and pathological findings in cats experimentally infected with feline coronavirus (FCoV) type I and in naturally FCoV-infected cats. *J. Feline Med. Surg.* **2004**, *6*, 69–81. [CrossRef] [PubMed]

35. Fonfara, S.; Hetzel, U.; Hahn, S.; Kipar, A. Age- and gender-dependent myocardial transcription patterns of cytokines and extracellular matrix remodelling enzymes in cats with non-cardiac diseases. *Exp. Gerontol.* **2015**, *72*, 117–123. [CrossRef] [PubMed]

36. Leutenegger, C.M.; Mislin, C.N.; Sigrist, B.; Ehrengruber, M.U.; Hofmann-Lehmann, R.; Lutz, H. Quantitative real-time PCR for the measurement of feline cytokine mRNA. *Vet. Immunol. Immunopathol.* **1999**, *71*, 291–305. [CrossRef]

37. Kipar, A.; Leutenegger, C.M.; Hetzel, U.; Akens, M.K.; Mislin, C.N.; Reinacher, M.; Lutz, H. Cytokine mRNA levels in isolated feline monocytes. *Vet. Immunol. Immunopathol.* **2001**, *78*, 305–315. [CrossRef]

38. Cummings, M.; McGinley, C.V.; Wilkinson, N.; Field, S.L.; Duffy, S.R.; Orsi, N.M. A robust RNA integrity-preserving staining protocol for laser capture microdissection of endometrial cancer tissue. *Anal. Biochem.* **2011**, *416*, 123–125. [CrossRef]

39. Pfaffl, M.W. A new mathematical model for relative quantification in real-time RT-PCR. *Nucleic Acids Res.* **2001**, *29*, e45. [CrossRef]

40. Frontera-Acevedo, K.; Sakamoto, K. Local pulmonary immune responses in domestic cats naturally infected with Cytauxzoon felis. *Vet. Immunol. Immunopathol.* **2015**, *163*, 1–7. [CrossRef]

41. Kipar, A.; Meli, M.L. Feline infectious peritonitis: Still an enigma? *Vet. Pathol.* **2014**, *51*, 505–526. [CrossRef] [PubMed]

42. Giambelluca, M.S.; Laflamme, C.; Pouliot, M. Post-transcriptional regulation of tumour necrosis factor alpha biosynthesis: Relevance to the pathophysiology of rheumatoid arthritis. *OA Inflamm.* **2013**, *1*, 1–6. [CrossRef]

43. Kipar, A.; Meli, M.L.; Baptiste, K.E.; Bowker, L.J.; Lutz, H. Sites of feline coronavirus persistence in healthy cats. *J. Gen. Virol.* **2010**, *91*, 1698–1707. [CrossRef] [PubMed]

44. de Groot-Mijnes, J.D.F.; Van Dun, J.M.; Van Der Most, G.; De Groot, R.J. Natural History of a Recurrent Feline Coronavirus Infection and the Role of Cellular Immunity in Survival and Disease. *J. Virol.* **2005**, *79*, 1036–1044. [CrossRef]

45. Abbas, A.K.; Lichtman, A.H.; Pillai, S. *Cellular and Molecular Immunology*, 9th ed.; Saunders Elsevier: Amsterdam, The Netherlands, 2017; ISBN 9780323479783.

46. Olyslaegers, D.A.J.; Dedeurwaerder, A.; Desmarets, L.M.B.; Vermeulen, B.L.; Dewerchin, H.L.; Nauwynck, H.J. Altered expression of adhesion molecules on peripheral blood leukocytes in feline infectious peritonitis. *Vet. Microbiol.* **2013**, *166*, 438–449. [CrossRef]

47. Watanabe, H.; Nakanishi, I.; Yamashita, K.; Hayakawa, T.; Okada, Y. Matrix metalloproteinase-9 (92 kDa gelatinase/type IV collagenase) from U937 monoblastoid cells: Correlation with cellular invasion. *J. Cell Sci.* **1993**, *104 Pt 4*, 991–999.

48. Sarén, P.; Welgus, H.G.; Kovanen, P.T. TNF-alpha and IL-1beta selectively induce expression of 92-kDa gelatinase by human macrophages. *J. Immunol.* **1996**, *157*, 4159–4165.

49. Robinson, S.C.; Scott, K.A.; Balkwill, F.R. Chemokine stimulation of monocyte matrix metalloproteinase-9 requires endogenous TNF-alpha. *Eur. J. Immunol.* **2002**, *32*, 404–412. [CrossRef]

50. Kent, L.W.; Rahemtulla, F.; Hockett, R.D.; Gilleland, R.C.; Michalek, S.M. Effect of lipopolysaccharide and inflammatory cytokines on interleukin-6 production by healthy human gingival fibroblasts. *Infect. Immun.* **1998**, *66*, 608–614.

51. Takano, T.; Ohyama, T.; Kokumoto, A.; Satoh, R.; Hohdatsu, T. Vascular endothelial growth factor (VEGF), produced by feline infectious peritonitis (FIP) virus-infected monocytes and macrophages, induces vascular permeability and effusion in cats with FIP. *Virus Res.* **2011**, *158*, 161–168. [CrossRef]

52. Pedersen, N.C. An update on feline infectious peritonitis: Virology and immunopathogenesis. *Vet. J.* **2014**, *201*, 123–132. [CrossRef] [PubMed]

53. Loeffler, S.; Fayard, B.; Weis, J.; Weissenberger, J. Interleukin-6 induces transcriptional activation of vascular endothelial growth factor (VEGF) in astrocytes in vivo and regulates VEGF promoter activity in glioblastoma cells via direct interaction between STAT3 and Sp1. *Int. J. Cancer* **2005**, *115*, 202–213. [CrossRef] [PubMed]

54. Feurino, L.W.; Zhang, Y.; Bharadwaj, U.; Zhang, R.; Li, F.; Fisher, W.E.; Brunicardi, F.C.; Chen, C.; Yao, Q.; Min, L. IL-6 stimulates Th2 type cytokine secretion and upregulates VEGF and NRP-1 expression in pancreatic cancer cells. *Cancer Biol. Ther.* **2007**, *6*, 1096–1100. [CrossRef] [PubMed]

55. Gurkan, O.U.; He, C.; Zielinski, R.; Rabb, H.; King, L.S.; Dodd-o, J.M.; D'Alessio, F.R.; Aggarwal, N.; Pearse, D.; Becker, P.M. Interleukin-6 mediates pulmonary vascular permeability in a two-hit model of ventilator-associated lung injury. *Exp. Lung Res.* **2011**, *37*, 575–584. [CrossRef] [PubMed]

56. Kishimoto, T. The biology of interleukin-6. *Blood* **1989**, *74*, 1–10. [CrossRef] [PubMed]

57. Iwasaki, H.; Takeuchi, O.; Teraguchi, S.; Matsushita, K.; Uehata, T.; Kuniyoshi, K.; Satoh, T.; Saitoh, T.; Matsushita, M.; Standley, D.M.; et al. The IκB kinase complex regulates the stability of cytokine-encoding mRNA induced by TLR-IL-1R by controlling degradation of regnase-1. *Nat. Immunol.* **2011**, *12*, 1167–1175. [CrossRef]

58. Buchwald, U.K.; Geerdes-Fenge, H.F.; Vöckler, J.; Ziege, S.; Lode, H. Interleukin-10: Effects on phagocytosis and adhesion molecule expression of granulocytes and monocytes in a comparison with prednisolone. *Eur. J. Med. Res.* **1999**, *4*, 85–94.

59. de Waal Malefyt, R.; Abrams, J.; Bennett, B.; Figdor, C.G.; de Vries, J.E. Interleukin 10 (IL-10) inhibits cytokine synthesis by human monocytes: An autoregulatory role of IL-10 produced by monocytes. *J. Exp. Med.* **1991**, *174*, 1209–1220. [CrossRef]

60. Cao, S.; Liu, J.; Chesi, M.; Bergsagel, P.L.; Ho, I.-C.; Donnelly, R.P.; Ma, X. Differential regulation of IL-12 and IL-10 gene expression in macrophages by the basic leucine zipper transcription factor c-Maf fibrosarcoma. *J. Immunol.* **2002**, *169*, 5715–5725. [CrossRef]

61. Watson, D.C.; Sargianou, M.; Panos, G. Interleukin-12 (IL-12)/IL-10 ratio as a marker of disease severity in Crimean-Congo hemorrhagic fever. *Clin. Vaccine Immunol.* **2012**, *19*, 823–824. [CrossRef]

62. Lasarte, J.J.; Corrales, F.J.; Casares, N.; López-Díaz de Cerio, A.; Qian, C.; Xie, X.; Borrás-Cuesta, F.; Prieto, J. Different doses of adenoviral vector expressing IL-12 enhance or depress the immune response to a coadministered antigen: The role of nitric oxide. *J. Immunol.* **1999**, *162*, 5270–5277. [PubMed]

63. Lee, K.; Overwijk, W.W.; O'Toole, M.; Swiniarski, H.; Restifo, N.P.; Dorner, A.J.; Wolf, S.F.; Sturmhoefel, K. Dose-dependent and schedule-dependent effects of interleukin-12 on antigen-specific CD8 responses. *J. Interf. Cytokine Res.* **2000**, *20*, 589–596.

64. Glansbeek, H.L.; Haagmans, B.L.; te Lintelo, E.G.; Egberink, H.F.; Duquesne, V.; Aubert, A.; Horzinek, M.C.; Rottier, P.J.M. Adverse effects of feline IL-12 during DNA vaccination against feline infectious peritonitis virus. *J. Gen. Virol.* **2002**, *83*, 1–10. [CrossRef] [PubMed]

Prevalence of the Mutations Responsible for Glanzmann Thrombasthenia in Horses in Brazil

Raíssa O. Leite [1], **Júlia F. Ferreira** [1], **César E. T. Araújo** [1], **Diego J. Z. Delfiol** [2], **Regina K. Takahira** [1]⊙, **Alexandre S. Borges** [1] and **Jose P. Oliveira-Filho** [1,*]⊙

[1] São Paulo State University (Unesp), School of Veterinary Medicine and Animal Science, Department of Veterinary Clinical Science,18618-681 Botucatu, Brazil; raissaleitevet@hotmail.com (R.O.L.); julia.franco.ferreira@gmail.com (J.F.F.); cesararaujovet@hotmail.com (C.E.T.A.); regina.takahira@unesp.br (R.K.T.); alexandre.s.borges@unesp.br (A.S.B.)

[2] School of Veterinary Medicine, Universidade Federal de Uberlândia, 38405-320 Uberlândia, Brazil; djzdelfiol@ufu.br

* Correspondence: jose.oliveira-filho@unesp.br

Simple Summary: Hereditary bleeding disorders occur in different species due to mutations in genes coding specific hemostatic proteins leading to alterations in their synthesis, or to the production of non-functional proteins which leads to impairment of hemostasis. Some of these disorders have been described in horses, i.e., Von Willebrand disease (VWD), hemophilia A, and Glanzmann's thrombasthenia (GT). GT is an inherited disease characterized by hemorrhage and has been described in different species including horses of varied breeds (Thoroughbred, Standardbred, Oldenburg, Peruvian Paso, and Quarter Horse). There are two different mutations described in horses a single guanine to cytosine substitution (CGG for CCG) and a 10 base pair deletion in the *ITGA2B* gene.

Abstract: Glanzmann's thrombasthenia (GT) is an autosomal recessive inherited disorder characterized by changes in platelet aggregation, leading to hemorrhage and epistaxis. To date, two independent mutations have been described in horses and associated with this disorder, a point mutation (c.122G > C) and a 10-base-pair deletion (g.1456_1466del) in the Integrin subunit alpha2β gene (*ITGA2B*) of horses of different breeds (Quarter Horse, Thoroughbred, Oldenburg, and Peruvian Paso). *ITGA2B* codifies the αIIb subunit of the αIIbβ3 integrin, also termed platelet fibrinogen receptor. Horses with GT have been diagnosed in the USA, Canada, Japan, and Australia. However, there are no studies on the prevalence of GT in horses. The aim of this study is to evaluate the prevalence of the mutations responsible for GT in horses in Brazil. A total of 1053 DNA samples of clinically healthy Quarter Horse (n = 679) and Warmblood horses (n = 374) were used. DNA fragments were amplified by PCR and sequenced. The genotype of each animal was analyzed and compared to the nucleotide sequence of the *ITGA2B* gene found on GenBank™. There were no carriers in the analyzed samples, that is, all animals tested were wild type. Therefore, under the conditions in which this study was carried out, it can be inferred that GT seems to be extremely rare in the population of Quarter Horses and Warmbloods in Brazil, although it is not possible to affirm that there are no horses carrying mutated alleles in Brazil.

Keywords: genetic disease; prevalence study; fibrinogen receptor; epidemiology

---

1. Introduction

Hereditary bleeding disorders occur due to mutations in genes coding specific hemostatic proteins, leading to alterations in their synthesis, or to the production of non-functional proteins [1]. Some of these disorders have been described in horses, i.e., Von Willebrand deficiency (VWD) [2], hemophilia A [3], and Glanzmann's thrombasthenia (GT) [4–9].

GT occurs due to quantitative or qualitative changes in the glycoprotein IIb-IIIa complex, also known as αIIbβ3 integrin or fibrinogen receptor, which is found on the surface of the platelets and has an essential role in platelet aggregation and clot retraction [1,5,6,10]. Mutations involving the genes that encode the subunits αIIb (ITGA2B) or β3 (ITGB3) can result in GT. In animal domestic species, mutations have only been noted in the ITGA2 gene [5,6,9], whereas in humans', mutations have been documented in both genes [10]. Clinically GT is characterized by cutaneous, mucosal, and gastrointestinal hemorrhages, and epistaxis is the most frequent clinical sign [6]. Laboratory tests of affected animals demonstrate normal coagulation screening tests, normal platelet counts, and normal Von Willebrand factor antigen levels, with clot retraction and platelet aggregation responses impaired; and also, a reduction in αIIbβ3 integrin indicated by flow cytometry [5,6,9,11]. This disorder has been described in Thoroughbred [4,7,8,11,12], Peruvian Paso [10] Standardbred [12], Oldenburg [13], and Quarter Horse breeds [8].

In horses, GT has an autosomal recessive inheritance pattern [5,6,9,11,13] and has been associated with two independent mutations, a point mutation (c.122G > C) [5,9] and a 10-base-pair deletion (g.1456_1466del) [6,11], in the Integrin subunit alpha2β gene (ITGA2B) of horses of different breeds (Quarter Horse [5,6], Thoroughbred [5], Oldenburg [9] and Peruvian Paso [11]). The point mutation leads to the substitution of a proline for an arginine in a highly conserved region of the encoded protein [5], and the deletion mutation leads to a lack of splicing, and inclusion of a premature stop codon 50 bp downstream of the mutation in the incompletely spliced messenger ribonucleic acid (mRNA) [6]. In horses, studies of the prevalence of theses mutated alleles have not been performed, therefore, the aim of this study was to evaluate the prevalence of the mutations describe as responsible for Glanzmann's Thrombasthenia in horses in Brazil.

2. Materials and Methods

This study was approved on 21 January 2019 by the Institutional Animal Care and Use Committee (262/2011-CEUA-UNESP) and samples were collected under a strict confidentiality agreement to ensure the anonymity of establishments, owners and animals. Since the allele frequencies of the two mutations are unknown, we used the anticipated frequency of heterozygotes of 50% [14], a population of Quarter Horse (QM) (500,000) and Warmblood (WB) horses (14,000) registered in Brazil, using a 5% margin of error, and 95% confidence interval to calculate the sample size (OpenEpi software). The sample size recommended for QM was 384, and 374 for the WB horses.

A total of 1053 horses DNA samples were used in this study. These samples were obtained from a genetic material database belonging to the Laboratory of Molecular Biology of the Veterinary Clinic at São Paulo State University (Unesp), School of Veterinary Medicine and Animal Science Botucatu/Brazil. This genetic database is composed by DNA samples (stored at −80 °C) which were extracted from whole blood samples obtained from adult horses (males and females), duly registered in the breeds associations (Brazilian Association of Quarter Horses Breeders and Brazilian Sport Horse Association). The samples from QHs were collected from 41 different farms and the WB samples from seven different farms or horses training centers.

Genotype analysis was performed using specific primers previously described for detection of the ITGA2B g.1456_1466del mutation [6] and for detection of the ITGA2B c.122G > C mutation [9]. Polymerase chain reactions were performed in a total volume of 25 μL, which contained 20 ng/μL (2.5 μL) of template DNA, 0.3 μM each forward and reverse primer, 12.5 μL of GoTaq® Green PCR Master Mix (Promega©, Madison, WI, USA), and 8.5 μL of nuclease-free water. In addition, a no-template control reaction was performed to check for the possible presence of contamination in the PCR preparations. The amplification conditions were as follows: initial denaturation at 95 °C for 2 min, followed by 40 cycles of denaturation at 95 °C for 30 s, 64 °C for 30 s, and 72 °C for 1 min, and final extension at 72 °C for 5 min. Amplicons (241 bp for the deletion mutation and 359 bp for the substitution mutation) were analyzed via 1.5% agarose gel electrophoresis, purified, and subjected to

Sanger direct sequencing. The obtained sequences and the electropherograms were analyzed using Geneious® 10.0.9 (Biomatters©, Auckland, New Zealand).

3. Results and Discussion

A total of 1053 horses DNA samples were analyzed, i.e., 679 QH (483 females and 196 males) and 374 WB horses (203 females and 171 males). All horses assessed in this study were identified as wild-type for both mutations. That is, there were no carriers in these populations.

The present study is the first report of the prevalence of the mutations (c.122G > C and g.1456_1466del) responsible for GT in horses. Although this disease has not been described in Brazil, studies in other countries may contribute to define the importance of GT for this species, since hemorrhage is a common clinical sign in horses and its genetic causes remain poorly elucidated [15]. In addition, the knowledge of the allele frequency of a genetic disease in a population and the identification of homozygous or heterozygous animals, enables the establishment of the impact and importance of these disorders to the species, especially for specific breeds [16].

Other studies on prevalence of different diseases with hereditary patterns that affect horses, but no related to hemostasis alterations, have been performed in Brazil: Hereditary equine regional dermal asthenia [17], Hyperkalemic periodic paralysis [18], Type 1 polysaccharide storage myopathy mutation [18], Malignant hyperthermia [19], Glycogen branching enzyme deficiency [20], and Warmblood fragile foal syndrome [21]. Many of these studies demonstrated similar results as found in other countries, such as the USA [16,22]. This may be related to the fact that lineages of the main horses of Brazil are often closely correlated with American herds, and it is suggested that the same situation for GT may be found in other countries, since the USA is the largest exporter of breeds like QHs, and Brazil is the fifth largest breeder.

The prevalence of GT in humans is higher in populations where inbreeding is commonly practiced and may have a frequency similar to other hemostatic diseases, such as hemophilia and VWD [10]. Considering that inbreeding is a common practice in horses [23], there may be differences between the frequencies of occurrence of GT in some horses' populations.

4. Conclusions

In summary, the mutations responsible for GT were not detected in this prevalent in the Brazilian horse population. Under the conditions in which this study was carried out, it can be inferred that although it is not possible to affirm that GT do not occurs in horses in Brazil, this disease seems to be extremely rare in the population of QH and WB.

Author Contributions: For Conceptualization, R.O.L., C.E.T.A., A.S.B. and J.P.O.-F.; Methodology, R.O.L. and J.P.O.-F.; Formal Analysis, R.O.L., J.F.F., C.E.T.A., D.J.Z.D., R.K.T., A.S.B. and J.P.O.-F.; Investigation, R.O.L., J.F.F. and J.P.O.-F.; Writing—Original Draft Preparation, R.O.L. and J.P.O.-F.; Writing—Review and Editing, R.O.L., J.F., C.E.T.A., D.J.Z.D., R.K.T., A.S.B. and J.P.O.-F.; Supervision, J.P.O.-F.; Funding Acquisition R.O.L., J.F.F. and J.P.O.-F.

References

1.   Patrushev, L.I. Genetic mechanisms of hereditary hemostasis disorders. *Biochemistry* **2002**, *67*, 33–46. [PubMed]
2.   Rathgeber, R.A.; Brooks, M.B.; Bain, F.T.; Byars, T.D. Clinical vignette. Von Willebrand disease in a Thoroughbred mare and foal. *J. Vet. Intern. Med.* **2001**, *15*, 63–66. [CrossRef] [PubMed]
3.   Norton, E.M.; Wooldridge, A.A.; Stewart, A.J.; Cusimano, L.; Schwartz, D.D.; Johnson, C.M.; Boudreaux, M.K.; Christopherson, P.W. Abnormal coagulation factor VIII transcript in a Tennessee Walking Horse colt with hemophilia A. *Vet. Clin. Pathol.* **2016**, *45*, 96–102. [CrossRef] [PubMed]
4.   Miura, N.; Senba, H.; Ogawa, H.; Sasaki, N.; Oishi, H.; Ohashi, F.; Takeuchi, A.; Usui, K. A case of equine thrombasthenia. *Nihon Juigaku Zasshi.* **1987**, *49*, 155–158. [CrossRef]
5.   Christopherson, P.W.; Insalaco, T.A.; van Santen, V.L.; Livesey, L.; Bourne, C.; Boudreaux, M.K. Characterization of the cDNA encoding alphaIIb and beta3 in normal horses and two horses with Glanzmann Thrombasthenia. *Vet. Pathol.* **2006**, *43*, 78–82. [CrossRef]

6. Christopherson, P.W.; van Santen, V.L.; Livesey, L.; Boudreaux, M.K. A 10-base-pair deletion in the gene encoding platelet glycoprotein IIb associated with Glanzmann thrombasthenia in a horse. *J. Vet Intern. Med.* **2007**, *21*, 196–198. [CrossRef]

7. Fry, M.M.; Walker, N.J.; Blevins, G.M.; Magdesian, K.G.; Tablin, F. Platelet function defect in a thoroughbred filly. *J. Vet Intern. Med.* **2005**, *19*, 359–362. [CrossRef]

8. Livesey, L.; Christopherson, P.; Hammond, A.; Perkins, J.; Toivio-Kinnucan, M.; Insalaco, T.; Boudreaux, M.K. Platelet dysfunction (Glanzmann's thrombasthenia) in horses. *J. Vet Intern. Med.* **2005**, *19*, 917–919. [CrossRef]

9. Macieira, S.; Lussier, J.; Bédard, C. Characterization of the cDNA and genomic DNA sequence encoding for the platelet integrin alpha IIB and beta III in a horse with Glanzmann thrombasthenia. *Can. J. Vet. Res.* **2011**, *75*, 222–227.

10. George, J.N.; Caen, J.P.; Nurden, A.T. Glanzmann's thrombasthenia: The spectrum of clinical disease. *Blood* **1990**, *75*, 1383–1395. [CrossRef]

11. Sanz, M.G.; Wills, T.B.; Christopherson, P.; Hines, M.T. Glanzmann thrombasthenia in a 17-year-old Peruvian Paso mare. *Vet. Clin. Pathol.* **2011**, *40*, 48–51. [CrossRef]

12. Sutherland, R.J.; Cambridge, H.; Bolton, J.R. Functional and morphological studies on blood platelets in a thrombasthenic horse. *Aust. Vet. J.* **1989**, *66*, 366–370. [CrossRef] [PubMed]

13. Macieira, S.; Rivard, G.E.; Champagne, J.; Lavoie, J.P.; Bédard, C. Glanzmann thrombasthenia in an Oldenbourg filly. *Vet. Clin. Pathol.* **2007**, *36*, 204–208. [CrossRef] [PubMed]

14. Dean, A.G.; Sullivan, K.M.; Soe, M.M. Open Source Epidemiologic Statistics for Public Health. OpenEpi, 2014. Available online: https://www.openepi.com/Menu/OE_Menu.htm (accessed on 10 October 2017).

15. Harrison, P.; Mackie, I.; Mumford, A.; Briggs, C.; Liesner, R.; Winter, M.; Machin, S. Guidelines for the laboratory investigation of heritable disorders of platelet function. *Br. J. Haematol.* **2011**, *155*, 30–44. [CrossRef] [PubMed]

16. Tryon, R.C.; Penedo, M.C.; McCue, M.E.; Valberg, S.J.; Mickelson, J.R.; Famula, T.R.; Wagner, M.L.; Jackson, M.; Hamilton, M.J.; Nooteboom, S.; et al. Evaluation of allele frequencies of inherited disease genes in subgroups of American Quarter Horses. *J. Am. Vet. Med. Assoc.* **2009**, *234*, 120–125. [CrossRef] [PubMed]

17. Badial, P.R.; Oliveira-Filho, J.P.; Pantoja, J.C.; Moreira, J.C.; Conceição, L.G.; Borges, A.S. Dermatological and morphological findings in quarter horses with hereditary equine regional dermal asthenia. *Vet. Dermatol.* **2014**, *25*, 547–554. [CrossRef]

18. Delfiol, D.J.Z.; Oliveira-Filho, J.P.; Battazza, A.; Souza, C.P.; Badial, P.R.; Araujo-Junior, J.P.; Borges, A.S. Prevalence of the hypercalemic periodic paralysis mutation in Quarter Horses in Brazil. *Cienc. Rural* **2015**, *45*, 854–857. [CrossRef]

19. Delfiol, D.J.Z.; Oliveira-Filho, J.P.; Badial, P.R.; Battazza, A.; Araujo-Junior, J.P.; Borges, A.S. Estimation of the allele frequency of type 1 polysaccharide storage myopathy and malignant hyperthermia in Quarter Horses in Brazil. *J. Equine Vet. Sci.* **2018**, *70*, 38–41. [CrossRef]

20. Araújo, C.E.T.; Delfiol, D.J.Z.; Badial, P.R.; Oliveira-Filho, J.P.; Araujo-Junior, J.P.; Borges, A.S. Prevalence of the glycogen branching enzyme deficiency mutation in Quarter Horses in Brazil. *J. Equine Vet. Sci.* **2018**, *62*, 81–84. [CrossRef]

21. Dias, N.M.; de Andrade, D.G.A.; Teixeira-Neto, A.R.; Trinque, C.M.; Oliveira-Filho, J.P.; Winand, N.J.; Araújo, J.P., Jr.; Borges, A.S. Warmblood fragile foal syndrome causative single nucleotide polymorphism frequency in Warmblood horses in Brazil. *Vet. J.* **2019**, *248*, 101–102. [CrossRef]

22. McCue, M.E.; Ribeiro, W.P.; Valberg, S.J. Prevalence of polysaccharide storage myopathy in horses with neuromuscular disorders. *Equine Vet. J. Suppl.* **2006**, *36*, 340–344. [CrossRef] [PubMed]

23. Norris, J.W.; Pratt, S.M.; Auh, J.H.; Wilson, S.J.; Clutter, D.; Magdesian, K.G.; Ferraro, G.L.; Tablin, F. Investigation of a novel, heritable bleeding diathesis of Thoroughbred horses and development of a screening assay. *J. Vet. Intern. Med.* **2006**, *20*, 1450–1456. [CrossRef] [PubMed]

Deleterious *AGXT* Missense Variant Associated with Type 1 Primary Hyperoxaluria (PH1) in Zwartbles Sheep

Anna Letko [1], Reinie Dijkman [2], Ben Strugnell [3], Irene M. Häfliger [1], Julia M. Paris [1], Katrina Henderson [4], Tim Geraghty [4], Hannah Orr [4], Sandra Scholes [4,†] and Cord Drögemüller [1,*,†]

1   Institute of Genetics, Vetsuisse Faculty, University of Bern, 3012 Bern, Switzerland; anna.letko@vetsuisse.unibe.ch (A.L.); irene.haefliger@vetsuisse.unibe.ch (I.M.H.); julia.paris@vetsuisse.unibe.ch (J.M.P.)
2   Royal GD, Postbus 9, 7400 AA Deventer, The Netherlands; r.dijkman2@gddiergezondheid.nl
3   Farm Post Mortems Ltd., Hamsterley, Bishop Auckland, County Durham DL13 3QF, UK; ben@farmpostmortems.co.uk
4   SRUC Consulting Veterinary Services, Pentlands Science Park, Bush Estate Loan, Penicuik, Midlothian EH26 0PZ, UK; katrina.henderson@sruc.ac.uk (K.H.); timothy.geraghty@sruc.ac.uk (T.G.); hannah.orr@sruc.ac.uk (H.O.); sandra.scholes@sruc.ac.uk (S.S.)
*   Correspondence: cord.droegemueller@vetsuisse.unibe.ch
†   These authors contributed equally to this work.

Abstract: Severe oxalate nephropathy has been previously reported in sheep and is mostly associated with excessive oxalate in the diet. However, a rare native Dutch breed (Zwartbles) seems to be predisposed to an inherited juvenile form of primary hyperoxaluria and no causative genetic variant has been described so far. This study aims to characterize the phenotype and genetic etiology of the inherited metabolic disease observed in several purebred Zwartbles sheep. Affected animals present with a wide range of clinical signs including condition loss, inappetence, malaise, and, occasionally, respiratory signs, as well as an apparent sudden unexpected death. Histopathology revealed widespread oxalate crystal deposition in kidneys of the cases. Whole-genome sequencing of two affected sheep identified a missense variant in the ovine *AGXT* gene (c.584G>A; p.Cys195Tyr). Variants in *AGXT* are known to cause type I primary hyperoxaluria in dogs and humans. Herein, we present evidence that the observed clinicopathological phenotype can be described as a form of ovine type I primary hyperoxaluria. This disorder is explained by a breed-specific recessively inherited pathogenic *AGXT* variant. Genetic testing enables selection against this fatal disorder in Zwartbles sheep as well as more precise diagnosis in animals with similar clinical phenotype. Our results have been incorporated in the Online Mendelian Inheritance in Animals (OMIA) database (OMIA 001672-9940).

Keywords: *Ovis aries*; oxalate nephropathy; whole-genome sequencing; metabolic disease; precision medicine; genetic test

1. Introduction

Primary hyperoxaluria is a rare autosomal recessive metabolic disease that leads to an accumulation of calcium oxalate in various tissues that finally result in renal failure [1]. In human patients, three types of primary hyperoxaluria are known and caused by homozygous or compound heterozygous variants in three different genes [1]. Variants in the gene encoding alanine-glyoxylate aminotransferase (*AGXT*) are responsible for type I primary hyperoxaluria (PH1; OMIM 259900), type II (PH2; OMIM 260000) is caused by variants in the glyoxylate reductase/hydroxypyruvate reductase gene (*GRHPR*), and type III (PH3; OMIM 613616) is caused by variants in the mitochondrial dihydrodipicolinate synthase-like gene (*HOGA1*).

In veterinary medicine, PH1 has been described in dogs (OMIA 001672-9615) with a breed-specific homozygous missense variant in *AGXT* (XP_003639939.1:p.Gly102Ser) and identified as a cause in the Coton de Tulear breed [2]. PH2 has been reported in cats (OMIA 000821-9685) with a splice site variant in *GRHPR* found in the affected kittens [3]. In cattle, rare cases of neonatal oxalate nephropathy in purebred calves with no known exposure to exogenous oxalates were reported [4,5]. In Zwartbles sheep, severe oxalate nephropathy was previously described with suspicion of hereditary predisposition on the basis of epidemiological findings in Great Britain and Northern Ireland [6,7]. The observed age of onset was quite variable (three weeks to three years) but the clinical signs and histopathology were similar in all the studied cases [6]. The prevalence of PH in sheep has not been studied prospectively, but data from the 2002–2009 period suggested that the incidence of all forms of urinary system disease in Zwartbles sheep is higher (7.2%, 13/179 submissions) compared to all other breeds (0.86%, 909/105,176 submissions) [6]. Additionally, our own data from ovine diagnostic submissions to SRUC Veterinary services during the period January 2015–end of August 2020 indicated that lesions of PH were detected only in pedigree Zwartbles sheep, comprising 6.5% (3/46 submissions) of purebred Zwartbles sheep.

The aim of this study is to describe the phenotype and to identify the underlying genetic variant in several purebred Zwartbles sheep affected by a recessively inherited metabolic disease. Herein, we present evidence that an ovine type I primary hyperoxaluria is due to a missense variant in the *AGXT* gene.

2. Materials and Methods

2.1. Ethics Statement

This study did not require official or institutional ethical approval as 'non-experimental clinical veterinary practices' are specifically excluded from being considered regulated procedures under The Animals (Scientific Procedures) Act, 1986, Section 2(8) as well as the Directive 2010/63/EU on the protection of animals used for scientific purposes, 2010, Article 1(5). All animals in this study were examined with the consent of their owners. All samples were obtained at postmortem examination of affected animals that had died and were submitted by the owner for laboratory diagnostic investigation.

2.2. Animals and DNA Samples

Tissue samples including kidney were collected for further analyses postmortem from nine purebred Zwartbles sheep suspected to be affected by primary hyperoxaluria in Scotland (*n* = 3), northern England (*n* = 1), and the Netherlands (*n* = 5) (Supplementary Table S1). Genomic DNA was isolated from the samples using the standard protocols of Maxwell RSC DNA Tissue and FFPE kits (Promega, Dübendorf, Switzerland).

2.3. Histopathology

Samples of kidneys from all Zwartbles sheep were fixed in 10% neutral buffered formalin and routinely processed to paraffin wax. Histopathological analyses were undertaken on hematoxylin and eosin-stained 5 μm sections. The characteristics of the crystals present were assessed also by viewing the sections with polarized light.

2.4. Whole-Genome Sequencing

In order to identify the causative variant, a whole-genome sequence (WGS) was generated after the preparation of a PCR-free fragment library for two PH1-affected sheep (case 1 and case 2).

The sequence data mapping to the ovine reference genome assembly Oar_rambouillet_v1.0 and the calling of single nucleotide and small indel variants including the prediction of functional effects were described previously [8]. PLINK v1.9 software [9] was used for homozygosity mapping of possible disease-associated intervals shared by both cases. The overlapping homozygous regions were determined by the option –homozyg group while allowing four heterozygous markers per window in order to account for possible calling errors as suggested by Ceballos et al. [10]. Private protein-changing variants shared by the two PH1-affected animals were identified by comparison with 79 publicly available control genomes, including 21 domestic sheep breeds unrelated to Zwartbles as well as two wild sheep subspecies (Supplementary Table S2). In addition, the Sheep Genomes Project Variant Database of further 453 samples of 54 other sheep breeds [11] available from the European Nucleotide Archive (ENA) was searched for the presence of the identified variants. The integrative genomics viewer (IGV) software [12] was used for visual inspection and screening for structural variants.

2.5. Candidate Variant Validation

Polymerase chain reaction (PCR) and Sanger sequencing were used to validate and genotype the variant identified from the WGS results. Primers were designed using Primer-BLAST [13] and PCR products from genomic DNA were amplified using AmpliTaqGold360 MasterMix (Thermo Fisher Scientific, Waltham, MA, USA). The purified PCR amplicons were directly sequenced on an ABI3730 capillary sequencer (Thermo Fisher Scientific). The *AGXT* missense variant (XM_027966918.1: c.584G>A) was genotyped using the following primers: GCTCACCTGTGGGTATGGG (forward) and ACAAGCCAGTGCTCCTGTTC (reverse). The obtained sequences were analyzed using Sequencher 5.1 software (GeneCodes, Ann Arbor, MI, USA).

2.6. Protein Predictions

PROVEAN [14] and MutPred2 [15], in silico prediction tools, were used to predict the biological consequences of the discovered variants on the protein. The default scores of ≤2.5 and ≥0.68 were considered to predict a variant as deleterious by PROVEAN and MutPred2, respectively. All references to the ovine *AGXT* gene correspond to the accessions NC_040252.1 (NCBI accession), XM_027966918.1 (mRNA), and XP_027822719.1 (protein). The genome aggregation database (gnomAD) v2.1.1 [16] was searched for the corresponding variant in the human AGXT.

2.7. Availability of Data and Material

The whole-genome data has been made freely available at the ENA under study accession number PRJEB30931 (sample accessions SAMEA6531513, SAMEA6531514). All accession numbers of the used genomes are available in Supplementary Table S2. The sheep genomes project variant database of further 453 samples is deposited in ENA under accession number PRJEB14685.

3. Results

3.1. Clinical Findings

Several purebred Zwartbles sheep of both sexes were submitted for laboratory investigation with a suspicion of breed-specific oxalate nephropathy in Scotland (*n* = 3), northern England (*n* = 1), and the Netherlands (*n* = 5) (Supplementary Table S1).

Two 1–2-month-old lambs (case 1 and case 2) that died suddenly were submitted for laboratory investigation from a small flock in Scotland. The first had a history of intermittent dullness while the second had been unwell for several days with coughing noted by the owner. Two other lambs of similar age from this flock died but were not further investigated. Case 3 was a 10-day-old lamb originating from a different small flock that appeared stiff and then fitted and died. Two 3–4 week-old Zwartbles lambs had previously died suddenly on the same farm but were not submitted for further investigation.

A 4-year old Zwartbles ewe (case 4) from a farm in northern England was presented with progressive condition loss and malaise over about three weeks, followed by death. The owner noticed it to be often near the water trough, suggesting polydipsia. Biochemical analysis of a urine sample from case 4 revealed an increased result of 84 μmol/mmol oxalate:creatinine ratio. This is probably higher than background levels in sheep [17], which suggested a defect in oxalate metabolism in this animal.

Five more Zwartbles sheep from the Netherlands were submitted for postmortem investigation with suspected hereditary nephropathy because of the known purebred pedigree. A 3-month old lamb (case 5) showed retarded growth without improvement on antibiotics treatment, and 1.5 week of increasing weakness followed by death. A 4-month old lamb (case 6) died suddenly, with no previous health problems reported in the flock. A 2-month old lamb (case 7) died after a period of shortness of breath and fever with initial improvement on antibiotics. A 1-month old lamb (case 8) suddenly died and was sent in by the owner because five more lambs on the same farm had succumbed without prior clinical signs. Additionally, a 2.5-month old lamb (case 9) suddenly died without further health history. More details about each animal are reported in Supplementary Table S1.

3.2. Macroscopic and Histopathological Findings

Postmortem examination of the examined sheep revealed moderate to good body condition and a urine-like smell (Supplementary Table S1). Kidneys of seven cases had pale firm cortices with a varying loss of cortico-medullary demarcation and prominent dilation of calyces and pelvices (Figure 1a). Histopathological analysis revealed severe chronic tubulointerstitial crystalline nephropathy with numerous intralesional oxalate crystals (Figure 1b) in most of the affected sheep (cases 1, 2, 3, 5, 6, 7, and 8). Limited purulent pyelonephritis associated with extension from omphalitis was also present in case 3. Figure 1 shows representative images of one case (case 3) in comparison with case 4. The kidneys of case 4 had pale cortices with clear demarcation from the purple medulla, with variable patency of renal calyces (Figure 1c). Histopathology of case 4 showed dilated tubules containing necrotic cell debris and purple-grey-black granular to crystalline deposits (Figure 1d). There was no evidence of end-stage renal disease, and the crystals were much less frequent than in the other cases with crystalline nephropathy. Case 9 had a purulent tubular and pyelonephritis with intralesional bacteria, *Escherichia coli* was cultured from the lesion.

Finally, on the basis of the comparison of clinicopathological findings, severe chronic fibrosing tubulointerstitial crystalline nephropathy with extensive oxalate crystal deposition was diagnosed in all but two cases (case 4 and case 9). In case 9, severe pyelonephritis due to *E. coli* has been found and no oxalate crystals were seen by histology, therefore disproving the initially suspected hyperoxaluria.

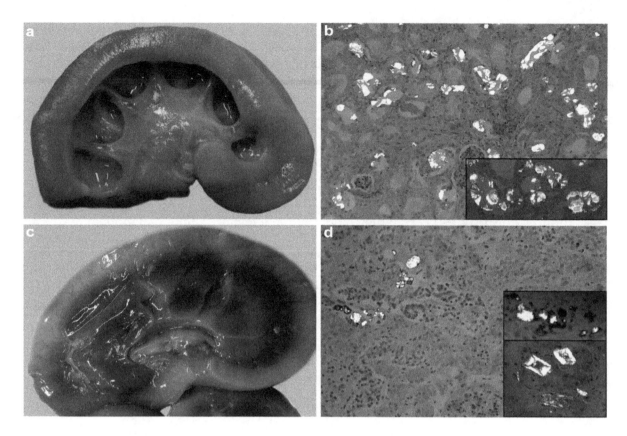

Figure 1. Macroscopic and histopathological findings in two Zwartbles sheep. (**a**) Kidney of case 3 showing the near-complete loss of corticomedullary demarcation and prominent dilation of the pelvis. (**b**) Numerous crystals in the renal tubules of case 3 are brightly birefringent when viewed by polarized light; the morphology is typical of oxalate (inset). (**c**) Kidney of case 4 showing cortical pallor and clear corticomedullary demarcation. (**d**) Sparse birefringent crystals in the renal tubules of case 4; the morphology is variable with some not typical of oxalate crystals (inset).

3.3. Identification of the Causative Variant

On the basis of the purebred pedigree history of the analyzed sheep and the recessive mode of inheritance described in other species for PH1, we hypothesized that a rare breed-specific deleterious variant is responsible for the described phenotype in the Zwartbles breed. Homozygosity mapping was used to identify intervals of extended homozygosity shared across both cases with available WGS (case 1 and case 2). This revealed 40 genomic regions representing 1.7% of the ovine reference sequence (Figure 2a). Visual inspection of the regions in the WGS of the affected sheep revealed no obvious structural variants. Filtering of the WGS data yielded 2,486 homozygous variants shared by both PH1-affected Zwartbles sheep and absent from the 79 controls (Supplementary Table S3). Out of those, 23 variants were protein-coding and only 10 of them were located within the detected homozygous intervals (Table 1). Beside three synonymous, seven missense variants in seven genes were found (Table 1). Two variants were also present heterozygously with low frequency in an independent control cohort of 453 genomes of unrelated sheep breeds [11]. Finally, only two variants in *ERICH3* and *AGXT* were predicted deleterious of which the *ERICH3* variant occurred rarely in other breeds (Table 1).

Moreover, the Zwartbles-specific missense variant in the *AGXT* gene (Figure 2b) was predicted as deleterious by both prediction tools (Table 1) and was subsequently pursued as a functional candidate, due to the gene's previous involvement in human primary hyperoxaluria [18]. The ovine variant (chr1: g.801189C>T; c.584G>A; p.Cys195Tyr) is located in exon 4 of the *AGXT* gene (Figure 2c) and affects a highly conserved amino acid residue within the large N-terminal domain of the AGXT protein (Figure 2d). MutPred2 [15] also predicted the probability (Pr) of the *AGXT* variant's impact on the following molecular mechanisms: altered metal binding (Pr = 0.72, *p*-value = 0.0009), gain of relative solvent accessibility (Pr = 0.30, p-value = 0.008), loss of allosteric site at H196 (Pr = 0.20, p-value = 0.04), altered transmembrane protein (Pr = 0.10, p-value = 0.04), and loss of pyrrolidone carboxylic acid at Q199 (Pr = 0.06, p-value = 0.03).

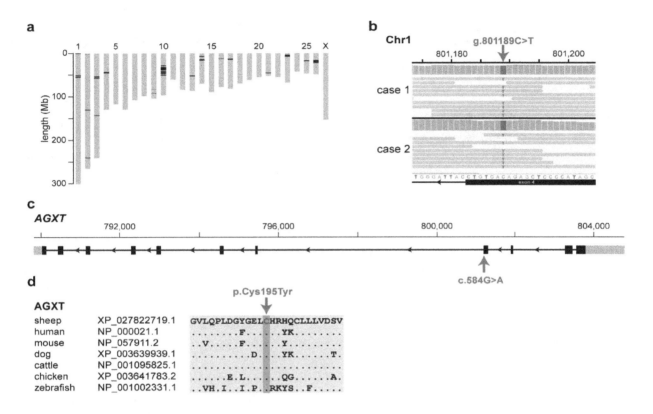

Figure 2. A missense variant in the alanine-glyoxylate aminotransferase (*AGXT*) gene is associated with type I primary hyperoxaluria (PH1) in Zwartbles sheep. (**a**) Representation of ovine chromosomes (grey bars) with highlighted regions of shared homozygosity (in black) in the two PH1-affected sheep with whole-genome sequence (WGS) data. (**b**) IGV [12] screenshot of the PH1-affected sheep WGS shows the missense variant present in both cases. (**c**) Schematic representation of the *AGXT* gene showing the variant location in exon 4. (**d**) Conservation of the affected amino acid in the AGXT protein across multiple species.

Table 1. Private protein-coding variants detected in the shared homozygous regions from whole-genome sequence (WGS) of two type I primary hyperoxaluria-affected Zwartbles sheep.

Variant Position [1]	Gene	Protein Change	Allele Frequency [2]	PROVEAN Score [3]	MutPred2 Score [4]
chr1:652874	*SNED1*	p.Glu747Lys	0	−1.279	0.628
chr1:801189	*AGXT*	p.Cys195Tyr	0	−9.768	0.891
chr1:54671486	*ERICH3*	p.Gly23Glu	0.0099	−4.526	0.852
chr10:36256345	*SPATA13*	p.Asp1073=	0.0036	NA	NA
chr10:38336210	*MPHOSPH8*	p.Arg426Gln	0	−0.638	0.085
chr14:14488283	*ZNF469*	p.Glu2351Lys	0	−1.756	0.271
chr17:13778922	*ZNF827*	p.Asn694Ser	0	−0.462	0.098
chr26:16667329	*CCDC110*	p.Asn649=	0	NA	NA
chr26:16820162	*SORBS2*	p.Pro394Leu	0	−0.301	0.121
chr26:17153454	*TLR3*	p.Leu244=	0	NA	NA

[1] All positions refer to the Oar_rambouillet_v1.0 reference sequence assembly. Additional descriptive details are given in full in Supplementary Table S3. [2] The variant allele frequency detected in the 453 sheep Genomes Project Variant Database [11]. [3] PROVEAN score ≤−2.5 predicts a variant as deleterious [14]. [4] MutPred2 score ≥0.68 predicts a variant as deleterious [15].

A different heterozygous missense variant (p.Cys173Trp, rs180177232) at the corresponding position of the human AGXT transcript was found in gnomAD [16] in a single genome. Further literature search revealed that a pathogenic missense variant with the same amino acid exchange in humans (p.Cys173Tyr, rs180177231) was associated with severely decreased catalytic activity and negative immunoreactivity in vitro and was found heterozygous in one PH1 patient [19]. Recently, another variant at the same position (p.Cys173Arg) was described in two closely related human PH1 patients exhibiting compound heterozygosity [20].

3.4. Targeted Genotyping

To experimentally confirm the AGXT missense variant (NC_040252.1: g.801189C>T), all nine available Zwartbles sheep were genotyped using Sanger sequencing. All seven PH1-affected sheep were homozygous for the variant (Supplementary Table S1). Case 4 was a heterozygous carrier and case 9, diagnosed with pyelonephritis, was homozygous for the wild type allele.

4. Discussion

On the basis of the presented clinicopathological data, an inherited form of type I primary hyperoxaluria characterized by severe chronic crystalline (oxalate) nephropathy was diagnosed in seven Zwartbles sheep homozygous for the AGXT missense variant. In contrast, an adult Zwartbles sheep with tubular necrosis and low grade tubular crystal formation was heterozygous for the variant. A ninth Zwartbles lamb that was suspected to have the disease was shown to have a bacterial pyelonephritis on postmortem examination and did not carry the identified variant. A WGS-based precision medicine approach was used to identify the underlying genetic variant in AGXT responsible for the described phenotype.

PH1 is caused by a loss of activity of the liver peroxisomal enzyme, which leads to a formation of insoluble calcium oxalate crystals. In human patients, the disease has a heterogeneous clinical phenotype with a very variable age of onset (early infancy to the 6th decade) as well as a severity of the disease [21]. Even within one family, the presentation may vary from infantile renal failure to occasional stone formation and a mild-to-moderate reduction in kidney function in adults. However, all patients are at an increased risk of developing end-stage renal disease eventually leading to death [21]. Molecular genetic testing is commonly used to identify pathogenic variants in the AGXT gene, an obvious functional candidate.

There are about 200 variants described in the human AGXT gene and the causative mutations were found in more than 99% of patients. The majority of pathological mutations for human PH1 are single nucleotide changes [18]. The missense mutations primarily affect the folding of the AGXT protein, which leads to its decreased stability [19]. A mouse model of PH1 showed that the Agxt-null mice, despite almost normal histology, develop hyperoxaluria and crystalluria with males having a higher concentration of urinary oxalate than females [22].

The interstitial lesions in all three Scottish cases and four Dutch cases with crystalline nephropathy indicated that the oxalate crystal deposition was associated with a chronic progressive renal disease similar to that reported in human PH1 [23]. The WGS of two PH1-affected sheep were used to map the disease-associated locus and to identify the most likely pathogenic AGXT variant (p.Cys195Tyr), which was absent from 532 unrelated control sheep. This amino acid exchange affects a residue highly conserved across multiple species and the ovine position Cys195 corresponds to amino acid position Cys173 of human AGXT protein. Several mutations affecting this residue have been previously reported in humans affected by PH1 [18,20,24]. Most recently, two missense heterozygous variants (AGXT: p.Cys173Arg; p.Ser223Arg) were identified in two patients from one family [20]. Interestingly, while the two probands suffering from a severe infantile form of PH1 carried both variants, all four heterozygous carriers of only the p.Cys173Arg variant were affected by kidney stones. On the other hand, five heterozygous carriers of only the p.Ser223Arg variant showed no signs of disease [20]. Furthermore, a pathogenic p.Cys173Tyr variant showed severely decreased catalytic activity and negative immunoreactivity in vitro [19]. PH1 likely remains underdiagnosed because of the wide variability in its clinical presentation as well as patients with only one heterozygous variant found [21,24].

While seven of the nine Zwartbles sheep available in this study were genotyped homozygous for the described AGXT:p.Cys195Tyr variant, a single sheep was a heterozygous carrier. Even though both renal injury and crystal formation were present in this case, the oxalate crystal accumulation was relatively minor and might have been a result of renal failure rather than a cause. However, further research is needed to investigate if heterozygotes for *AGXT* variants are possibly more prone to oxalate deposition in a range of conditions. Detection of greater than background levels of oxalate crystals, even if not associated with end-stage renal pathology, might raise suspicion of carrier status, and this might potentially predispose to development of oxalate nephrosis on high oxalate diets. Lastly, one initially suspected case of oxalate nephrosis, but finally diagnosed with kidney inflammation due to a bacterial infection, was genotyped homozygous wild type. This example shows the difficulties of a precise phenotypic diagnosis based on signalment and clinical examination alone.

5. Conclusions

In conclusion, we identified a non-synonymous variant in a highly plausible functional candidate gene through WGS data analyses. Our results combined with the current knowledge on AGXT function in other species provide strong evidence for a breed-specific missense variant affecting a conserved residue of AGXT as the most likely causative genetic variant for recessively inherited type 1 primary hyperoxaluria in Zwartbles sheep. This is the first report of the underlying pathogenesis of PH1 in sheep that supports the efficiency of the chosen method in rare metabolic disease gene discovery and enables the development of a genetic test for veterinary diagnostic and breeding purposes. Identification of this variant should bring about improvements in animal welfare by enabling the screening of breeding animals to determine and reduce the prevalence of the PH1 in the Zwartbles sheep population.

Author Contributions: Conceptualization, A.L., S.S., and C.D.; methodology, A.L., R.D., and S.S.; formal analysis, A.L., R.D., and S.S.; software, A.L. and I.M.H.; investigation, A.L., B.S., R.D., and S.S.; resources, B.S., K.H., T.G., H.O., R.D., S.S., and C.D.; data curation, I.M.H.; visualization, A.L., J.M.P., and S.S.; supervision, C.D. and S.S.; project administration, A.L., S.S. and C.D.; funding acquisition, S.S. and C.D.; writing—original draft, A.L., B.S. and S.S.; writing—review and editing, A.L., B.S., J.M.P., R.D., S.S., and C.D. All authors have read and agreed to the published version of the manuscript.

Acknowledgments: The authors are grateful to the owners of all sheep who provided samples and shared valuable information. We thank Nathalie Besuchet Schmutz for expert technical assistance. The Next Generation Sequencing Platform and the Interfaculty Bioinformatics Unit of the University of Bern are acknowledged for performing the WGS and providing high-performance computational infrastructure. The authors thank Marie Walker, Beth Armstrong, Mark Wessels, and John Fundter for excellent histotechnological inputs.

References

1. Cochat, P.; Rumsby, G. Primary hyperoxaluria. *N. Engl. J. Med.* **2013**, *369*, 649–658. [CrossRef]
2. Vidgren, G.; Vainio-Siukola, K.; Honkasalo, S.; Dillard, K.; Anttila, M.; Vauhkonen, H. Primary hyperoxaluria in Coton de Tulear. *Anim. Genet.* **2012**, *43*, 356–361. [CrossRef] [PubMed]
3. Goldstein, R.E.; Narala, S.; Sabet, N.; Goldstein, O.; McDonough, S.P. Primary hyperoxaluria in cats is caused by a mutation in the feline GRHPR gene. *J. Hered.* **2009**, *100*, S2–S7. [CrossRef]
4. Rhyan, J.C.; Sartin, E.A.; Powers, R.D.; Wolfe, D.F.; Dowling, P.M.; Spano, J.S. Severe renal oxalosis in five young Beefmaster calves. *J. Am. Vet. Med. Assoc.* **1992**, *201*, 1907–1910.
5. Yavuz Gülbahar, M.; Kaya, A.; Gölen, Ý. Renal oxalosis in a calf. *Turkish J. Vet. Anim. Sci.* **2002**, *26*, 1197–1200.
6. Strugnell, B.W.; Gaudie, C.M.; Wessels, M.; Schock, A.; Davies, I. Sheep: Severe oxalate nephropathy in zwartbles sheep. *Vet. Rec.* **2011**, *169*, 81. [CrossRef] [PubMed]
7. Barley, J.; Hanna, R.; McConnell, S. Oxalate nephrosis in Zwartble sheep. *Vet. Irel. J.* **2015**, *5*, 46–48.

8.   Paris, J.M.; Letko, A.; Häfliger, I.M.; Ammann, P.; Flury, C.; Drögemüller, C. Identification of two TYRP1 loss-of-function alleles in Valais Red sheep. *Anim. Genet.* **2019**, *50*, 778–782. [CrossRef]

9.   Chang, C.C.; Chow, C.C.; Tellier, L.C.A.M.; Vattikuti, S.; Purcell, S.M.; Lee, J.J. Second-generation PLINK: Rising to the challenge of larger and richer datasets. *Gigascience* **2015**, *4*, 1–16. [CrossRef]

10. Ceballos, F.C.; Joshi, P.K.; Clark, D.W.; Ramsay, M.; Wilson, J.F. Runs of homozygosity: Windows into population history and trait architecture. *Nat. Rev. Genet.* **2018**, *19*, 220–234. [CrossRef]

11. Naval-Sanchez, M.; Nguyen, Q.; McWilliam, S.; Porto-Neto, L.R.; Tellam, R.; Vuocolo, T.; Reverter, A.; Perez-Enciso, M.; Brauning, R.; Clarke, S.; et al. Sheep genome functional annotation reveals proximal regulatory elements contributed to the evolution of modern breeds. *Nat. Commun.* **2018**, *9*, 1–13. [CrossRef] [PubMed]

12. Thorvaldsdóttir, H.; Robinson, J.T.; Mesirov, J.P. Integrative Genomics Viewer (IGV): High-performance genomics data visualization and exploration. *Brief. Bioinform.* **2013**, *14*, 178–192. [CrossRef] [PubMed]

13. Ye, J.; Coulouris, G.; Zaretskaya, I.; Cutcutache, I.; Rozen, S.; Madden, T.L. Primer-BLAST: A tool to design target-specific primers for polymerase chain reaction. *BMC Bioinform.* **2012**, *13*. [CrossRef] [PubMed]

14. Choi, Y.; Chan, A.P. PROVEAN web server: A tool to predict the functional effect of amino acid substitutions and indels. *Bioinformatics* **2015**, *31*, 2745–2747. [CrossRef] [PubMed]

15. Pejaver, V.; Urresti, J.; Lugo-Martinez, J.; Pagel, K.A.; Lin, G.N.; Nam, H.-J.; Mort, M.; Cooper, D.N.; Sebat, J.; Iakoucheva, L.M.; et al. MutPred2: Inferring the molecular and phenotypic impact of amino acid variants. *BioRxiv* **2017**, 134981. [CrossRef]

16. Karczewski, K.J.; Francioli, L.C.; Tiao, G.; Cummings, B.B.; Alföldi, J.; Wang, Q.; Collins, R.L.; Laricchia, K.M.; Ganna, A.; Birnbaum, D.P.; et al. Variation across 141,456 human exomes and genomes reveals the spectrum of loss-of-function intolerance across human protein-coding genes. *BioRxiv* **2019**. [CrossRef]

17. McIntosh, G.H.; Belling, G.B. An isotopic study of oxalate excretion in sheep. *Aust. J. Exp. Biol. Med. Sci.* **1975**, *53*, 479–487. [CrossRef]

18. Williams, E.L.; Acquaviva, C.; Amoroso, A.; Chevalier, F.; Coulter-Mackie, M.; Monico, C.G.; Giachino, D.; Owen, T.; Robbiano, A.; Salido, E.; et al. Primary hyperoxaluria type 1: Update and additional mutation analysis of the AGXT gene. *Hum. Mutat.* **2009**, *30*, 910–917. [CrossRef]

19. Williams, E.; Rumsby, G. Selected exonic sequencing of the AGXT gene provides a genetic diagnosis in 50% of patients with primary hyperoxaluria type I. *Clin. Chem.* **2007**, *53*, 1216–1221. [CrossRef]

20. Lu, X.; Chen, W.; Li, L.; Zhu, X.; Huang, C.; Liu, S.; Yang, Y.; Zhao, Y. Two novel AGXT mutations cause the infantile form of primary hyperoxaluria type I in a Chinese family: Research on missed mutation. *Front. Pharmacol.* **2019**, *10*, 1–9. [CrossRef]

21. Cochat, P.; Groothoff, J. Primary hyperoxaluria type 1: Practical and ethical issues. *Pediatr. Nephrol.* **2013**, *28*, 2273–2281. [CrossRef] [PubMed]

22. Salido, E.C.; Li, X.M.; Lu, Y.; Wang, X.; Santana, A.; Roy-Chowdhury, N.; Torres, A.; Shapiro, L.J.; Roy-Chowdhury, J. Alanine-glyoxylate aminotransferase-deficient mice, a model for primary hyperoxaluria that responds to adenoviral gene transfer. *Proc. Natl. Acad. Sci. USA* **2006**, *103*, 18249–18254. [CrossRef] [PubMed]

23. Salido, E.; Pey, A.L.; Rodriguez, R.; Lorenzo, V. Primary hyperoxalurias: Disorders of glyoxylate detoxification. *Biochim. Biophys. Acta Mol. Basis Dis.* **2012**, *1822*, 1453–1464. [CrossRef] [PubMed]

24. Van Woerden, C.S.; Groothoff, J.W.; Wijburg, F.A.; Annink, C.; Wanders, R.J.A.; Waterham, H.R. Clinical implications of mutation analysis in primary hyperoxaluria type 1. *Kidney Int.* **2004**, *66*, 746–752. [CrossRef] [PubMed]

A Deletion in *GDF7* is Associated with a Heritable Forebrain Commissural Malformation Concurrent with Ventriculomegaly and Interhemispheric Cysts in Cats

Yoshihiko Yu [1,2,†], Erica K. Creighton [1,†], Reuben M. Buckley [1], Leslie A. Lyons [1,*] and 99 Lives Consortium [‡]

[1] Department of Veterinary Medicine and Surgery, College of Veterinary Medicine, University of Missouri, Columbia, MO 65211, USA; yoshi.yu@nvlu.ac.jp (Y.Y.); erica-creighton@idexx.com (E.K.C.); buckleyrm@missouri.edu (R.M.B.)

[2] Laboratory of Veterinary Radiology, Nippon Veterinary and Life Science University, Musashino, Tokyo 180-8602, Japan

* Correspondence: lyonsla@missouri.edu

† The authors contributed equally to this work.

‡ Membership of the 99 Lives Consortium is provided in the Acknowledgments.

Abstract: An inherited neurologic syndrome in a family of mixed-breed Oriental cats has been characterized as forebrain commissural malformation, concurrent with ventriculomegaly and interhemispheric cysts. However, the genetic basis for this autosomal recessive syndrome in cats is unknown. Forty-three cats were genotyped on the Illumina Infinium Feline 63K iSelect DNA Array and used for analyses. Genome-wide association studies, including a sib-transmission disequilibrium test and a case-control association analysis, and homozygosity mapping, identified a critical region on cat chromosome A3. Short-read whole genome sequencing was completed for a cat trio segregating with the syndrome. A homozygous 7 bp deletion in *growth differentiation factor 7* (*GDF7*) (c.221_227delGCCGCGC [p.Arg74Profs]) was identified in affected cats, by comparison to the 99 Lives Cat variant dataset, validated using Sanger sequencing and genotyped by fragment analyses. This variant was not identified in 192 unaffected cats in the 99 Lives dataset. The variant segregated concordantly in an extended pedigree. In mice, *GDF7* mRNA is expressed within the roof plate when commissural axons initiate ventrally-directed growth. This finding emphasized the importance of *GDF7* in the neurodevelopmental process in the mammalian brain. A genetic test can be developed for use by cat breeders to eradicate this variant.

Keywords: feline; *Felis catus*; brain malformation; BMP12; neurodevelopment; genetics; genomics; mendelian traits; genome-wide association study; whole genome sequencing

1. Introduction

Congenital brain malformations in humans are caused by genetic variants, in utero infection, or other environmental factors. Dogs and cats are also occasionally diagnosed with congenital brain malformations (reviewed in [1]), which are noted as breed predispositions, familial aggregations, or sporadic cases, especially in dogs [2–6]. Congenital hydrocephalus is common in toy and brachycephalic dog breeds, such as the Maltese, Yorkshire terrier, Chihuahua, toy poodle and pug dogs [7]. Widespread in Cavalier King Charles Spaniels, Chiari-like malformation is a common cause of foramen magnum obstruction, and results in the secondary syringomyelia in dogs, characterized by the mismatch of size between the brain and the skull [8].

Similarly, high grades of brachycephaly in cats are also associated with malformations of the calvarial and facial bones, as well as dental malformations or respiratory abnormalities [9–12]. A familial craniofacial malformation with meningoencephalocele has been recognized in Burmese cats [13], which is caused by *ALX Homeobox 1* (*ALX1*) variant [14]. However, feline brain malformations with (suspected) idiopathic nature are mostly reported as sporadic events [15–20]. Overall, the genetic factors contributing to brain (mal) formation and structural congenital brain disease in dogs and cats are largely unknown.

In an effort to develop a breed of cats having similar phenotypes to a tiger, including a small rounded ear, a mixed breed cat derived from the Oriental cat breed was discovered to have small rounded ears and hence, was used as a foundation sire for a breeding program. Outcross and backcross breeding indicated the phenotype was autosomal recessive [21]. However, a magnetic resonance imaging (MRI) examination of a kitten with the desired ear phenotype, which had an accidental head injury from a fall, indicated the presence of congenital hydrocephalus. Additional MRIs of the breeding stock suggested cats with the ear phenotype had congenital brain malformations. These cats have small rounded ear pinnae and doming of the head (Figure 1). This extended family of mixed-breed cats derived from the Oriental breed has been characterized clinically and histopathologically with forebrain commissural malformation concurrent with ventriculomegaly and interhemispheric cysts [21]. The forebrain malformations include dysgenesis of the septum pellucidum, interthalamic adhesion, and all the midline commissures, excluding the rostral white commissure, as well as hippocampal hypoplasia. Clinical symptoms include mild generalized ataxia when walking, and mild to marked postural reaction deficits, although cranial nerve examination and segmental reflexes are within normal limits. All the cats with neurological signs have midline and limbic structure abnormalities, dilated ventricles and hemispheral cysts with or without a suprapineal cyst. These findings resemble a mild variant of holoprosencephaly (HPE) in human (OMIM: 236,100 and others). Although variations in the severity of the forebrain commissural malformation were seen, most affected cats are hydrocephalic. No chromosomal abnormalities are noted in a karyotypic analysis of the cats. Segregation analysis suggests an autosomal recessive mode of inheritance; however, the causal variant remained unknown [21].

As a result of the potentially harmful impacts associated with the trait, the breeder promptly discontinued the breeding program and altered subsequent cats. However, some carriers for the trait had already been adopted for other breeding programs. A group of affected cats were presented to the researchers for pathological and genetic studies. Sample collection from the cats in the owner's breeding program and cats from controlled breeding within the university colony supported the genetic investigation of the abnormal brain development and mode of inheritance.

Genome-wide association studies (GWAS), using a sib-transmission disequilibrium test (sib-TDT) and a case-control analysis, and homozygosity mapping were conducted to detect an associated genomic region for the syndrome using genotypes from a feline single nucleotide polymorphism (SNP) DNA array [22]. Whole genome sequencing (WGS) was conducted on a cat trio segregating for the syndrome to define the location and identify candidate variants.

2. Materials and Methods

2.1. Sampling and Pedigree

All procedures were performed with an approved University of Missouri (MU) Institutional Animal Care and Use Committee protocol (ACUC protocol # 8292). Four affected and two carrier cats were donated and housed at the MU colony for controlled breeding. Additional buccal swab and cadaver samples from an external breeding program were provided voluntarily by the breeder/owner (N = 129). DNA samples were extracted using DNeasy Blood & Tissue Kit (Qiagen, Valencia, CA, USA). The quality of the DNA samples was visualized and confirmed by agarose gel electrophoresis. DNA samples whose concentration was insufficient were whole genome amplified, using the REPLI-g Mini Kit (Qiagen). The relationship of the ascertained cats was confirmed using short tandem repeat

(STR) markers, as previously described [23]. Parentage analysis was performed using the computer program COLONY [24,25]. Clinical and histopathological features of the syndrome were characterized previously [21]. Although some cats were phenotyped based on MRI and/or histopathology, most cats were assumed to have the brain malformation based on the ear morphology, since clinically healthy cats had elongated (normal) ears and clinically affected cats had the small, rounded ear type [21] (Figure 1). Images or cadavers of cats were not always available.

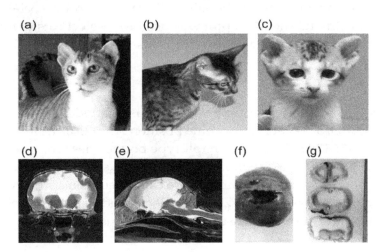

Figure 1. Domestic cats with heritable forebrain commissural malformation. Note the abnormal presentation of the pinnae used to determine affection status. (**a**) Frank—affected sire (left). (**b**) Camilla—carrier dam. (**c**) Bobble—affected offspring. These three cats (**a**–**c**) were whole genome sequenced. (**d**) Transverse plane of T2-weighted magnetic resonance imaging of an affected cat at the level of the thalamus. Severe ventriculomegaly, thinning of the cerebral parenchyma and midline structure deficits are seen. A part of the parietal lobe is deficient. (**e**) Mid-sagittal plane of T2-weighted magnetic resonance imaging of an affected cat (the same cat as (**d**)). Midline structure deficits are recognized. Note that the spinal cord is formed normally. Interhemispheric cysts are also seen at the rostrotentorial region and the quadrigeminal cistern. Due to the presence of cysts, cerebellar herniation is seen. (**f**) Gross dorsal view of the dissected head at necropsy. The skin was removed, and the skull was exposed. (**g**) Transverse sections of formalin-fixed brain tissue at the level of frontal lobe and thalamus. Severe ventriculomegaly, thinning of the cerebral parenchyma and midline structure deficits are seen. Note that a cat whose magnetic resonance imaging of (**d**) and (**e**) are presented here is different from cats whose gross pathological pictures of (**f**) and (**g**) are provided here.

2.2. DNA Array Genotyping

Fifty-two genomic DNA samples (~600 ng each) were submitted to GeneSeek (Neogene, Lincoln, NE, USA) for SNP genotyping on the Illumina Infinium Feline 63K iSelect DNA Array (Illumina, San Diego, CA, USA) [22]. The original SNP positions were based on an early assembly of the cat genome [26], and have been since relocalized to the latest feline genome assembly, Felis_catus_9.0. The SNP positions based on the Felis_catus_9.0 assembly were used for the analyses and the required map file is available. [27]. Quality control of the SNP data was performed using PLINK (v1.07) [28]. The following criteria were applied: (i) individuals with genotyping success rate of <80% were removed (–mind 0.2); (ii) SNP markers with a genotyping rate <80% were removed (–geno 0.2); and (iii) SNPs with a minor allele frequency of 0.05 or less were removed (–maf 0.05). Furthermore, SNPs that were previously reported to have missing ≥10% of genotypes and Mendelian errors [22], and that remained after quality controls were excluded.

2.3. Genome-Wide Association Studies

After the SNP pruning described above, GWAS were conducted using PLINK. Sib-TDT [29] was performed using the DFAM procedure in PLINK (–dfam). This method implements sib-TDT and also includes unrelated individuals in the analysis. A case-control association analysis was performed (–assoc). The genomic inflation factor was calculated using the function (–adjust). Multi-dimensional scaling (MDS) analysis was conducted (–genome) and MDS plots were generated to visualize the population stratification, using PLINK and R software (version 3.3.3; R Foundation for Statistical Computing, Vienna, Austria), respectively. A quantile-quantile (QQ) plot was created using R. Genome-wide significance for both analyses, which was determined using 100,000 permutations (–mperm 100000). Manhattan plots from the sib-TDT, case-control association and permutation analyses were generated using R. The MDS plot was used to reselect cats to minimize stratification between cases and controls for the secondary case-control association analysis, by visual interpretation.

2.4. Haplotype Analysis

An approximately 6 Mb region surrounding highly associated SNPs was extracted, including 81 SNPs, from SNP chrA3.163737349 at chromosome position A3: 123,014,546 to SNP chrA3.156620632 at chromosome position A3: 128,837,125. The haplotype boundaries were visually confirmed using Haploview (version 4.2) [30]. Linkage disequilibrium (LD) blocks were identified using the solid spine of LD method in Haploview. Haplotype sequences are estimated using an accelerated EM algorithm, as implemented in Haploview. When analyzing LD blocks and haplotypes, SNPs with MAF of 0% were allowed and included, because most cases showed the consistent genotypes at each SNP.

2.5. Homozygosity Analysis

Homozygosity analysis was performed using PLINK. SNPs within a 1000 kb window, containing at least 25, were investigated for runs of homozygosity (–homozyg-window-kb 1000, –homozyg-snp 25). In each window, five missing genotypes (20%) and a single heterozygote (2%) were tolerated (–homozyg-window-missing 5, –homozyg-window-het 1). The threshold of homozygosity match was set as 0.99 (–homozyg-match 0.99). A homozygous block was characterized by five SNPs (~200–250 kb). Consensus homozygosity blocks were identified as overlaps between individual homozygosity blocks (–consensus-match, –homozyg-group).

2.6. Whole Genome Sequencing

A trio of cats including an affected sire, a carrier dam and an affected offspring was selected for WGS as part of the 99 Lives Cat Genome Sequencing Initiative (http://felinegenetics.missouri.edu/99lives). These cats were produced at the MU colony; thus, the parentage was known. DNA extraction and library preparation were conducted as previously described [31]. A minimum of 4 μg genomic DNA was submitted for WGS to the MU DNA Core Facility. Two PCR-free libraries with insertion sizes of 350 bp and 550 bp were constructed for each cat using the TruSeq DNA PCR Free library preparation kit (Illumina). The Illumina HiSeq 2000 (Illumina) was used to generate sequence data.

Sequence reads were mapped to the latest feline genome assembly, Felis_catus_9.0, and processed as previously described [27]. Briefly, read mapping was conducted with Burrows-Wheeler Aligner (BWA) version 0.7.17 [32]. Duplicates were marked using Picard tool MarkDuplicates (http://broadinstitute. github.io/picard/). Potential insertions or deletions (indels) realignment was performed using the Genome Analysis Tool Kit (GATK version 3.8) [33] IndelRealigner. Variants were called using GATK HaplotypeCaller in gVCF mode [34]. VarSeq v2.0.2 (Golden Helix, Bozeman, MT, USA) was used to annotate variants with Ensembl 99 gene annotations and identify variants unique to the trio cats and absent from 192 unaffected unrelated domestic cats. Exonic variants were extracted from the dataset, including variants 21 bp flanking the exons to ensure inclusion of variants that may affect splice donor and accept sites. Candidate variants segregating across the trio were visualized using Integrative Genomics Viewer (IGV) [35].

2.7. Variant Validation and Genotyping

PCR and Sanger sequencing were performed to validate the 7 bp deletion in the candidate gene *GDF7* for cats that were submitted to WGS. The primer sequences were: forward primer: 5′-AGCGACATCATGAACTGGTG-3′, reverse primer: 5′-CCACGGAGCCCATGGACC-3′. PCR was performed using AccuPrime GC-Rich DNA Polymerase (Invitrogen, Carlsbad, CA, USA). PCR was performed following the manufacturer's instructions, with the annealing temperature of 61 °C and 35 cycles. PCR amplicon was purified using QIAquick Gel Extraction Kit (Qiagen), or using ExoSAP-IT PCR Product Cleanup Reagent (Thermo Fisher Scientific, Waltham, MA, USA). Sanger sequencing was conducted at the MU DNA Core Facility using an Applied Biosystems 3730xl DNA Analyzer (Applied Biosystems, Foster City, CA, USA) with BigDye Terminator v3.1 Cycle Sequencing Kit (Applied Biosystems).

Fragment analysis was conducted for population screening. PCR conditions and reagents used were the same as above, except the forward primer was fluorescein amidite [FAM] labeled at the 5′ end. Fragment analysis was conducted at the MU DNA Core Facility using an Applied Biosystems 3730xl DNA Analyzer (Applied Biosystems). The expected wildtype fragment size was 294 bp, while the mutant fragment size was expected as 287 bp. Amplicons were analyzed using STRand software [36].

3. Results

3.1. Pedigree and Genotyping

Using 18 STRs, the parentage for 69 of 129 cats was determined with a high likelihood using the COLONY software [24,25] (data not shown), producing a pedigree of 79 cats (Figure S1). For GWAS, 52 cats were selected using owner provided and pedigree information, including 26 cases, and 26 controls, in which 43 cats were included in the pedigree (Figure S1). Cat DNA samples were genotyped on Feline 63K SNP array (File S1). Selection criteria for genotyping focused on cats that were as unrelated as possible. Nine cats with call rates below 80% were removed, and 478 SNPs were removed with missingness rates > 20%. An additional 22,297 SNPs were also removed with minor allele frequencies < 0.05. After filtering, 20 cases and 23 controls remained with a genotyping rate of 0.977 across 40,263 SNPs. Furthermore, 372 SNPs were excluded, due to missing ≥10% of genotypes and Mendelian errors previously reported [22]. The GWAS was conducted with 39,891 SNPs.

3.2. Association Studies

Sib-TDT was conducted on the pedigree formed by the 20 cases and 23 controls. After permutation testing, no SNPs were significant; however, nine SNPs with the highest, the second-highest, or the third-highest association were localized to cat chromosome A3:123,055,238–128,667,138 on the Felis_catus_9.0, extending approximately 5.6 Mb (Table 1). The result of the sib-TDT analysis was presented as a Manhattan plot (Figure 2a). In the initial case-control association analysis, 65 SNPs had genome-wide significance and were located cat chromosome A3: 116,714,934–129,668,450, extending ~13.0 Mb and C1: 105,429,018–115,412,315, extending ~10.0 Mb (Table 1). However, the genomic inflation factor was 1.89; thus, the MDS plot (Figure S2) was used to reselect cases and controls for the analysis. A second case-control association analysis was performed with 14 cases and nine controls, and the genomic inflation factor was reduced to one. Seventeen SNPs showed genome-wide significance and were located cat chromosome A3: 119,105,247–129,372,537, encompassing ~10.3 Mb (Figure 2b, Table 1). This chromosome A3 region encompassed the entire region suggested by the sib-TDT, and was within the initial case-control association analysis.

Table 1. Single nucleotide polymorphism (SNP) associations for cats with heritable forebrain commissural malformation in the sib-transmission disequilibrium test (sib-TDT) and case-control association analyses.

SNP *	Chr	Position †	Sib-TDT	Case-Control (Initial)	Case-Control (2nd)
chrA3.164724433	A3	123353491	>0.6	0.0001	0.0045
chrA3.164567500	A3	122318611	>0.6	0.0001	0.0045
chrA3.164340161	A3	122513677	>0.6	0.0001	0.0045
chrA3.164113252	A3	122698750	>0.6	0.0001	0.0045
chrA3.163320257	A3	123353491	0.5639	0.0001	0.0045
chrA3.162970354	A3	123644765	>0.6	0.0001	0.0045
chrA3.162343840	A3	124176474	>0.6	0.0004	0.0045
chrA3.158624618	A3	127189752	>0.6	0.0001	0.0045
chrA3.159621145	A3	126377299	0.5639	0.0001	0.0082
chrA3.162413594	A3	124100380	>0.6	0.0014	0.0137
chrA3.156826206	A3	128667138	0.5639	0.0001	0.0169
chrA3.156620632	A3	128837125	>0.6	0.0001	0.0169
chrA3.155936886	A3	129372537	>0.6	0.0004	0.0169
chrA3.168960567	A3	119105247	>0.6	0.0128	0.0261
chrA3.168031908	A3	119810207	>0.6	0.0264	0.0261
chrA3.167492986	A3	120088757	>0.6	0.0061	0.0261
chrA3.167322483	A3	120215597	>0.6	0.0292	0.0261
chrA3.162621987	A3	123934341	0.5521	0.0014	>0.05
chrA3.163679766	A3	123055238	0.5639	0.0004	>0.05
chrA3.161984351	A3	124475589	0.5639	0.0002	>0.05
chrA3.161943004	A3	124509146	0.5639	0.0002	>0.05
chrA3.161399869	A3	124945294	0.5639	0.0020	>0.05
chrA3.160673309	A3	125511595	0.5639	0.0002	>0.05

p-values were presented with up to four decimal places. * SNP IDs are based on an early cat genome assembly [26]
† Positions based on current cat genome assembly [27].

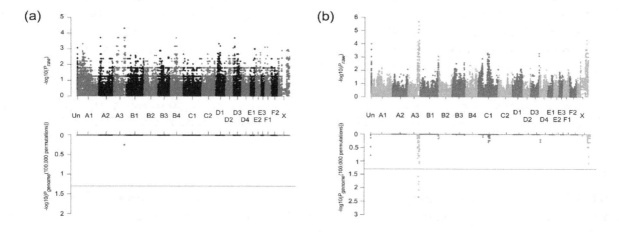

Figure 2. Manhattan plot of the genome-wide association studies (GWAS) for heritable forebrain commissural malformation in cats. Cats (20 cases and 23 controls) were genotyped on the Illumina Infinium Feline 63K iSelect DNA Array (Illumina, San Diego, CA, USA) and used for GWAS. In both panels of (**a**) and (**b**), the upper plots exhibit the P_{raw} value of the analysis, while the lower exhibits the P_{genome} values after 100,000 permutations. Red horizontal lines indicate genome-wide significance ($P_{genome} = 0.05$, $-\log_{10} = 1.3$). (**a**) Sib-TDT analysis. Genome-wide significance was not achieved. (**b**) Case-control association analysis. Significant association is localized to chromosome A3 for 17 SNPs. The genomic inflation was 1.

3.3. Haplotype Analysis

The 6 Mb region, on chrA3: from approximately 123 to 129 Mb and encompassing the overlapped region identified in GWAS, was visually inspected for common haplotypes using Haploview. In affected cats, a large extended LD block encompassing approximately 4.3 Mb (A3: 123,082,369–127,348,216) was identified with a 95% frequency of the sequential haplotype. Considering that two cats had 82.7% and 91.4% genotyping rate, one cat had 98.8% and the others had 100% genotyping rate in this area, a few missing produced the remaining haplotypes (File S2). Short and discontinuous LD blocks are identified by Haploview in controls. There are various haplotype sequences and frequencies approximately within the 6 Mb regions in unaffected cats.

3.4. Homozygosity Analysis

Homozygosity mapping was performed on 20 cases and 23 controls. The homozygosity analysis identified the same location on chromosome A3 in 18 of 20 affected cats, excluding the same two cases that did not have sufficiently high genotyping rates, with A3: 125,601,560–127,684,693, spanning approximately 2.1 Mb, and no unaffected cats were homozygosity (Table S1). The region was identified by the two genome-wide association analyses (Table 1). Although other ROHs were identified, none were specific to cases or as extensive.

3.5. Whole Genome Sequencing

Cat genomes have been submitted to the NCBI short read archive under BioProject: PRJNA528515; Accessions PRJNA343385; SRX2654400 (Sire), SRX2654398 (dam) and SRX2654399 (offspring). Genome sequence analyses and variant calling for the 99 Lives project has been previously described [37]. Approximately 2.5 million variants were ascertained across 195 cats in the exonic portion of the dataset, which included 21 bp of exon flank sequence. No candidate genes were identified on cat chromosome A3 during the initial analysis, when considering the sire and offspring to be homozygous affected, and considering the dam as an obligate carrier for an alternative allele (Table 2). Only an intergenic variant (C1:106,990,675) and an intronic variant in *sperm antigen with calponin homology and coiled-coil domains* (*SPECC1*) (E1:9,973,078) met the segregation criteria. Using relaxed constraints, where affected cats were allowed to also be considered as carriers, four more variants were identified (C1:96,095,693, C1:96,839,645 and D2:33,368,378) with only one variant located within the critical region and also in a gene coding region (Table 2). This variant was a 7 bp deletion in the coding region of *GDF7* (c.221_227delGCCGCGC [p.Arg74Profs*17]) at the position A3:127002233 (ENSFCAT00000063603). The variant was identified as homozygous in the affected sire, heterozygous in the obligate carrier dam, heterozygous in the affected offspring, and absent from the other 192 domestic cats. Although each cat in the trio had an average of ~30× genome coverage, the sire had 18× coverage within the region, the dam had ~14× coverage with seven reads per allele, and the affected offspring had ~16× coverage, with only one of the reads representing the reference allele, likely misrepresenting the offspring as heterozygous, and visual inspection with IGV suggested the affected offspring was instead very likely homozygous for the variant (Figure 3). The affected cat was confirmed as a homozygote for the alternate allele by genotyping. The *GDF7* variant was predicted to cause a truncated protein with 89 amino acids, while the wildtype protein has 455 amino acids (Figure S3). Feline *GDF7* amino acid sequence is predicted to be 86.2%, 90.1%, 84.6%, 77.8% and 77.2% identical to human, horse, cow, rat and mouse, respectively (Figure S3). In addition, comparison of the *GDF7* locus between the Felis_catus_9.0 and Felis_catus_8.0 genome assemblies, revealed the region containing the *GDF7* candidate variant is absent from the Felis_catus_8.0 assembly, indicating the importance of the updated reference genome for trait discovery.

Table 2. Variants identified in 99 Lives whole genome sequence dataset considering segregation within the trio.

Chr:Pos	Ref/Alt	No. Het *	No. Homo	Gene Name	Sequence Ontology	Effect	HGVS c. (Clinically Relevant)
A3:127002233	GCGCGGC/-	2	1	GDF7	frameshift	LoF	ENSFCAT00000063603: c.221_227delGCCGCGC
C1:96095693	C/T	2	1		intergenic	Other	
C1:96839645	C/T	2	1		intergenic	Other	
D2:33368378	C/A	2	1		intergenic	Other	
C1:106990675	C/A	1	2		intergenic	Other	
E1:9973078	C/T	1	2	SPECC1	Intron	Other	ENSFCAT00000005195: c.2850 + 13572G > A

* Only the dam should be heterozygous for the variant in the dataset and the sire and offspring homozygous for the variant. Sequence data was poor within the critical region on cat Chromosome A3, and the affected offspring was erroneously considered heterozygous by the Genome Analysis Tool Kit (GATK version 3.8). Four variants are identified when the offspring is considered heterozygous.

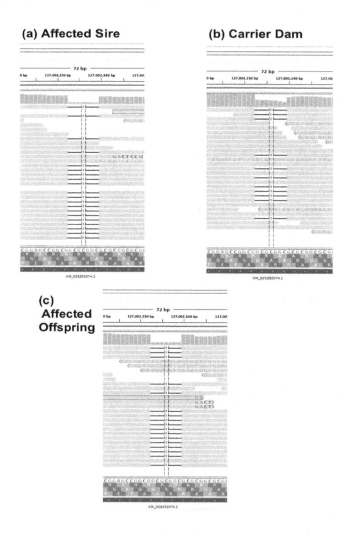

Figure 3. Depiction of the whole genome sequence reads using the Integrated Genome Viewer (IGV) of (**a**) affected sire, (**b**) carrier dam, and (**c**) affected offspring for the *GDF7* variant. Grey horizontal bars represent individual reads, while grey vertical bars at the top of each sub figure represent depth of coverage. Notice in affected individuals (**a,c**), coverage is close to zero in the deleted region, while, in the carrier sequencing (**b**), coverage is approximately 50%. Additionally, in affected individuals (**a,c**), reads with high numbers of mismatches are indicative of the misidentification of an indel, and tend to occur near the ends of reads.

3.6. Variant Validation and Genotyping

Sanger sequencing was performed to confirm the identified *GDF7* c.221_227delGCCGCGC in affected and obligate carrier cats, including the cats in the WGS trio. The 7 bp deletion in *GDF7* was screened in 25 affected, 39 unaffected, and two cats with unknown phenotype in the extended pedigree using fragment analysis (Figure S4). Both unknown cats were homozygous for the variant allele. Overall, 13 of 14 suspected wildtype cats in the extended pedigree were concordant, and one cat genotyped as a heterozygote. Of 25 suspected carriers, 23 genotyped as heterozygote and two as wildtype normal. Of 22 suspected affected cats, 20 genotyped as homozygous for the variant, one as heterozygous and one as wildtype normal.

4. Discussion

Brain malformations are occasionally identified in veterinary practice. However, little is known about the genetic causes and interactions for brain malformation. Due to the health concerns associated with breed development, particularly in dog breeds [38,39], many breeders have become more vigilant to health-associated consequences of selection based on morphological phenotypes. Feline brain malformation syndrome seen in this extended family happened to be generated in the course of breeding selection for the ear morphological phenotype.

Most of the cat samples had been archived as frozen cadavers by the breeder, and later provided to the researchers. As a result of poor documentation of relationships and disease status, a pedigree was established by determining parentage using STRs, age, and gender of the cats and from interviews with the breeder. Ear phenotypes, which were used as a proxy for disease, were difficult to determine from frozen cadavers. Due to the significant inbreeding and backcrossing required to maintain the phenotype, 18 STRs were often insufficient to determine parentage. However, some known breedings were available from the university colony. Overall, an extended pedigree was developed, and was expected to be sufficient for GWAS and WGS investigations for the causal variant. Furthermore, a variant dataset from WGS of domestic cats, the 99 Lives Cat Genome Sequencing Initiative, which has revealed the causative variants for several cat diseases and traits in the last several years [31,40–46], was considered to facilitate the variant filtering to find the private variants.

In humans, HPE is the most common malformation of the prosencephalon, and its prevalence is approximate 1 in 10,000 births [47]. A common feature of HPE includes the incomplete separation of the anterior part of the forebrain or telencephalon. The previous study indicated this feline heritable brain malformation syndrome resembled a mild form of HPE [21]. Many genes have been reported to cause HPE in humans (reviewed in [48–50]). However, *GDF7*, also known as *bone morphogenetic protein 12 (BMP12)*, has not been reported to be associated with HPE in humans. Initially, *GDF7* activity was shown to be required for the specification of neuronal identity in the spinal cord [51]. *GDF7* mRNA is expressed within the roof plate, when commissural axons initiate to grow ventrally-directed. Furthermore, *GDF7*-null mutant mice show hydrocephalus, and they show considerable variation in the location of the dilated ventricle [51]. This evidence supports these findings that the frameshift mutation in *GDF7* causing the truncated protein is highly likely to be associated with this heritable brain malformation syndrome in cats. Transcriptomic and proteomic analyses would be essential to ascertain that this *GDF7* variant causes heritable forebrain commissural malformation in cats.

The variable severity of this syndrome in the cat pedigree was reported previously [21]. In humans, heterogeneity in familial HPE is also identified even if different individuals are carrying the same mutation [52–54]. The influence of environmental or teratogenic factors or modifier genes have been suggested for the spectrum (reviewed in [47,48,50]). Assuming no exposure to teratogen and relatively homogeneous living environment, the presence of modifier genes is suspected for the variable severity of the dilated ventricles and supratentorial cysts in cats presented here.

Bone morphogenetic proteins (BMPs) belong to the transforming growth factor-β (TGF-β) superfamily of proteins that are involved in many functions such as cell proliferation, differentiation, apoptosis, cell fate determination and morphogenesis [55]. The BMPs also play various roles in the neural development [56]. Among them, *GDF7* also known as BMP12, plays an essential role in bone and cartilage formation as well [57]. Except for hydrocephalus seen in *GDF7*-null mutant mice [51], several phenotypes caused by *GDF7* deficient mice have been reported, including the subtle effect on Achilles tendon [58], increased endochondral bone growth [59], seminal vesicle defects and sterility [60], and smaller bone cross-sectional geometric parameters [61]. In addition, a variant in *GDF7* (rs3072) has been reported to increase risk for Barrett's esophagus and esophageal adenocarcinoma [62,63]. Although, to the authors' knowledge, there was no report about the involvement of *GDF7* in ear or skull morphology, there is a possibility that small rounded pinnae and/or domed craniums may be influenced by the *GDF7* variant, because *GDF7*, also known as BMP12, has been considered to play a negative role on chondrogenesis [59], and to be involved in the structural integrity of bone [61].

In conclusion, the combination of GWAS, homozygosity mapping and WGS identified a 7 bp deletion in *GDF7* (c.221_227delGCCGCGC), which is the most likely variant causing feline forebrain commissural malformation, concurrent with ventriculomegaly and interhemispheric cysts in this domestic cat lineage, although the functional analysis has not been achieved to prove the deterministic mechanism. Furthermore, this study highlights the importance of *GDF7* in the neurodevelopmental course in cats, and brings new insight into neurodevelopmental biology. Cat breeders can now perform a genetic test to eradicate the *GDF7* mutation from the breeding population.

Supplementary Materials:
Table S1: Regions of homozygosity was unique to 18 cats with the inherited forebrain commissural malformation, and were absent in all the unaffected cats. Figure S1: Pedigree of cats segregating for an autosomal recessive forebrain commissural malformation. Relationships of 79 cats (27 nuclear families) provided by the breeder and confirmed with genetic testing of short tandem repeats when possible. Arrow indicates the proband. Circles indicate females, squares indicate males, and diamonds indicate unknown sex. Filled symbols represent cats with small rounded ears, which were suspected to have forebrain commissural malformation concurrent with ventriculomegaly and interhemispheric cysts. Half-filled represent obligate carriers. Symbols with question marks represent cats with unknown phenotype. A symbol with no fill indicates the cat is known to be completely unrelated and not expected to be a carrier. The cats genotyped on the DNA array and used for genome-wide association studies and homozygosity mapping are indicated by a "T" on the upper left of the symbol (The nine cats removed by quality control are not indicated). A black filled circle at the left bottom of symbol are individuals that were whole genome sequenced. Cats with a bar above the symbol were confirmed by magnetic resonance imaging. Cats with an open circle to the upper right had histology performed at necropsy. The cats' ID/name is indicated below the symbol. Size in basepairs of the genotypes for the 7 bp *GDF7* indel are indicated below each cat available. Figure S2: Multi-dimensional scaling plot and quantile-quantile plot of cases and controls for genome-association analyses. (a) Multi-dimensional scaling (MDS) plot of cats used for the initial case-control association analysis. The genomic inflation was 1.89. Therefore, cats clustered within the blue rectangular area were selected for the second case-control association analysis as visual inspection suggests less stratification between cases and controls. The genomic inflation factor was reduced to 1. (b,c) The quantile-quantile plots of cats used for the initial (b) and second (c) analyses demonstrate the observed versus expected–log(p) values. Figure S3: Protein sequence alignment of *GDF7* in cats (*Felis catus*) and other species. GDF7 protein sequences are aligned from wildtype cat (*Felis catus*), GDF7 mutant cat, cow (*Bos Taurus*: NP_001193030.1 [ARS-UCD1.2]), horse (*Equus caballus*: XP_023475218.1 [EquCab3.0]), mouse (*Mus musculus*: NP_001299805.1 [GRCm38.p4]), and rat (*Rattus norvegicus*: XP_006239940.1 [Rnor_6.0]). Identical amino acids to those of Felis catus sequence are represented as a dot (.). Deleted amino acids are represented as a dash (–). A 7 bp deletion causes a frameshift and changes the amino acid sequence from 74th position (highlighted in yellow), starting with an arginine to a proline change, which results in the truncated protein with a stop codon 17 amino acids downstream. Figure S4. Variant validation by Sanger sequencing and fragment analysis. (a) Sanger sequence of a wildtype and homozygous affected cat for the 7 bp *GDF7* variant (boxed region). (b) Fluorescence-based fragment analysis using an ABI 3730XL for the *GDF7* variant. Left—homozygous wildtype with 294 bp fragment, middle—heterozygous with 287 and 294 bp fragments, and right—affected with 287 bp fragment. LIZ standard (Applied Biosystems, Foster City, CA, USA) was used to size DNA fragments. File S1: Ped file for PLINK of cats genotyped using Illumina Infinium Feline 63K iSelect DNA Array. File S2: SNPs (*n* = 81) forming common haplotype for cats in the association studies.

Author Contributions: Conceptualization, L.A.L.; Methodology, L.A.L.; Software, R.M.B., Y.Y.; Validation, Y.Y.; Formal Analysis, E.K.C., Y.Y.; Investigation, E.K.C., Y.Y., R.M.B.; Resources, L.A.L., E.K.C.; Data Curation, L.A.L., R.M.B.; Writing—Original Draft Preparation, Y.Y., E.K.C.; Writing—Review & Editing, Y.Y., R.M.B., E.K.C., L.A.L.; Visualization, Y.Y., R.M.B., E.K.C.; Supervision, L.A.L.; Project Administration, L.A.L.; Funding Acquisition, L.A.L. All authors have read and agreed to the published version of the manuscript.

Acknowledgments: We also thank Barbara Gandolfi and Thomas R. Juba for technical assistance and assistance with figures from Karen Clifford. 99 Lives Consortium (2019 cat analysis—99Lives195) Organizer: Leslie A. Lyons [1]; Data analyst: Reuben M. Buckley [1]; Each member of the 99 Lives Consortium (2019 cat analysis – 99Lives195) has provided at least one >15x coverage genome of the domestic cat or a wild felid to support the analyses of the dataset. Members: Reuben M. Buckley [1], Danielle Aberdein [2], Paulo C. Alves [3,4], Gregory S. Barsh [5,6], Rebecca R. Bellone [7], Tomas F. Bergström [8], Adam R. Boyko [9], Jeffrey A. Brockman [10], Margret L. Casal [11], Marta G. Castelhano [12], Ottmar Distl [13], Nicholas H. Dodman [14], N. Matthew Ellinwood [15], Jonathan E. Fogle [16], Oliver P. Forman [17], Dorian J. Garrick [2,15], Edward I. Ginns [18], Jens Häggström [19], Robert J. Harvey [20], Daisuke Hasegawa [21], Bianca Haase [22], Christopher R. Helps [23], Isabel Hernandez [24], Marjo K. Hytönen [25], Maria Kaukonen [25], Christopher B. Kaelin [5,6], Tomoki Kosho [26], Emilie Leclerc [27], Teri L. Lear [28], Tosso Leeb [29], Ronald H.L. Li [30], Hannes Lohi [25], Maria Longeri [31], Mark A. Magnuson [32], Richard Malik [33], Shrinivasrao P. Mane [34], John S. Munday [2], William J. Murphy [35], Niels C. Pedersen [36], Simon M. Peterson-Jones [37], Max F. Rothschild [15], Clare Rusbridge [38], Beth Shapiro [39], Joshua A. Stern [36], William F. Swanson [40], Karen A. Terio [41], Rory J. Todhunter [12], Wesley C. Warren [42], Elizabeth A. Wilcox [12], Julia H. Wildschutte [43], Yoshihiko Yu [21], Leslie A. Lyons [1].

[1]   Department of Veterinary Medicine and Surgery, College of Veterinary Medicine, University of Missouri, Columbia, MO 65211, USA

[2]   School of Veterinary Science, Massey University, Palmerston North 4442, New Zealand

[3]   CIBIO/InBIO, Centro de Investigação em Biodiversidade e Recursos Genéticos/InBIO Associate Lab & Faculdade de Ciências, Universidade do Porto, Campus e Vairão, 4485–661 Vila do Conde, Portugal

[4]   Wildlife Biology Program, University of Montana, Missoula, MT 59812, USA

[5]   HudsonAlpha Institute for Biotechnology, Huntsville, AL 35806, USA

[6]   Department of Genetics, Stanford University, Stanford, CA 94305 USA

[7]   Veterinary Genetics Laboratory, University of California, Davis, CA 95616, USA

[8]   Department of Animal Breeding and Genetics, Swedish University of Agricultural Sciences, 750 07 Uppsala, Sweden

[9]   Department of Biomedical Sciences, College of Veterinary Medicine, Cornell University, Ithaca, NY 14853, USA

[10]   Hill's Pet Nutrition Inc., Topeka, KS 66601, USA

[11]   Reproduction, and Pediatrics, School of Veterinary Medicine, University of Pennsylvania, Philadelphia, PA 19104, USA

[12]   Department of Clinical Sciences, College of Veterinary Medicine, Cornell University, Ithaca, NY 14853, USA

[13]   Institute for Animal Breeding and Genetics, University of Veterinary Medicine, Hannover, 30559 Hannover, Germany

[14]   Department of Clinical Sciences, Cummings School of Veterinary Medicine, Tufts University, Grafton, MA 01536, USA

[15]   Department of Animal Science, College of Agriculture and Life Sciences, Iowa State University, Ames, IA 50011, USA

[16]   College of Veterinary Medicine, North Carolina State University, Raleigh, NC 27607, USA

[17]   WALTHAM Centre for Pet Nutrition, Freeby Lane, Waltham on the Wolds, Leicestershire LE14 4RT, UK

[18]   Department of Psychiatry, University of Massachusetts Medical School, Worcester, MA 01655, USA

[19]   Department of Clinical Sciences, Faculty of Veterinary Medicine and Animal Science, Swedish University of Agricultural Sciences, SE-750 07 Uppsala, Sweden

[20]   School of Health and Sport Sciences, University of the Sunshine Coast, Sippy Downs, QLD 4558, Australia

[21]   Laboratory of Veterinary Radiology, Nippon Veterinary and Life Science University, Tokyo 180-8602, Japan

[22]   Sydney School of Veterinary Science, Faculty of Science, University of Sydney, Sydney, NSW 2006, Australia

[23]   Langford Vets, University of Bristol, Langford, Bristol BS40 5DU, UK

[24]   Pediatrics and Medical Genetics Service, College of Veterinary Medicine, Cornell University, Ithaca, NY 14853, USA

[25]   Department of Veterinary Biosciences; Department of Medical Genetics, University of Helsinki and Folkhälsan Research Center, 00014 Helsinki, Finland

[26]   Department of Medical Genetics, Center for Medical Genetics, Shinshu University Hospital, Matsumoto, Nagano 390-8621, Japan

[27]   SPF-Diana Pet food-Symrise Group-56250 Elven, France

[28]   Department of Veterinary Science, University of Kentucky - Lexington, Lexington, KY 40506, USA (*In memoriam*)

[29]   Vetsuisse Faculty, Institute of Genetics, University of Bern, 3001 Bern, Switzerland

[30]   Department of Surgical and Radiological Sciences, School of Veterinary Medicine, University of California Davis, One Shields Ave, Davis, CA 95616, USA

[31]   Dipartimento di Medicina Veterinaria, University of Milan, 20122 Milan, Italy

32   Departments of Molecular Physiology and Biophysics, Cell and Developmental Biology, and Medicine, Vanderbilt University, School of Medicine, Nashville, TN 37232, USA

33   Centre for Veterinary Education, University of Sydney, Sydney, NSW 2006, Australia

34   Elanco Animal Health, Greenfield, IN 46140, USA

35   Department of Veterinary Integrative Biosciences, College of Veterinary Medicine, Texas A&M University, College Station, TX 77845, USA

36   Department of Medicine and Epidemiology, School of Veterinary Medicine, University of California at Davis, Davis, CA 95616, USA

37   Department of Small Animal Clinical Sciences, Veterinary Medical Center, Michigan State University, East Lansing, MI 48824, USA

38   School of Veterinary Medicine, Faculty of Health & Medical Sciences, Univesity of Surrey, Guildford, Surrey GU2 7AL, UK

39   Department of Ecology and Evolutionary Biology, University of California, Santa Cruz, Santa Cruz, CA 95064, USA

40   Center for Conservation and Research of Endangered Wildlife (CREW), Cincinnati Zoo & Botanical Garden, Cincinnati, OH 45220, USA

41   Zoological Pathology Program, University of Illinois, Brookfield, IL 60513, USA

42   Division of Animal Sciences, College of Agriculture, Food and Natural Resources; School of Medicine, University of Missouri, Columbia, MO 65211, USA

43   Department of Biological Sciences, Bowling Green State University, Bowling Green, OH 43403, USA

References

1.   MacKillop, E. Magnetic resonance imaging of intracranial malformations in dogs and cats. *Vet. Radiol. Ultrasound.* **2011**, *52*, S42–S51. [CrossRef] [PubMed]

2.   Jurney, C.; Haddad, J.; Crawford, N.; Miller, A.D.; Van Winkle, T.J.; Vite, C.H.; Sponenberg, P.; Inzana, K.D.; Cook, C.R.; Britt, L.; et al. Polymicrogyria in standard poodles. *J. Vet. Intern. Med.* **2009**, *23*, 871–874. [CrossRef] [PubMed]

3.   Goncalves, R.; Volk, H.; Smith, P.M.; Penderis, J.; Garosi, L.; MacKillop, E.; de Stefani, A.; Cherubini, G.; McConnell, J.F. Corpus callosal abnormalities in dogs. *J. Vet. Intern. Med.* **2014**, *28*, 1275–1279. [CrossRef] [PubMed]

4.   Bernardino, F.; Rentmeister, K.; Schmidt, M.J.; Bruehschwein, A.; Matiasek, K.; Matiasek, L.A.; Lauda, A.; Schoon, H.A.; Fischer, A. Inferior cerebellar hypoplasia resembling a Dandy-Walker-like malformation in purebred Eurasier dogs with familial non-progressive ataxia: A retrospective and prospective clinical cohort study. *PLoS ONE* **2015**, *10*, e0117670. [CrossRef] [PubMed]

5.   Gerber, M.; Fischer, A.; Jagannathan, V.; Drogemuller, M.; Drogemuller, C.; Schmidt, M.J.; Bernardino, F.; Manz, E.; Matiasek, K.; Rentmeister, K.; et al. A deletion in the VLDLR gene in Eurasier dogs with cerebellar hypoplasia resembling a Dandy-Walker-like malformation (DWLM). *PLoS ONE* **2015**, *10*, e0108917. [CrossRef]

6.   Estey, C.M. Congenital Hydrocephalus. *Vet. Clin. North. Am. Small Anim. Pract.* **2016**, *46*, 217–229. [CrossRef]

7.   Selby, L.A.; Hayes, H.M., Jr.; Becker, S.V. Epizootiologic features of canine hydrocephalus. *Am. J. Vet. Res.* **1979**, *40*, 411–413.

8.   Knowler, S.P.; Galea, G.L.; Rusbridge, C. Morphogenesis of Canine Chiari Malformation and Secondary Syringomyelia: Disorders of Cerebrospinal Fluid Circulation. *Front. Vet. Sci.* **2018**, *5*, 171. [CrossRef]

9.   Schmidt, M.J.; Kampschulte, M.; Enderlein, S.; Gorgas, D.; Lang, J.; Ludewig, E.; Fischer, A.; Meyer-Lindenberg, A.; Schaubmar, A.R.; Failing, K.; et al. The Relationship between Brachycephalic Head Features in Modern Persian Cats and Dysmorphologies of the Skull and Internal Hydrocephalus. *J. Vet. Intern. Med.* **2017**, *31*, 1487–1501. [CrossRef]

10.   Schlueter, C.; Budras, K.D.; Ludewig, E.; Mayrhofer, E.; Koenig, H.E.; Walter, A.; Oechtering, G.U. Brachycephalic feline noses: CT and anatomical study of the relationship between head conformation and the nasolacrimal drainage system. *J. Feline Med. Surg.* **2009**, *11*, 891–900. [CrossRef]

11.   Farnworth, M.J.; Chen, R.; Packer, R.M.; Caney, S.M.; Gunn-Moore, D.A. Flat feline faces: Is brachycephaly associated with respiratory abnormalities in the domestic cat (*Felis catus*)? *PLoS ONE* **2016**, *11*, e0161777. [CrossRef] [PubMed]

12. Mestrinho, L.A.; Louro, J.M.; Gordo, I.S.; Niza, M.; Requicha, J.F.; Force, J.G.; Gawor, J.P. Oral and dental anomalies in purebred, brachycephalic Persian and exotic cats. *J. Am. Vet. Med. Assoc.* **2018**, *253*, 66–72. [CrossRef] [PubMed]

13. Sponenberg, D.P.; Graf-Webster, E. Hereditary meningoencephalocele in Burmese cats. *J. Hered.* **1986**, *77*, 60. [CrossRef] [PubMed]

14. Lyons, L.A.; Erdman, C.A.; Grahn, R.A.; Hamilton, M.J.; Carter, M.J.; Helps, C.R.; Alhaddad, H.; Gandolfi, B. Aristaless-Like Homeobox protein 1 (ALX1) variant associated with craniofacial structure and frontonasal dysplasia in Burmese cats. *Dev. Biol.* **2016**, *409*, 451–458. [CrossRef] [PubMed]

15. Lowrie, M.; Wessmann, A.; Gunn-Moore, D.; Penderis, J. Quadrigeminal cyst management by cystoperitoneal shunt in a 4-year-old Persian cat. *J. Feline Med. Surg.* **2009**, *11*, 711–713. [CrossRef]

16. Reed, S.; Cho, D.Y.; Paulsen, D. Quadrigeminal arachnoid cysts in a kitten and a dog. *J. Vet. Diagn. Invest.* **2009**, *21*, 707–710. [CrossRef]

17. Herrmann, A.; Hecht, W.; Herden, C. Lissencephaly and microencephaly combined with hypoplasia of corpus callosum and cerebellum in a domestic cat. *Tierarztl Prax Ausg K Kleintiere Heimtiere* **2011**, *39*, 116–120.

18. Shimbo, G.; Tagawa, M.; Yanagawa, M.; Miyahara, K. MRI of lobar holoprosencephaly in a cat with hypodipsic hypernatraemia. *JFMS Open Rep.* **2018**, *4*. [CrossRef]

19. Boccanera, C.; Stabile, F.; Corvi, R.; Mariscoli, M.; Mandara, M.T. Hydrocephalus, supratentorial diverticulum and agenesis of the interthalamic adhesion and corpus callosum in a cat: MRI findings, treatment and follow-up. *Vet. Record Case Rep.* **2018**, *6*, e000416. [CrossRef]

20. Woerde, D.J.; Hoffmann, K.L.; Brown, N.L. Frontoethmoidal encephalocele in a cat. *JFMS Open Rep.* **2018**, *4*. [CrossRef]

21. Keating, M.K.; Sturges, B.K.; Siso, S.; Wisner, E.R.; Creighton, E.K.; Lyons, L.A. Characterization of an Inherited Neurologic Syndrome in Toyger Cats with Forebrain Commissural Malformations, Ventriculomegaly and Interhemispheric Cysts. *J. Vet. Intern. Med.* **2016**, *30*, 617–626. [CrossRef] [PubMed]

22. Gandolfi, B.; Alhaddad, H.; Abdi, M.; Bach, L.H.; Creighton, E.K.; Davis, B.W.; Decker, J.E.; Dodman, N.H.; Ginns, E.I.; Grahn, J.C.; et al. Applications and efficiencies of the first cat 63K DNA array. *Sci Rep.* **2018**, *8*, 7024. [CrossRef] [PubMed]

23. Lipinski, M.J.; Amigues, Y.; Blasi, M.; Broad, T.E.; Cherbonnel, C.; Cho, G.J.; Corley, S.; Daftari, P.; Delattre, D.R.; Dileanis, S.; et al. An international parentage and identification panel for the domestic cat (Felis catus). *Anim Genet.* **2007**, *38*, 371–377. [CrossRef] [PubMed]

24. Jones, O.R.; Wang, J. COLONY: A program for parentage and sibship inference from multilocus genotype data. *Mol. Ecol. Resour.* **2010**, *10*, 551–555. [CrossRef]

25. Wang, J. A simulation module in the computer program COLONY for sibship and parentage analysis. *Mol. Ecol. Resour.* **2013**, *13*, 734–739. [CrossRef]

26. Mullikin, J.C.; Hansen, N.F.; Shen, L.; Ebling, H.; Donahue, W.F.; Tao, W.; Saranga, D.J.; Brand, A.; Rubenfield, M.J.; Young, A.C.; et al. Light whole genome sequence for SNP discovery across domestic cat breeds. *BMC Genom.* **2010**, *11*, 406. [CrossRef]

27. Buckley, R.M.; Davis, B.W.; Brashear, W.A.; Farias, F.H.G.; Kuroki, K.; Graves, T.; Hillier, L.W.; Kremitzki, M.; Li, G.; Middleton, R.; et al. A new domestic cat genome assembly based on long sequence reads empowers feline genomic medicine and identifies a novel gene for dwarfism. *bioRxiv* **2020**. [CrossRef]

28. Purcell, S.; Neale, B.; Todd-Brown, K.; Thomas, L.; Ferreira, M.A.; Bender, D.; Maller, J.; Sklar, P.; de Bakker, P.I.; Daly, M.J.; et al. PLINK: A tool set for whole-genome association and population-based linkage analyses. *Am. J. Hum. Genet.* **2007**, *81*, 559–575. [CrossRef]

29. Spielman, R.S.; Ewens, W.J. A sibship test for linkage in the presence of association: The sib transmission/disequilibrium test. *Am. J. Hum. Genet.* **1998**, *62*, 450–458. [CrossRef]

30. Barrett, J.C.; Fry, B.; Maller, J.; Daly, M.J. Haploview: Analysis and visualization of LD and haplotype maps. *Bioinformatics* **2005**, *21*, 263–265. [CrossRef]

31. Lyons, L.A.; Creighton, E.K.; Alhaddad, H.; Beale, H.C.; Grahn, R.A.; Rah, H.; Maggs, D.J.; Helps, C.R.; Gandolfi, B. Whole genome sequencing in cats, identifies new models for blindness in AIPL1 and somite segmentation in HES7. *BMC Genom.* **2016**, *17*, 265. [CrossRef] [PubMed]

32. Li, H.; Durbin, R. Fast and accurate short read alignment with Burrows-Wheeler transform. *Bioinformatics* **2009**, *25*, 1754–1760. [CrossRef] [PubMed]

33. McKenna, A.; Hanna, M.; Banks, E.; Sivachenko, A.; Cibulskis, K.; Kernytsky, A.; Garimella, K.; Altshuler, D.; Gabriel, S.; Daly, M.; et al. The Genome Analysis Toolkit: A MapReduce framework for analyzing next-generation DNA sequencing data. *Genome Res.* **2010**, *20*, 1297–1303. [CrossRef] [PubMed]

34. Van der Auwera, G.A.; Carneiro, M.O.; Hartl, C.; Poplin, R.; Del Angel, G.; Levy-Moonshine, A.; Jordan, T.; Shakir, K.; Roazen, D.; Thibault, J.; et al. From FastQ data to high confidence variant calls: The Genome Analysis Toolkit best practices pipeline. *Curr. Protoc. Bioinform.* **2013**, *43*, 11.10.1–11.10.33. [CrossRef]

35. Thorvaldsdottir, H.; Robinson, J.T.; Mesirov, J.P. Integrative Genomics Viewer (IGV): High-performance genomics data visualization and exploration. *Brief. Bioinform.* **2013**, *14*, 178–192. [CrossRef]

36. Toonen, R.J.; Hughes, S. Increased throughput for fragment analysis on an ABI PRISM 377 automated sequencer using a membrane comb and STRand software. *Biotechniques* **2001**, *31*, 1320–1324. [PubMed]

37. Buckley, R.M.; Gandolfi, B.; Creighton, E.K.; Pyne, C.A.; Leroy, M.L.; Senter, D.A.; Bouhan, D.M.; Gobble, J.R.; Abitbol, M.; Lyons, L.A.; et al. Werewolf, there wolf: Variants in *Hairless* associated wih hypotrichia and roaning in the lykoi cat breed. *bioRxiv* **2020**. [CrossRef]

38. Ancot, F.; Lemay, P.; Knowler, S.P.; Kennedy, K.; Griffiths, S.; Cherubini, G.B.; Sykes, J.; Mandigers, P.J.J.; Rouleau, G.A.; Rusbridge, C.; et al. A genome-wide association study identifies candidate loci associated to syringomyelia secondary to Chiari-like malformation in Cavalier King Charles Spaniels. *BMC Genet.* **2018**, *19*, 16. [CrossRef] [PubMed]

39. Marchant, T.W.; Dietschi, E.; Rytz, U.; Schawalder, P.; Jagannathan, V.; Hadji Rasouliha, S.; Gurtner, C.; Waldvogel, A.S.; Harrington, R.S.; Drogemuller, M.; et al. An ADAMTS3 missense variant is associated with Norwich Terrier upper airway syndrome. *PLoS Genet.* **2019**, *15*, e1008102. [CrossRef] [PubMed]

40. Aberdein, D.; Munday, J.S.; Gandolfi, B.; Dittmer, K.E.; Malik, R.; Garrick, D.J.; Lyons, L.A.; Lives, C. A FAS-ligand variant associated with autoimmune lymphoproliferative syndrome in cats. *Mamm Genome* **2017**, *28*, 47–55. [CrossRef] [PubMed]

41. Gandolfi, B.; Grahn, R.A.; Creighton, E.K.; Williams, D.C.; Dickinson, P.J.; Sturges, B.K.; Guo, L.T.; Shelton, G.D.; Leegwater, P.A.; Longeri, M.; et al. COLQ variant associated with Devon Rex and Sphynx feline hereditary myopathy. *Anim Genet.* **2015**, *46*, 711–715. [CrossRef] [PubMed]

42. Mauler, D.A.; Gandolfi, B.; Reinero, C.R.; O'Brien, D.P.; Spooner, J.L.; Lyons, L.A.; 99 Lives Consortium. Precision Medicine in Cats: Novel Niemann-Pick Type C1 Diagnosed by Whole-Genome Sequencing. *J. Vet. Intern. Med.* **2017**, *31*, 539–544. [CrossRef] [PubMed]

43. Oh, A.; Pearce, J.W.; Gandolfi, B.; Creighton, E.K.; Suedmeyer, W.K.; Selig, M.; Bosiack, A.P.; Castaner, L.J.; Whiting, R.E.; Belknap, E.B.; et al. Early-Onset Progressive Retinal Atrophy Associated with an IQCB1 Variant in African Black-Footed Cats (Felis nigripes). *Sci. Rep.* **2017**, *7*, 43918. [CrossRef] [PubMed]

44. Ontiveros, E.S.; Ueda, Y.; Harris, S.P.; Stern, J.A.; Lives, C. Precision medicine validation: Identifying the MYBPC3 A31P variant with whole-genome sequencing in two Maine Coon cats with hypertrophic cardiomyopathy. *J. Feline Med. Surg.* **2019**, *21*, 1086–1093. [CrossRef]

45. Jaffey, J.A.; Reading, N.S.; Giger, U.; Abdulmalik, O.; Buckley, R.M.; Johnstone, S.; Lyons, L.A.; Lives Cat Genome, C. Clinical, metabolic, and genetic characterization of hereditary methemoglobinemia caused by cytochrome b5 reductase deficiency in cats. *J. Vet. Intern. Med.* **2019**, *33*, 2725–2731. [CrossRef]

46. Buckley, R.M.; Grahn, R.A.; Gandolfi, B.; Herrick, J.R.; Kittleson, M.D.; Bateman, H.L.; Newsom, J.; Swanson, W.F.; Prieur, D.J.; Lyons, L.A. Assisted reproduction mediated resurrection of a feline model for Chediak-Higashi syndrome caused by a large duplication in LYST. *Sci. Rep.* **2020**, *10*, 64. [CrossRef]

47. Summers, A.D.; Reefhuis, J.; Taliano, J.; Rasmussen, S.A. Nongenetic risk factors for holoprosencephaly: An updated review of the epidemiologic literature. *Am. J. Med. Genet. C Semin Med. Genet.* **2018**, *178*, 151–164. [CrossRef]

48. Dubourg, C.; Kim, A.; Watrin, E.; de Tayrac, M.; Odent, S.; David, V.; Dupe, V. Recent advances in understanding inheritance of holoprosencephaly. *Am. J. Med. Genet. C Semin Med. Genet.* **2018**, *178*, 258–269. [CrossRef]

49. Kruszka, P.; Martinez, A.F.; Muenke, M. Molecular testing in holoprosencephaly. *Am. J. Med. Genet. C Semin Med. Genet.* **2018**, *178*, 187–193. [CrossRef]

50. Roessler, E.; Hu, P.; Muenke, M. Holoprosencephaly in the genomics era. *Am. J. Med. Genet. C Semin Med. Genet.* **2018**, *178*, 165–174. [CrossRef]

51. Lee, K.J.; Mendelsohn, M.; Jessell, T.M. Neuronal patterning by BMPs: A requirement for GDF7 in the generation of a discrete class of commissural interneurons in the mouse spinal cord. *Genes Dev.* **1998**, *12*, 3394–3407. [CrossRef] [PubMed]

52. Heussler, H.S.; Suri, M.; Young, I.D.; Muenke, M. Extreme variability of expression of a Sonic Hedgehog mutation: Attention difficulties and holoprosencephaly. *Arch. Dis Child.* **2002**, *86*, 293–296. [CrossRef] [PubMed]

53. Marini, M.; Cusano, R.; De Biasio, P.; Caroli, F.; Lerone, M.; Silengo, M.; Ravazzolo, R.; Seri, M.; Camera, G. Previously undescribed nonsense mutation in SHH caused autosomal dominant holoprosencephaly with wide intrafamilial variability. *Am. J. Med. Genet. A* **2003**, *117A*, 112–115. [CrossRef] [PubMed]

54. Hehr, U.; Gross, C.; Diebold, U.; Wahl, D.; Beudt, U.; Heidemann, P.; Hehr, A.; Mueller, D. Wide phenotypic variability in families with holoprosencephaly and a sonic hedgehog mutation. *Eur. J. Pediatr.* **2004**, *163*, 347–352. [CrossRef]

55. Hogan, B.L. Bone morphogenetic proteins: Multifunctional regulators of vertebrate development. *Genes Dev.* **1996**, *10*, 1580–1594. [CrossRef]

56. Mehler, M.F.; Mabie, P.C.; Zhang, D.; Kessler, J.A. Bone morphogenetic proteins in the nervous system. *Trends Neurosci.* **1997**, *20*, 309–317. [CrossRef]

57. Wang, R.N.; Green, J.; Wang, Z.; Deng, Y.; Qiao, M.; Peabody, M.; Zhang, Q.; Ye, J.; Yan, Z.; Denduluri, S.; et al. Bone Morphogenetic Protein (BMP) signaling in development and human diseases. *Genes Dis* **2014**, *1*, 87–105. [CrossRef]

58. Mikic, B.; Bierwert, L.; Tsou, D. Achilles tendon characterization in GDF-7 deficient mice. *J. Orthop Res.* **2006**, *24*, 831–841. [CrossRef]

59. Mikic, B.; Ferreira, M.P.; Battaglia, T.C.; Hunziker, E.B. Accelerated hypertrophic chondrocyte kinetics in GDF-7 deficient murine tibial growth plates. *J. Orthop Res.* **2008**, *26*, 986–990. [CrossRef]

60. Settle, S.; Marker, P.; Gurley, K.; Sinha, A.; Thacker, A.; Wang, Y.; Higgins, K.; Cunha, G.; Kingsley, D.M. The BMP family member Gdf7 is required for seminal vesicle growth, branching morphogenesis, and cytodifferentiation. *Dev. Biol.* **2001**, *234*, 138–150. [CrossRef]

61. Maloul, A.; Rossmeier, K.; Mikic, B.; Pogue, V.; Battaglia, T. Geometric and material contributions to whole bone structural behavior in GDF-7-deficient mice. *Connect. Tissue Res.* **2006**, *47*, 157–162. [CrossRef] [PubMed]

62. Palles, C.; Chegwidden, L.; Li, X.; Findlay, J.M.; Farnham, G.; Castro Giner, F.; Peppelenbosch, M.P.; Kovac, M.; Adams, C.L.; Prenen, H.; et al. Polymorphisms near TBX5 and GDF7 are associated with increased risk for Barrett's esophagus. *Gastroenterology* **2015**, *148*, 367–378. [CrossRef] [PubMed]

63. Becker, J.; May, A.; Gerges, C.; Anders, M.; Schmidt, C.; Veits, L.; Noder, T.; Mayershofer, R.; Kreuser, N.; Manner, H.; et al. The Barrett-associated variants at GDF7 and TBX5 also increase esophageal adenocarcinoma risk. *Cancer Med.* **2016**, *5*, 888–891. [CrossRef] [PubMed]

LAMB3 Missense Variant in Australian Shepherd Dogs with Junctional Epidermolysis Bullosa

Sarah Kiener [1,2,†], Aurore Laprais [3,†], Elizabeth A. Mauldin [4], Vidhya Jagannathan [1,2], Thierry Olivry [5,*] and Tosso Leeb [1,2,*]

[1]   Institute of Genetics, Vetsuisse Faculty, University of Bern, 3001 Bern, Switzerland; sarah.kiener@vetsuisse.unibe.ch (S.K.); vidhya.jagannathan@vetsuisse.unibe.ch (V.J.)
[2]   Dermfocus, University of Bern, 3001 Bern, Switzerland
[3]   The Ottawa Animal Emergency and Specialty Hospital, Ottawa, ON K1K 4C1, Canada; alaprais@oaesh.com
[4]   School of Veterinary Medicine, University of Pennsylvania, Philadelphia, PA 19104, USA; emauldin@vet.upenn.edu
[5]   Department of Clinical Sciences, College of Veterinary Medicine, North Carolina State University, Raleigh, NC 27607, USA
[*]   Correspondence: tolivry@ncsu.edu (T.O.); tosso.leeb@vetsuisse.unibe.ch (T.L.);
[†]   These authors contributed equally to this work (shared first authors).

Abstract: In a highly inbred Australian Shepherd litter, three of the five puppies developed widespread ulcers of the skin, footpads, and oral mucosa within the first weeks of life. Histopathological examinations demonstrated clefting of the epidermis from the underlying dermis within or just below the basement membrane, which led to a tentative diagnosis of junctional epidermolysis bullosa (JEB) with autosomal recessive inheritance. Endoscopy in one affected dog also demonstrated separation between the epithelium and underlying tissue in the gastrointestinal tract. As a result of the severity of the clinical signs, all three dogs had to be euthanized. We sequenced the genome of one affected puppy and compared the data to 73 control genomes. A search for private variants in 37 known candidate genes for skin fragility phenotypes revealed a single protein-changing variant, *LAMB3*:c.1174T>C, or p.Cys392Arg. The variant was predicted to change a conserved cysteine in the laminin β3 subunit of the heterotrimeric laminin-322, which mediates the binding of the epidermal basement membrane to the underlying dermis. Loss-of-function variants in the human *LAMB3* gene lead to recessive forms of JEB. We confirmed the expected co-segregation of the genotypes in the Australian Shepherd family. The mutant allele was homozygous in two genotyped cases and heterozygous in three non-affected close relatives. It was not found in 242 other controls from the Australian Shepherd breed, nor in more than 600 other controls. These data suggest that *LAMB3*:c.1174T>C represents the causative variant. To the best of our knowledge, this study represents the first report of a *LAMB3*-related JEB in domestic animals.

Keywords: dog; *Canis lupus familiaris*; whole genome sequence; wgs; dermatology; genodermatosis; skin; laminin; precision medicine

1. Introduction

When a human or animal, usually at or soon after birth, develops erosions and epithelial sloughing on the mucosae, areas of friction, and extremities, a genetic disorder of skin fragility is to be considered. A consensus reclassification of skin fragility disorders was published recently, which separates those that affect the basement membrane itself or the basal keratinocytes (i.e., hereditary epidermolysis bullosa (EB) variants) from others, in which the separation occurs more superficially in the epidermis [1]. In this reclassification, four main categories of inherited "classical" EB are proposed, which reflect the differences in the level of cleavage in the basement membrane zone [1]. Also included in this reclassification are four new categories of epidermal disorders of skin fragility associated with 20 possibly mutated genes, namely: peeling skin disorders, erosive skin fragility disorders, keratinopathic ichthyoses, and pachyonychia congenita [1]. Finally, a single syndromic connected tissue disorder with (dermal) skin fragility associated with *PLOD3* variants and a lysyl hydroxylase-3 deficiency was also included in this group of diseases [1]. All of the known 37 candidate genes for these human diseases are summarized in Table 1.

Table 1. Consensus reclassification of epidermolysis bullosa and other disorders with epidermal fragility and their known functional candidate genes, as of 2020 [1].

Disorder	Level of Cleavage	Gene	Protein	Inheritance [1]
Classical Epidermolysis Bullosa (EB)				
EB simplex (EBS)	Basal epidermal	*CD151*	CD151 molecule (Raph blood group)	AR
		DST	dystonin	AR
		EXPH5	exophilin 5	AR
		KLHL24	kelch like family member 24	AD
		KRT5	keratin 5	AD, AR
		KRT14	keratin 14	AD, AR
		PLEC	plectin	AR
Junctional EB (JEB)	Junctional	*COL17A1*	collagen type XVII, α 1 chain	AR
		ITGA3	integrin subunit α 3	AR
		ITGA6	integrin subunit α 6	AR
		ITGB4	integrin subunit β 4	AR
		LAMA3	laminin subunit α 3	AR
		LAMB3	laminin subunit β 3	AR
		LAMC2	laminin subunit γ 2	AR
Dystrophic EB (DEB)	Dermal	*COL7A1*	collagen type VII, α 1 chain	AD, AR
Kindler EB	Mixed	*FERMT1*	fermitin family homolog 1	AR
Other Disorders with Skin Fragility				
Peeling skin disorders	Intraepidermal	*CAST*	calpastatin	AR
		CSTA	cystatin A	AR
		CTSB	cystatin B	AR
		DSG1	desmoglein 1	AR
		FLG2	filaggrin family member 2	AR
		SERPINB8	serpin family B member 8	AR
		SPINK5	serine peptidase inhibitor Kazal type 5	AR
Erosive skin fragility disorders	Intraepidermal	*DSC3*	desmocollin 3	AR
		DSG3	desmoglein 3	AR
		DSP	desmoplakin	AR
		JUP	junction plakoglobin	AR
		PKP1	plakophilin 1	AR
Keratinopathic ichthyoses	Intraepidermal	*KRT1*	keratin 1	AD
		KRT2	keratin 2	AD
		KRT10	keratin 10	AD, AR
Pachyonychia congenita	Intraepidermal	*KRT6A*	keratin 6A	AD
		KRT6B	keratin 6B	AD
		KRT6C	keratin 6C	AD
		KRT16	keratin 16	AD
		KRT17	keratin 17	AD
Syndromic connective tissue disorder with skin fragility	Dermal	*PLOD3*	procollagen-lysine,2-oxoglutarate 5-dioxygenase 3	AR

[1] AD—autosomal dominant; AR—autosomal recessive.

In domestic dogs, only two other epidermal disorders of skin fragility have been reported, namely: epidermolytic ichthyosis associated with a *KRT10* variant in Norfolk terriers [2], and ectodermal dysplasia/skin fragility syndrome with a *PKP1* variant in Chesapeake Bay Retrievers [3] (Table S1). In contrast, cases of hereditary EB have been recognized for decades, and the causative genetic variants have now been characterized in three canine, one feline, two equine, two ovine, and five bovine EB variants (Table S1).

In dogs, there is at least one example for each of the three main subtypes of classical EB in which the genetic defect has been reported, namley: a *PLEC* variant in the EB simplex of Eurasier dogs in the USA [4]; a *LAMA3* variant in the junctional EB of German Shorthaired Pointers in France [5]; and *COL7A1* variants in the dystrophic EB (mild) in Golden Retrievers, also in France [6], or severe in Central Asian Shepherds [7].

Laminin-332, a rod-like heterotrimer composed of the laminin α3, β3, and γ2 chains, is a critical component of hemidesmosomes, adhesion complexes that attach the basal epidermal keratinocytes to the underlying dermal connective tissue [8–10]. The prominent role of laminin-332 for skin integrity stems from its ability to link two important molecules—one in the epidermis and the other in the dermis. Via its carboxy-terminus, laminin α3 binds to the external domains of the integrin α6β4 that protrude from the basal keratinocytes. At the other end of the laminin trimer, the amino-terminal domains of the laminin β3 and γ2 chains bind to the NC1 amino-terminus of the superficial dermal collagen type VII [11].

Genetic variants in the *LAMA3, LAMB3,* and *LAMC2* genes that encode the laminin α3, β3, and γ2 chains are causative for the intermediate and severe forms of junctional EB (JEB), not only in humans [1], but also in animals (Table S1). Variants in any one of these genes can lead to a similar phenotype, as the abnormal expression or function of either of the three individual laminin chains is expected to impair the assembly or the function of the entire laminin-332. A good example of this phenomenon is the near identical phenotype exhibited by American Saddlebred horses with severe JEB associated with a *LAMA3* variant [12], and that found in Belgian, Breton, Comtois, and Italian draft horses caused by a *LAMC2* variant [13–15].

While JEB subsets associated with *LAMB3* variants are common in humans [16–18], they have not yet been reported in animals. So far, an abnormal epidermal expression of laminin β3—without investigation of the underlying molecular genetics—has only been shown in a single cat exhibiting a phenotype of mild EB [19].

Herein, we report a missense variant in *LAMB3,* which we believe is causative of a JEB phenotype with intermediate severity in a litter of Australian Shepherds in Ontario, Canada. Of clinical interest is the demonstration, for the first time or so it seems, of intestinal epithelial sloughing in a case of animal JEB.

2. Materials and Methods

2.1. Ethics Statement

The affected Australian Shepherds in this study were privately owned, and skin and biopsy samples were collected with the consent of their owners. The collection of all other blood samples was approved by the "Cantonal Committee for Animal Experiments" (Canton of Bern; permits 75/16 and 71/19).

2.2. Animal Selection

This study included 247 Australian Shepherds. Genomic DNA was either isolated from EDTA blood samples with the Maxwell RSC Whole Blood Kit, or from formalin-fixed paraffin-embedded (FFPE) tissue samples with the Maxwell RSC DNA FFPE Kit using a Maxwell RSC instrument (Promega, Dübendorf, Switzerland).

2.3. Histopathological Examinations

Skin punch biopsies (8 mm) were obtained under general anesthesia. The samples were fixed in 10% neutral buffered formalin and routinely processed, including staining with hematoxylin and eosin.

2.4. Whole Genome Sequencing

An Illumina TruSeq PCR-free DNA library with ~400 bp insert size of a JEB affected Australian Shepherd was prepared. We collected 175 million 2 × 150 bp paired-end reads or 18.9× coverage on a NovaSeq 6000 instrument. The reads were mapped to the dog reference genome assembly CanFam3.1 and were aligned as previously described [20]. The sequence data were submitted to the European Nucleotide Archive, with study accession number PRJEB16012 and sample accession number SAMEA6862980.

2.5. Variant Calling

Variant calling was performed as previously described [20]. To predict the functional effects of the called variants, SnpEff software [21], together with NCBI annotation release 105 for the CanFam 3.1 genome reference assembly, was used. For variant filtering, we used 73 control genomes (Table S2).

2.6. Gene Analysis

We used the dog reference genome assembly CanFam3.1 and NCBI annotation release 105. Numbering within the canine *LAMB3* gene corresponds to the NCBI RefSeq accession numbers XM_014115071.2 (mRNA) and XP_013970546.1 (protein). For a multiple species comparison of the *LAMB3* amino acid sequences, we used the following accessions: NP_000219.2 (*Homo sapiens*), NP_001075065.1 (*Bos taurus*), XP_023496552.1 (*Equus caballus*), NP_001264857.1 (*Mus musculus*), NP_001094311.1 (*Rattus norvegicus*), XP_425827.3 (*Gallus gallus*), XP_002933550.2 (*Xenopus tropicalis*), and XP_700808.6 (*Danio rerio*).

2.7. Sanger Sequencing

To confirm the candidate variant *LAMB3*:c.1174T>C, and to genotype all of the dogs in this study, Sanger Sequencing was used. A 403 bp PCR product was amplified from genomic DNA using AmpliTaqGold360Mastermix (Thermo Fisher Scientific, Waltham, MA, USA) and primers 5′-TCT TGT GCC AAG CAC TGT TC-3′ (Primer F) and 5′-GGC ATA GGT GAG TCC CGT AA-3′ (Primer R). A smaller PCR product of 153 bp size was amplified for FFPE-derived DNA with primers 5′-GGT GGC TGC TTT TCT GTC TC-3′ (Primer F) and 5′-GGT GAG TCC CGT AAA TCC TG-3′ (Primer R). After treatment with shrimp alkaline phosphatase and exonuclease I, PCR amplicons were sequenced on an ABI 3730 DNA Analyzer (Thermo Fisher Scientific). Sanger sequences were analyzed using the Sequencer 5.1 software (GeneCodes, Ann Arbor, MI, USA).

3. Results

3.1. Family Anamnesis, Clinical Examinations, and Histopathology

Three Australian Shepherd puppies with severe skin lesions were identified in a highly inbred litter resulting from a father–daughter mating. The litter consisted of three affected and two non-affected puppies that were born out of normal parents. The pedigree relationships were suggestive for a monogenic autosomal recessive inherited disease (Figure 1).

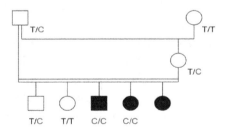

Figure 1. Pedigree of the investigated Australian Shepherd family. Squares represent males and circles represent females. The three affected puppies are indicated by the filled symbols. Note that the father of the litter was simultaneously the maternal grandfather. A close inbreeding loop greatly increases the risk for recessive hereditary defects. Genotypes at the *LAMB3*:c.1174T>C variant are indicated for all animals, from which a DNA sample is available (see Section 3.2).

At the time of their first presentation to the breeder's veterinarian for vaccination at 7 weeks of age, the three affected puppies were noted to have ulcers in the mouth, inner pinnae, and abdomen. The puppies reportedly also had marked lymph node enlargement. The average weight of the affected puppies was half that of their unaffected siblings.

At 17 weeks of age, one of the affected dogs, a blue merle with copper intact female was presented to the dermatologist for evaluation of severe ulceration of both the oral cavity and haired skin. Ulcers were located on the gingival and buccal mucosa, tongue, and hard and soft palates (Figure 2a). The concave pinnae, bilaterally, were also ulcerated, oozing, and covered with exudate (Figure 2b), but the otoscopic examination only revealed mild erythema in the ear canal. Several footpads, either digital or central, were also ulcerated (Figure 2c), and four claws were missing or misshapen. Erosions and ulcers were covered by thick crusts on the elbows, hocks, and the tip of the tail. The vulva and anus were grossly normal.

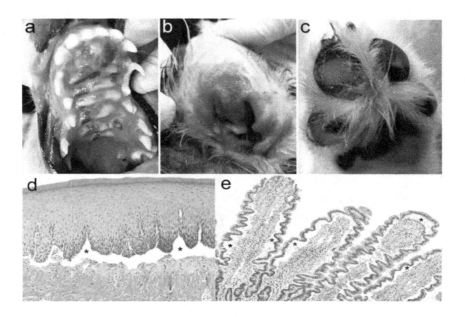

Figure 2. Clinical and histopathological phenotype. (**a**) Severe coalescing ulcers on the gingiva and hard and soft palate, (**b**) concave pinna (**c**) and footpads. Biopsy samples collected from the (**d**) oral cavity and (**e**) duodenum revealed widespread separation of the epithelium from the underlying connective tissue (asterisks).

Thoracic auscultation, abdominal, and lymph node palpation were all unremarkable. Blood was collected for a complete blood count and a serum chemistry panel, and the most relevant changes were a mild regenerative anemia (hemoglobin: 129 (reference range: 134–207 g/L); reticulocytes: 118 (10–110 k/μL)) and hypoproteinemia (total proteins: 46 (55–75 g/L); albumin: 23 (27–39 g/L); globulins: 23 (24–40 g/L)). To determine if these abnormal changes were due to digestive ulcers, an upper gastrointestinal endoscopy was performed under general anesthesia, two weeks after the original admission to the specialty clinic. The esophagus appeared normal, and the stomach and duodenum were hyperrhemic but did not show a visible loss of epithelium; endoscopic biopsies were nevertheless collected from the stomach and duodenum. During this general anesthesia, punch skin biopsies were collected from the concave pinnae, footpads, and oral cavity (hard palate, buccal mucosa, and tongue).

Microscopically, the skin and mucosal biopsy samples all exhibited limited-to-widespread epidermal detachment (Figure 2d), and ulcers were covered with serocellular crusts; inflammation was sparse in non-ulcerated areas. In some sections (as in Figure 2d), the basement membrane could be discerned at the base of the clefts, thus suggesting the diagnosis of JEB. The endoscopic biopsies from the stomach (pyloric and nonpyloric areas) and duodenum all showed mild-to-moderate inflammation with lymphocytes, plasma cells, and eosinophils, with a detachment of the epithelium from the underlying lamina propria (Figure 2e). Because of the severity of the lesions, the dog was euthanized at 7.5 months of age.

The medical records of the two other affected puppies were also reviewed. A blue merle with copper intact male puppy was noted to have ulcers on the tongue, gingiva, soft palate, pharynx, tonsils, and larynx. Skin ulcers were found on the concave pinnae and pressure points of one elbow, one hock, and both stifles. Because of the worsening lesions, this puppy was euthanized at 16 weeks of age, with biopsy samples of the tongue, soft palate ear, and footpad collected post-mortem. As for the samples obtained from the littermate described above, microscopic lesions consisted of subepidermal vesicles leading to dermo-epidermal separation, ulceration, and granulation tissue.

The third affected puppy, a blue merle female, had been euthanized at 5 months of age because of severe gingival, labial, oropharyngeal, and esophageal ulceration. The dog had crusts on the chin, ulcers and crusts on the concave pinnae and footpads, and exudate at the base of multiple claws; samples for histopathology were not collected.

Finally, both the sire and dam, as well as the two healthy siblings, were examined by veterinarians, and they were deemed to be free of skin lesions.

3.2. Genetic Analysis

In order to characterize the underlying causative genetic variant, we sequenced the genome of one affected dog at 18.9× coverage and searched for homozygous variants in the 37 genes known to cause human skin fragility (Table 1), which were exclusively present in the affected dog and absent from the genomes of 73 other dogs (Table 2, Tables S2 and S3).

Table 2. Results of variant filtering in the affected Australian Shepherd dog against 73 control genomes. Only homozygous variants are reported.

Filtering Step	Variants
All variants in the affected dog	3,111,811
Private variants	11,754
Protein-changing private variants	54
Protein-changing private variants in 37 candidate genes	1

This analysis identified a single homozygous private protein-changing variant in *LAMB3*, a known candidate gene for JEB in humans [1]. The variant can be designated as Chr7:8,286,613A>G (CanFam3.1 assembly). It is a missense variant, XM_014115071.2:c.1174T>C, predicted to change a highly conserved cysteine residue in the third EGF-like domain of laminin β3, XP_013970546.1:p.(Cys392Arg).

We confirmed the presence of the *LAMB3* missense variant by Sanger sequencing (Figure 3). The mutant allele showed the expected co-segregation with JEB in the available family. The two available DNA samples from the JEB affected puppies carried the mutant allele in a homozygous state, while their parents were heterozygous, as expected for obligate carriers (Figure 1).

We determined the genotypes at *LAMB3*:c.1174T>C in a cohort comprising 247 Australian Shepherd dogs, including the index family. The mutant *LAMB3* allele was not detected in the homozygous state in any of the 245 non-affected Australian Shepherd dogs or 663 dogs from other breeds. Three of these dogs, all members of the index family, carried the mutant *LAMB3* allele in a heterozygous state (Table 3).

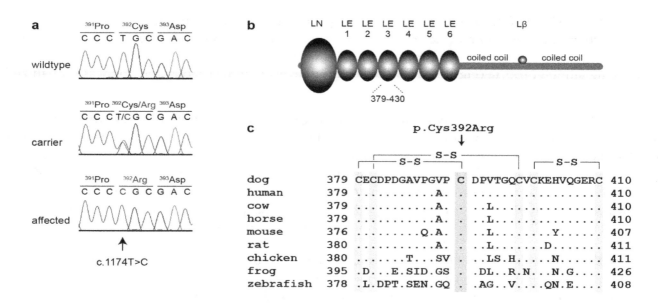

Figure 3. Details of the *LAMB3*:c.1174T>C, p.Cys392Arg variant. (**a**) Representative electropherograms of three dogs with different genotypes are shown. The variable position is indicated by an arrow, and the amino acid translations are shown. (**b**) Domain organization of the 1172 amino acid laminin β3 precursor [8]. The N-terminus consists of a globular domain (LN), followed by six laminin EGF-like (LE) domains. These N-terminal domains are located in the basement membrane and may be involved in binding to collagen VII. The C-terminal half of laminin β3 participates in two coiled-coil domains that mediate trimerization with the α3 and γ2 chains in the laminin-332 heterotrimer. The small Lβ domain mediates the binding of agrin. (**c**) Multiple-species alignment of the beginning of the LE3 domain harboring the p.Cys392Arg variant. The variant affects a highly conserved cysteine residue that forms a disulfide bridge with Cys-379 [22]. Note that all six cysteine residues in this region contribute to disulfide bonds, and are strictly conserved across vertebrates.

Table 3. Genotype-phenotype association of the *LAMB3*:c.1174T>C variant with JEB.

Dogs	T/T	T/C	C/C
Cases (n = 2) [1]	-	-	2
Controls, Australian Shepherd dogs (n = 245)	242	3	-
Controls, other breeds (n = 663) [1]	663	-	-

[1] These genotypes were derived from 590 genome sequences reported in the literature [20], and the 73 control genomes used in this study.

4. Discussion

In the affected Australian Shepherds described in this study, the age of lesion onset, as well as the presence of ulceration in the oral cavity and pressure points on the limbs with a loss of claws, all suggested the clinical diagnosis of a skin fragility disorder, of which EB is the most representative disease group in domestic animals and humans (Table S1). Because of the resembling phenotypes, clinical signs cannot alone reliably permit differentiation between the three main subtypes of animal EB (simplex, junctional, and dystrophic). For a more precise diagnosis, the specific location of the dermo-epidermal separation must be determined, for example, with a periodic acid Schiff (PAS) stain to visualize the glycoproteins in the basement membrane lamina densa [7], single or double antigen immunomapping [23], or transmission electron microscopy [4]. In this case, the routine histopathology enabled the visualization of the basement membrane delineating the contour of dermal imprints of the epidermal ridges, thus establishing that clefting occurred in a supra-lamina densa manner; this confirmed the diagnosis of JEB.

There is only one other occurrence of JEB in the canine species [5,23,24]. In the early 1990s, JEB was first discovered in German Shorthaired Pointers in the French Alps. The clinical signs were indistinguishable from those present in the Australian Shepherds described herein. Both the Pointer and Australian Shepherd puppies exhibited the first clinical signs weeks after, and not at, birth. In both cases, lesions consisted of ulcerative skin lesions affecting the inner (medial and concave) pinnae, footpads, and at pressure points of the extremities [23,24]. Shedding of the claws was also reported [24]. Of interest is that dental enamel abnormalities, a common finding in human JEB [1], were not recognized in either the German Shorthaired Pointers or the Australian Shepherds described in this study. A unique finding seen in one of the three Australian Shepherd puppies was the endoscopic observation of duodenal hyperrhemia, which was found on the histopathology to be associated with an extensive detachment of the digestive epithelium from its underlying connective tissue. Unfortunately, as ulceration of the duodenum was not seen during endoscopy, we cannot rule out that the digestive epithelial detachment seen on the histopathology might have been artifactual. Nevertheless, the *LAMA3*, *LAMB3*, and *LAMC2* genes, which encode the three laminin-332 chains, are all expressed in the small intestine [25]. As a result, based on our hypothesis, that the *LAMB3* missense variant affects the adhesive function of the laminin-332, it is conceivable that any trauma to the small intestine during the endoscopic biopsy process could result in a forced epithelial separation from the lamina propria, a phenomenon that normally does not happen to that extent in healthy individuals. To our knowledge, such a lesion has never been reported in a case of animal EB, and these are findings seen more often in the severe generalized than intermediate variants of human JEB; they are typically not found in localized JEB [26].

In this study, we identified a homozygous missense variant, *LAMB3*:p.Cys392Arg, as a candidate causative variant for a new JEB in Australian Shepherd dogs. *LAMB3* encodes the laminin β3 chain, which, together with the α3 and γ2 chains, forms the heterotrimer laminin-332. Laminin β3 has two coiled-coil domains for the heterotrimer formation with the α3 and γ2 chains at its C-terminal end. The N-terminus consists of a globular domain (LN) and six laminin-type epidermal growth factor-like (LE) repeats [8,22]. The LE domains have conserved disulfide bonds, which may be important for the tertiary structure of these domains [27,28]. The LN and LE domains form a short arm in the cross-shaped laminin-332 heterotrimer, and mediate binding to type VII collagen in hemidesmosomes, which are necessary for the stable association between the epithelium and the stroma underneath [8,11].

The p.Cys392Arg variant changes one of the highly conserved cysteine residues in the third LE domain, which prevents the formation of the disulfide bond between Cys-392 and Cys-379. We hypothesize that this may lead to a change in the tertiary structure of laminin β3, and impair the binding of laminin-322 to collagen type VII in hemidesmosomes. Further experiments at the protein level are required in order to confirm this putative pathomechanism.

With this description, we now have two variants of canine intermediate JEB due to variants in related genes (*LAMA3* in German Shorthaired Pointers and *LAMB3* in Australian Shepherds) encoding the laminin α3 and β3 chains that assemble with the γ2 chain to form the laminin-332 heterotrimer. In both of these breeds, the variants are predicted to result in some residual protein function (Australian Shepherds), or in the secretion of some normal laminin-332 trimers (German Shorthaired Pointers) [5], which may explain the similar absence of lesions at birth and the intermediate clinical phenotype.

In humans, the specific variants and their consequences at the mRNA and protein levels contribute to the spectrum of severity encountered in different subtypes of EB [10]. Severe forms of JEB are associated with nonsense, frameshift, or out-of-frame splicing variants that result in nonfunctional or complete loss of the protein. Intermediate JEB occurs when a laminin chain is mutated, but the LM-332 heterotrimer can still form, which is often the case for missense variants [16]. Missense variants affecting cysteine residues in the LE domains, *LAMB3*:p.Cys355Arg and p.Cys433Trp, have been reported in human patients with intermediate JEB [16–19]. The clinical phenotype observed in the investigated dogs homozygous for p.Cys392Arg can also be classified as JEB of intermediate severity, and corresponds well to the human spectrum of genotype–phenotype correlations.

5. Conclusions

We characterized a new recessive form of JEB in Australian Shepherd dogs. A precision medicine approach identified a missense variant in the *LAMB3* gene, c.1174T>C or p.Cys392Arg as likely candidate causative variant. Our data enable genetic testing to avoid the unintentional breeding of further affected dogs and provide the first spontaneous large animal model for JEB due to altered laminin β3.

Author Contributions: Conceptualization, T.O. and T.L.; data curation, V.J.; investigation, S.K., A.L., E.A.M., T.O., and T.L.; writing (original draft), S.K., A.L., T.O., and T.L.; writing (review and editing), S.K., A.L., E.A.M., V.J., T.O., and T.L. supervision, T.O. and T.L. All authors have read and agreed to the published version of the manuscript.

Acknowledgments: We thank Sophie Saati for collection of the endoscopic samples and Andrew Lowe for the skin biopsies. The authors are grateful to all dog owners and referring veterinarians who donated samples and shared health and pedigree data of their dogs. We thank Nathalie Besuchet Schmutz, Catia Coito, Marion Ernst, and Daniela Steiner for their expert technical assistance; the Next Generation Sequencing Platform of the University of Bern for performing the high-throughput sequencing experiments; and the Interfaculty Bioinformatics Unit of the University of Bern for providing high performance computing infrastructure. We thank the Dog Biomedical Variant Database Consortium (Gus Aguirre, Catherine André, Danika Bannasch, Doreen Becker, Brian Davis, Cord Drögemüller, Kari Ekenstedt, Kiterie Faller, Oliver Forman, Steve Friedenberg, Eva Furrow, Urs Giger, Christophe Hitte, Marjo Hytönen, Vidhya Jagannathan, Tosso Leeb, Frode Lingaas, Hannes Lohi, Cathryn Mellersh, Jim Mickelson, Leonardo Murgiano, Anita Oberbauer, Sheila Schmutz, Jeffrey Schoenebeck, Kim Summers, Frank van Steenbeek, and Claire Wade) for sharing the whole genome sequencing data from the control dogs. We also acknowledge all canine researchers who deposited dog whole genome sequencing data into public databases.

References

1. Has, C.; Bauer, J.W.; Bodemer, C.; Bolling, M.C.; Bruckner-Tuderman, L.; Diem, A.; Fine, J.D.; Heagerty, A.; Hovnanian, A.; Marinkovich, M.P.; et al. Consensus reclassification of inherited epidermolysis bullosa and other disorders with skin fragility. *Br. J. Dermatol.* **2020**. [CrossRef] [PubMed]
2. Credille, K.M.; Barnhart, K.F.; Minor, J.S.; Dunstan, R.W. Mild recessive epidermolytic hyperkeratosis associated with a novel keratin 10 donor splice-site mutation in a family of Norfolk terrier dogs. *Br. J. Dermatol.* **2005**, *153*, 51–58. [CrossRef] [PubMed]
3. Olivry, T.; Linder, K.E.; Wang, P.; Bizikova, P.; Bernstein, J.A.; Dunston, S.M.; Paps, J.S.; Casal, M.L. Deficient plakophilin-1 expression due to a mutation in *PKP1* causes ectodermal dysplasia-skin fragility syndrome in Chesapeake Bay Retriever dogs. *PLoS ONE* **2012**, *7*, e32072. [CrossRef]
4. Mauldin, E.A.; Wang, P.; Olivry, T.; Henthorn, P.S.; Casal, M.L. Epidermolysis bullosa simplex in sibling Eurasier dogs is caused by a *PLEC* non-sense variant. *Vet. Dermatol.* **2017**, *28*, 10-e3. [CrossRef] [PubMed]
5. Capt, A.; Spirito, F.; Guaguere, E.; Spadafora, A.; Ortonne, J.P.; Meneguzzi, G. Molecular basis of inherited junctional epidermolysis bullosa in the German pointer: Establishment of a large animal model for the condition. *J. Investig. Dermatol.* **2005**, *124*, 530–535. [CrossRef] [PubMed]
6. Baldeschi, C.; Gache, Y.; Rattenholl, A.; Bouille, P.; Danos, O.; Ortonne, J.P.; Bruckner-Tuderman, L.; Meneguzzi, G. Genetic correction of canine dystrophic epidermolysis bullosa mediated by retroviral vectors. *Hum. Mol. Genet.* **2003**, *12*, 1897–1905. [CrossRef] [PubMed]
7. Niskanen, J.; Dillard, K.; Arumilli, M.; Salmela, E.; Anttila, M.; Lohi, H.; Hytönen, M.K. Nonsense variant in *COL7A1* causes recessive dystrophic epidermolysis bullosa in Central Asian Shepherd dogs. *PLoS ONE* **2017**, *12*, e0177527. [CrossRef]
8. Domogatskaya, A.; Rodin, S.; Tryggvason, K. Functional diversity of laminins. *Annu. Rev. Cell Dev. Biol.* **2012**, *28*, 523–553. [CrossRef]
9. Pozzi, A.; Yurchenco, P.D.; Iozzo, R.V. The nature and biology of basement membranes. *Matrix Biol.* **2017**, *57*, 1–11. [CrossRef]
10. Has, C.; Nystrom, A.; Saeidian, A.H.; Bruckner-Tuderman, L.; Uitto, J. Epidermolysis bullosa: Molecular pathology of connective tissue components in the cutaneous basement membrane zone. *Matrix Biol.* **2018**, *71*, 313–329. [CrossRef]

11. Chen, M.; Marinkovich, M.P.; Jones, J.C.; O'Toole, E.A.; Li, Y.Y.; Woodley, D.T. NC1 domain of type VII collagen binds to the beta3 chain of laminin 5 via a unique subdomain within the fibronectin-like repeats. *J. Investig. Dermatol.* **1999**, *112*, 177–183. [CrossRef] [PubMed]

12. Graves, K.T.; Henney, P.J.; Ennis, R.B. Partial deletion of the *LAMA3* gene is responsible for hereditary junctional epidermolysis bullosa in the American Saddlebred Horse. *Anim. Genet.* **2009**, *40*, 35–41. [CrossRef] [PubMed]

13. Spirito, F.; Charlesworth, A.; Linder, K.; Ortonne, J.P.; Baird, J.; Meneguzzi, G. Animal models for skin blistering conditions: Absence of laminin 5 causes hereditary junctional mechanobullous disease in the Belgian horse. *J. Investig. Dermatol.* **2002**, *119*, 684–691. [CrossRef] [PubMed]

14. Milenkovic, D.; Chaffaux, S.; Taourit, S.; Guerin, G. A mutation in the *LAMC2* gene causes the Herlitz junctional epidermolysis bullosa (H-JEB) in two French draft horse breeds. *Genet. Sel. Evol.* **2003**, *35*, 249–256. [CrossRef]

15. Cappelli, K.; Brachelente, C.; Passamonti, F.; Flati, A.; Silvestrelli, M.; Capomaccio, S. First report of junctional epidermolysis bullosa (JEB) in the Italian draft horse. *BMC Vet. Res.* **2015**, *11*, 55. [CrossRef] [PubMed]

16. Nakano, A.; Chao, S.C.; Pulkkinen, L.; Murrell, D.; Bruckner-Tuderman, L.; Pfendner, E.; Uitto, J. Laminin 5 mutations in junctional epidermolysis bullosa: Molecular basis of Herlitz vs. non-Herlitz phenotypes. *Hum. Genet.* **2002**, *110*, 41–51. [CrossRef]

17. Varki, R.; Sadowski, S.; Pfendner, E.; Uitto, J. Epidermolysis bullosa. I. Molecular genetics of the junctional and hemidesmosomal variants. *J. Med. Genet.* **2006**, *43*, 641–652. [CrossRef]

18. Kiritsi, D.; Has, C.; Bruckner-Tuderman, L. Laminin 332 in junctional epidermolysis bullosa. *Cell Adh. Migr.* **2013**, *7*, 135–141. [CrossRef]

19. Alhaidari, Z.; Olivry, T.; Spadafora, A.; Thomas, R.C.; Perrin, C.; Meneguzzi, G.; Ortonne, J.P. Junctional epidermolysis bullosa in two domestic shorthaired kittens. *Vet. Dermatol.* **2005**, *16*, 69–73. [CrossRef]

20. Jagannathan, V.; Drögemüller, C.; Leeb, T.; Dog Biomedical Variant Database Consortium (DBVDC). A comprehensive biomedical variant catalogue based on whole genome sequences of 582 dogs and eight wolves. *Anim. Genet.* **2019**, *50*, 695–704. [CrossRef]

21. Cingolani, P.; Platts, A.; Wang, L.L.; Coon, M.; Nguyen, T.; Wang, L.; Land, S.J.; Lu, X.; Ruden, D.M. A program for annotating and predicting the effects of single nucleotide polymorphisms, SnpEff: SNPs in the genome of Drosophila melanogaster strain w1118; iso-2; iso-3. *Fly* **2012**, *6*, 80–92. [CrossRef] [PubMed]

22. UniProt Website, Entry Q13751. Available online: https://www.uniprot.org/uniprot/Q13751 (accessed on 20 May 2020).

23. Olivry, T.; Poujade-Delverdier, A.; Dunston, S.M.; Fine, J.-D.; Ortonne, J.-P. Absent expression of collagen XVII (BPAG2, BP180) in canine familial localized junctional epidermolysis bullosa. *Vet. Dermatol.* **1997**, *8*, 203–212. [CrossRef]

24. Guaguère, E.; Olivry, T.; Poujade-Delverdier, A.; Magnol, J.P. Epidermolyse bulleuse jonctionnelle familiale associée à une absence d'expression de collagène XVII chez le Braque Allemand: À propos de deux cas. *Prat. Méd. Chir. Anim. Comp.* **1997**, *32*, 471–480.

25. GeneCards: The Human Gene Database. Available online: https://www.genecards.org (accessed on 10 August 2020).

26. Fine, J.D.; Bruckner-Tuderman, L.; Eady, R.A.; Bauer, E.A.; Bauer, J.W.; Has, C.; Heagerty, A.; Hintner, H.; Hovnanian, A.; Jonkman, M.F.; et al. Inherited epidermolysis bullosa: Updated recommendations on diagnosis and classification. *J. Am. Acad. Dermatol.* **2014**, *70*, 1103–1126. [CrossRef] [PubMed]

27. Engel, J. EGF-like domains in extracellular matrix proteins: Localized signals for growth and differentiation? *FEBS Lett.* **1989**, *251*, 1–7. [CrossRef]

28. Beck, K.; Hunter, I.; Engel, J. Structure and function of laminin: Anatomy of a multidomain glycoprotein. *FASEB J.* **1990**, *4*, 148–160. [CrossRef] [PubMed]

NSDHL Frameshift Deletion in a Mixed Breed Dog with Progressive Epidermal Nevi

Matthias Christen [1,2], **Michaela Austel** [3], **Frane Banovic** [3], **Vidhya Jagannathan** [1,2] **and Tosso Leeb** [1,2,*]

[1]   Institute of Genetics, Vetsuisse Faculty, University of Bern, 3001 Bern, Switzerland; matthias.christen@vetsuisse.unibe.ch (M.C.); vidhya.jagannathan@vetsuisse.unibe.ch (V.J.)

[2]   Dermfocus, University of Bern, 3001 Bern, Switzerland

[3]   Department of Small Animal Medicine and Surgery, College of Veterinary Medicine, University of Georgia, Athens, GA 30602, USA; maustel@uga.edu (M.A.); fbanovic@uga.edu (F.B.)

*   Correspondence: tosso.leeb@vetsuisse.unibe.ch;

Abstract: Loss-of-function variants in the *NSDHL* gene have been associated with epidermal nevi in humans with congenital hemidysplasia, ichthyosiform nevi, and limb defects (CHILD) syndrome and in companion animals. The *NSDHL* gene codes for the NAD(P)-dependent steroid dehydrogenase-like protein, which is involved in cholesterol biosynthesis. In this study, a female Chihuahua cross with a clinical and histological phenotype consistent with progressive epidermal nevi is presented. All exons of the *NSDHL* candidate gene were amplified by PCR and analyzed by Sanger sequencing. A heterozygous frameshift variant, c.718_722delGAACA, was identified in the affected dog. In lesional skin, the vast majority of *NSDHL* transcripts lacked the five deleted bases. The variant is predicted to produce a premature stop codon truncating 34% of the encoded protein, p.Glu240Profs*17. The mutant allele was absent from 22 additionally genotyped Chihuahuas, as well as from 647 control dogs of diverse breeds and eight wolves. The available experimental data together with current knowledge about *NSDHL* variants and their functional impact in humans, dogs, and other species prompted us to classify this variant as pathogenic according to the ACMG guidelines that were previously established for human sequence variants. Therefore, we propose the c.718_722delGAACA variant as causative variant for the observed skin lesions in this dog.

Keywords: *Canis lupus familiaris*; animal model; genodermatosis; dermatology; skin; CHILD syndrome; ILVEN; epidermal nevus; precision medicine

1. Introduction

Congenital hemidysplasia, ichthyosiform nevi, and limb defects (CHILD) is a well-described syndrome in humans (OMIM #308050) [1–5]. CHILD patients typically have unilateral limb defects together with the characteristic skin lesions termed as CHILD nevi [2]. The severity of the limb defects ranges from aplasia of whole limbs to dystrophy of single finger- or toenails [1,6]. CHILD syndrome is an X-linked semidominant trait. Heterozygous females show the CHILD phenotype, while embryonic lethality is observed in hemizygous males. Due to the random X-chromosome inactivation in heterozygous females, the skin lesions often follow a characteristic pattern, the so-called Blaschko's lines [7].

To date, a wide range of variants in the *NSDHL* gene have been described as suspected causative variants for the pathogenesis of CHILD syndrome in humans [3,8]. In mice, variants in this gene are responsible for the bare patches (*Bpa*) and striated (*Str*) phenotypes [9]. *Bpa* and *Str* mice do not show limb defects, but their skin phenotype closely resembles CHILD nevi [9]. In veterinary medicine, congenital epidermal nevi without limb defects and candidate causative variants in the *NSDHL* gene have been described in two Labrador Retrievers [10], one purebred Chihuahua [11], and one cat [12] (OMIA 002117-9615, 002117-9685).

The *NSDHL* gene encodes the NAD(P)-dependent steroid dehydrogenase-like protein, which is involved in cholesterol biosynthesis and localized on ER membranes as well as on the surface of lipid droplets [8,13]. A deficiency of this enzyme leads to accumulation of metabolic products from the cholesterol biosynthetic pathway [14,15]. The combination of the toxic effect of those sterol precursors together with decreased cholesterol synthesis and secretion into the stratum corneum is ultimately responsible for the observed skin lesions in CHILD syndrome in humans [16,17].

The currently used therapy for the skin-associated changes in humans and companion animals is aimed at the incorrect cholesterol synthesis. Good results were achieved with topical application of early inhibitors of the cholesterol synthesis pathway in combination with cholesterol-ointments [11,18,19].

In a continuation of our earlier studies [10–12], the present study aimed to characterize the clinical and histopathological phenotype in a female Chihuahua cross with congenital progressive epidermal nevi and to identify the likely causative genetic variant.

2. Materials and Methods

2.1. Ethics Statement

All animal experiments were performed according to local regulations. The dog in this study was privately owned and was examined with the consent of the owner. The "Cantonal Committee for Animal Experiments" approved the collection of blood samples from control dogs (Canton of Bern; permit 71/19).

2.2. Animal Selection

A female spayed Chihuahua cross was investigated. The clinical and dermatological examinations were done by two board certified veterinary dermatologists (M.A. and F.B.). An EDTA blood sample was collected for genomic DNA isolation. Routine histopathological examination of skin biopsies was performed before and after euthanasia of the animal.

Additionally, 22 blood samples of purebred Chihuahuas, which had been donated to the Vetsuisse Biobank were used. They represented unrelated controls without skin lesions. The same 22 dogs had been used as controls in our earlier publication [11]. Furthermore, 655 publicly available canine genome sequences [20] were analyzed as control dataset (Table S1); 594 of these had been used in our earlier publication [11]. The skin phenotypes of these 655 control dogs were not consistently documented. As the investigated phenotype is rare and at the same time very striking and obvious, we assumed that these animals were all nonaffected. The available data on their phenotype are summarized in Table S1.

2.3. DNA and RNA Extraction

Genomic DNA was isolated from EDTA blood samples with the Maxwell RSC Whole Blood DNA Kit using a Maxwell RSC instrument (Promega, Dübendorf, Switzerland). Total RNA was extracted from skin biopsies using the RNeasy Mini Kit (Qiagen, Hilden, Germany). The RNA was cleared of genomic DNA contamination using the QuantiTect Reverse Transcription Kit (Qiagen). The same kit was used to synthetize cDNA, as described by the manufacturer.

2.4. Gene Analysis

The CanFam3.1 dog reference genome assembly and the NCBI annotation release 105 were used. Numbering within the canine *NSDHL* gene corresponds to the NCBI RefSeq accession numbers XM_014111859.2 (mRNA) and XP_013967334.1 (protein).

2.5. PCR and Sanger Sequencing

Primer pairs for the amplification of all ten exons of the *NSDHL* gene were described previously [8] and are given in Table S2. PCR products for each exon were amplified from genomic DNA using AmpliTaq Gold 360 Master mix (Thermo Fisher Scientific, Reinach, Switzerland). PCR products were visualized using a 5200 Fragment Analyzer instrument (Agilent, Basel, Switzerland), which uses capillary electrophoresis to enable accurate sizing and quantification of nucleic acids. All exons of the *NSDHL* gene were analyzed by direct Sanger sequencing of PCR amplicons. After treatment with exonuclease I and alkaline phosphatase, amplicons were sequenced on an ABI 3730 DNA Analyzer (Thermo Fisher Scientific, Reinach, Switzerland). Sanger sequences were analyzed using the Sequencher 5.1 software (Gene Codes, Ann Arbor, MI, USA). For the RT-PCR on skin cDNA, a forward primer located at the boundary of exons 6 and 7 together with a reverse primer located in exon 10 was used (Table S2). After an initial denaturation of 10 min at 95 °C, 35 cycles of 30 s at 95 °C, 30 s at 60 °C, and 60 s at 72 °C were performed, followed by a final extension step of 7 min at 72 °C. The RT-PCR products were analyzed on a Fragment Analyzer and sequenced as described above.

3. Results

3.1. Clinical Examination, Necropsy, and Histopathology

A female spayed Chihuahua mix was examined at 7 and 27 months of age. The dog presented with a history of band- to plaque-like cutaneous lesions affecting both sides of the body and head since adoption at 3 months of age. The lesions were sharply demarcated and characterized by alopecia, hyperpigmentation, verrucous hyperplasia with pronounced enlargement of follicular ostia, tan-colored scaling, brown to black crusting and, in some areas, peripheral erythema along with malodor (Figure 1a). Band-like lesions often followed the lines of Blaschko (Figure 1a,b). Although both sides of the body were affected, there was a striking lesion severity lateralization to the right side. A somewhat sharp linear demarcation of the lesions was noted along the ventral midline (Figure 1a,b). The paw pads of both front limbs exhibited severe hyperkeratosis, fissuring, and moderate tissue swelling.

Over the course from the first to the second examination, the severity and extent of epidermal nevi progressed to involve diffuse areas on head, both inner ear pinnae, neck, and dorsal and lateral trunk (Figure 1c,d). Pronounced lesional lateralization of the epidermal nevi on the right side of the body was still present (Figure 1c,d). Lesion-associated pruritus and right front limb lameness were initially not observed but became pronounced over time.

Multiple general physical examinations over time yielded findings within normal limits with the exception of the skin. Hematology results and biochemistry parameters showed mild anemia, leukocytosis, hypergammaglobulinemia, and hypoalbuminemia. Schirmer tear test results remained within normal limits over time. Multiple skin scrapes were negative for ectoparasites. Numerous skin cytologies at various points in time revealed mild to partially severe, chronic, secondary bacterial infections with mainly coccoid bacteria. A bacterial tissue culture grew methicillin-resistant *Staphylocoocus pseudintermedius* at one point in time.

Histopathological examination of multiple skin biopsies revealed massive parakeratotic hyperkeratosis mixed with compact lamellar orthokeratotic hyperkeratosis along with irregular, severe acanthosis with broad rete ridges extending deep into the superficial dermis (Figure 1e,f). The hyperkeratosis and acanthosis were also present in follicular infundibular epithelium and were associated with follicular distention supported by an underlying proliferative granular cell layer and stratum spinosum. There were small to large clusters of neutrophils within the stratum corneum and multilaminated, pustular crusts enclosing mixed bacteria covered portions of the epidermis. Hair follicles with sebaceous and apocrine glands were incarcerated in the dermis. Moderate numbers of melanocytes and melanin-filled macrophages were present at the dermal-epidermal junction with mild pigmentary incontinence in the superficial dermis. The dermis contained occasional periadnexal infiltrates of lymphocytes, plasma cells, and neutrophils with some dermal edema. When correlated with the description of the linear nature of the patient's lesions, the histopathological findings were consistent with an epidermal nevus.

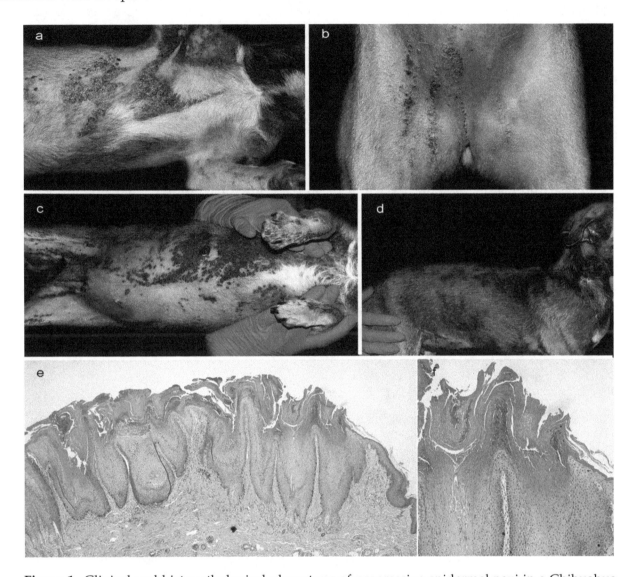

Figure 1. Clinical and histopathological phenotype of progressive epidermal nevi in a Chihuahua mix. (**a,b**) Clinical phenotype at 7 months of age. Pronounced lateralization of the skin lesions at the initial presentation on the right axillary area (**a**) and right side of ventral/inguinal area (**b**). (**c,d**) Clinical phenotype at 27 months of age. Progression of the severity and extent of epidermal nevi to involve diffuse areas in the axillae, ventral abdomen, and inguinal region (**c**) as well as head, both inner ear pinnae, neck, and dorsal and lateral trunk (**d**). (**e**) Histopathology of a skin biopsy taken at 27 months of age from the ventral neck showing severe parakeratotic hyperkeratosis and acanthosis with broad rete ridges extending deep into the superficial dermis. Follicular infundibula are similarly affected by acanthosis and hyperkeratosis and appear distended. (**f**) Details of the histopathology at higher magnification.

The patient's skin underwent histopathological evaluation of different body sites at three different points in time (at 4, 7, and 27 months of age), which all yielded similar results with variations only in regard to the severity of the observed changes and the extent and nature of secondary infections.

Treatments over time included systemic antibiotics (cephalexin, cefpodoxime, clindamycin, and amoxicillin/clavulanic acid), systemic antifungal (fluconazole), antimicrobial shampoos and sprays (chlorhexidine/miconazole), antiseborrheic shampoo and conditioner (gluconolactone-based), antibiotic ointment (mupirocin 2%), topical steroid (betamethasone dipropionate 0.05%), oral glucocorticoid (prednisone), oral vitamin A, oral isotretinoin, oral antihistamine (diphenhydramine), cryotherapy, and interleukin 31 antibody injections, which all yielded minimal to no improvement of clinical signs. Notable exceptions were the interleukin-31 antibody injections, which were accompanied by a reduction in the patient's pruritus, and oral prednisone, which correlated with significantly improved right front paw tissue swelling and lameness.

Due to the steady decline in the patient's overall quality of life, the client elected humane euthanasia at 2 years and 3 months of age. Upon necropsy, no pathologic abnormalities besides the cutaneous lesions and mild, generalized lymphadenopathy were found.

3.2. Genetic Analysis

As clinical and histopathological findings resembled previously published companion animals with congenital epidermal nevi [10–12], we hypothesized that the phenotype in the affected dog was due to a heterozygous variant in the NSDHL gene. Hence, NSDHL was investigated as the top functional candidate gene.

Sanger sequencing of all ten exons of the NSDHL gene of the examined dog identified a single variant in the coding sequence. The variant is a five base pair deletion in exon 9 of the NSDHL gene (Figure 2). The genomic variant designation is NC_006621.3:120,752,486_120,752,490delGAACA. It is a frameshift variant, XM_014111859.2:c.718_722delGAACA.

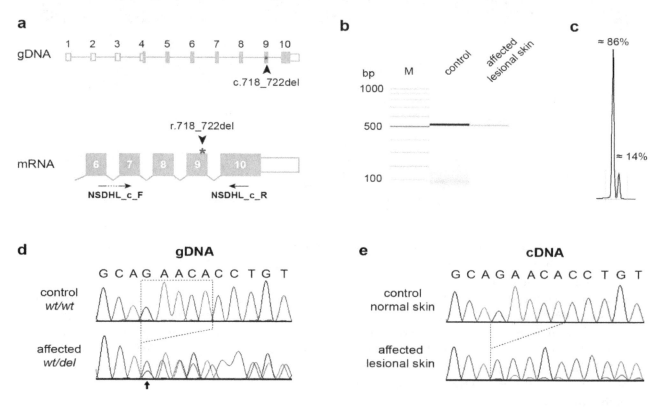

Figure 2. Details of the NSDHL:c.718_722delGAACA variant. (**a**) Genomic organization of the canine NSDHL gene with 10 annotated exons. The position of the variant on the genomic DNA and the mRNA level are indicated. The position of the primers used for the RT-PCR experiment are also indicated. (**b**) RT-PCR amplification products obtained from cDNA from skin of a healthy control and lesional skin from the affected dog. The samples were analyzed on a FragmentAnalyzer capillary gel electrophoresis instrument. The predominant band in the affected dog corresponds to a correctly spliced transcript

lacking 5 nucleotides of coding sequence (r.718_722del). The minor band that migrated slower than the main product most likely represents heteroduplex molecules consisting of one strand containing the 5-nucleotide deletion annealed to a wildtype strand. (c) Relative quantification of these two bands. Please note that the ratio of these end-point RT-PCR amplicons should only be seen as a semiquantitative proxy for the true ratio of transcripts. (d) Sanger electropherograms derived from genomic PCR products of a control dog and the affected dog. The five bases that are deleted in the affected animal are indicated with dotted lines. The arrow indicates the beginning of overlapping signals in the electropherogram of the affected dog. The intensities of the overlapping signals correspond well to the expected 50:50 allelic ratio for a heterozygous animal. (e) Analysis of mRNA. RT-PCR amplicons from the skin of a normal control dog and lesional skin of the affected dog were sequenced. The vast majority of *NSDHL* transcripts of the affected dog lacked 5 nucleotides corresponding to positions 718-722 in the coding sequence. Note the difference in relative signal intensity of the two alleles in the cDNA amplicon compared to the genomic sequence in the affected dog.

RT-PCR on RNA derived from a lesional skin biopsy of the affected dog yielded an amplicon of the expected size. Sanger sequencing confirmed that the transcripts were normally spliced. We observed pronounced allelic imbalance in lesional skin of the affected dog. The *NSDHL* transcripts were almost exclusively expressed from the mutant allele and lacked the five deleted nucleotides (XM_014111859.2:r.718_722del; Figure 2b,c,e). The frameshift deletion truncates 122 codons (34%) from the open reading frame of the wild-type *NSDHL* transcript, XP_013967334.1:p.(Glu240Profs*17).

We genotyped 22 unaffected Chihuahuas for the frameshift variant. None of these control dogs carried the mutant allele. The mutant allele was also absent from whole-genome sequence data of 647 control dogs of diverse breeds and eight wolves (Table S1).

4. Discussion

In this study, we identified a heterozygous *NSDHL*: c.718_722delGAACA frameshift variant in a mixed breed dog with a severe form of progressive epidermal nevi. The *NSDHL* gene encodes the enzyme NAD(P) dependent steroid dehydrogenase-like, which is involved in cholesterol biosynthesis and has been associated with human CHILD syndrome [8], as well as canine and feline congenital epidermal nevi [10–12].

In this single case investigation, we attempted to apply the American College of Medical Genetics and Genomics (ACMG) approved guidelines for the interpretation of sequence variants in human genetics to a dog with the *NSDHL*:c.718_722delGAACA variant [21]. Three arguments support the pathogenicity of the *NSDHL*:c.718_722delGAACA variant.

Computational and predictive data provide a very strong argument for pathogenicity (PVS1) as the frameshift variant is predicted to result in a loss-of-function (LOF) of the *NSDHL* gene [21]. *NSDHL* LOF variants in human and animal patients represent an established mechanism of disease [8–10].

Population data indicate that the mutant allele was only present in a single affected dog, while it was absent from more than 600 control dogs. We rate this as a moderate evidence for pathogenicity (PM2) [21].

Other data finally provide additional supporting evidence for pathogenicity (PP4) [21]. The clinical and histopathological skin phenotype is highly specific and *NSDHL* is the only known candidate gene for such a phenotype. Furthermore, the distribution of the skin lesions along Blaschko's lines and the female sex of the patient strongly point to an X-chromosomal causative variant.

According to the established ACMG criteria, the combinations of one very strong, one moderate, and one supporting type of evidence is sufficient to classify the *NSDHL*: c.718_722delGAACA variant as pathogenic.

To the best of our knowledge, the found variant is the third disease-causing *NSDHL* variant identified in dogs. Previous studies reported a 14 kb deletion spanning the last three exons of *NSDHL* gene [10] and a single missense variant p.Gly234Arg [11] in dogs with congenital epidermal nevi.

5. Conclusions

We identified a frameshift variant, *NSDHL*: c.718_722delGAACA as the probable causative variant for progressive epidermal nevi in a single mixed breed dog. Established guidelines for the interpretation of human sequence variants justify the classification of this variant as pathogenic.

Author Contributions: Conceptualization, T.L.; investigation, M.C., M.A., F.B., V.J., and T.L.; data curation, V.J.; writing—original draft preparation, M.C., M.A., and T.L.; writing—review and editing, M.C., M.A., F.B., V.J., and T.L.; supervision, T.L. All authors have read and agreed to the published version of the manuscript.

Acknowledgments: The authors are grateful to the dog owner who donated samples and participated in the study. We thank Nathalie Besuchet Schmutz for expert technical assistance, Jan Henkel for help with the RNA experiments, the Next Generation Sequencing Platform of the University of Bern for performing the high-throughput sequencing experiments, and the Interfaculty Bioinformatics Unit of the University of Bern for providing high-performance computing infrastructure.

References

1.   Happle, R.; Koch, H.; Lenz, W. The CHILD syndrome. Congenital hemidysplasia with ichthyosiform erythroderma and limb defects. *Eur. J. Pediatr.* **1980**, *134*, 27–33. [CrossRef]

2.   Happle, R.; Mittag, H.; Küster, W. The CHILD nevus: A distinct skin disorder. *Dermatology* **1995**, *191*, 210–216. [CrossRef] [PubMed]

3.   Bornholdt, D.; König, A.; Happle, R.; Leveleki, L.; Bittar, M.; Danarti, R.; Vahlquist, A.; Tilgen, W.; Reinhold, U.; Poiares Baptista, A.; et al. Mutational spectrum of NSDHL in CHILD syndrome. *J. Med. Genet.* **2005**, *42*, e17. [CrossRef] [PubMed]

4.   Avgerinou, G.P.; Asvesti, A.P.; Katsambas, A.D.; Nikolaou, V.A.; Christofidou, E.C.; Grzeschik, K.H.; Happle, R. CHILD syndrome: The NSDHL gene and its role in CHILD syndrome, a rare hereditary disorder. *J. Eur. Acad. Dermatol. Venereol.* **2010**, *24*, 733–736. [CrossRef] [PubMed]

5.   Garcias-Ladaria, J.; Cuadrado Rosón, M.; Pascual-López, M. Epidermal Nevi and Related Syndromes—Part 1: Keratinocytic Nevi. *Actas Dermosifiliogr.* **2018**, *109*, 677–686. [CrossRef] [PubMed]

6.   Bittar, M.; Happle, R.; Grzeschik, K.-H.; Leveleki, L.; Hertl, M.; Bornholdt, D.; König, A. CHILD syndrome in 3 generations. *Arch. Dermatol.* **2006**, *142*, 7–10. [CrossRef] [PubMed]

7.   Happle, R. X-chromosome inactivation: Role in skin disease expression. *Acta Paediatr. Suppl.* **2006**, *95*, 16–23. [CrossRef]

8.   König, A.; Happle, R.; Bornholdt, D.; Engel, H.; Grzeschik, K.H. Mutations in the NSDHL gene, encoding a 3β-hydroxysteroid dehydrogenase, cause CHILD syndrome. *Am. J. Med. Genet.* **2000**, *90*, 339–346. [CrossRef]

9.   Liu, X.Y.; Dangel, A.W.; Kelley, R.I.; Zhao, W.; Denny, P.; Botcherby, M.; Cattanach, B.; Peters, J.; Hunsicker, P.R.; Mallon, A.M.; et al. The gene mutated in bare patches and striated mice encodes a novel 3β-hydroxysteroid dehydrogenase. *Nat. Genet.* **1999**, *22*, 182–187. [CrossRef]

10. Bauer, A.; De Lucia, M.; Jagannathan, V.; Mezzalira, G.; Casal, M.L.; Welle, M.M.; Leeb, T. A large deletion in the *NSDHL* gene in Labrador Retrievers with a congenital cornification disorder. *G3 Genes Genomes Genet.* **2017**, *7*, 3115–3121. [CrossRef]

11. Leuthard, F.; Lehner, G.; Jagannathan, V.; Leeb, T.; Welle, M. A missense variant in the *NSDHL* gene in a Chihuahua with a congenital cornification disorder resembling inflammatory linear verrucous epidermal nevi. *Anim. Genet.* **2019**, *50*, 768–771. [CrossRef]

12. De Lucia, M.; Bauer, A.; Spycher, M.; Jagannathan, V.; Romano, E.; Welle, M.; Leeb, T. Genetic variant in the *NSDHL* gene in a cat with multiple congenital lesions resembling inflammatory linear verrucous epidermal nevi. *Vet. Dermatol.* **2019**, *30*, 64-e18. [CrossRef]

13. Caldas, H.; Herman, G.E. NSDHL, an enzyme involved in cholesterol biosynthesis, traffics through the Golgi and accumulates on ER membranes and on the surface of lipid droplets. *Hum. Mol. Genet.* **2003**, *12*, 2981–2991. [CrossRef]

14. Zettersten, E.; Man, M.Q.; Sato, J.; Denda, M.; Farrell, A.; Ghadially, R.; Williams, M.L.; Feingold, K.R.; Elias, P.M. Recessive x-linked ichthyosis: Role of cholesterol-sulfate accumulation in the barrier abnormality. *J. Investig. Dermatol.* **1998**, *111*, 784–790. [CrossRef] [PubMed]

15. Elias, P.M.; Williams, M.L.; Holleran, W.M.; Jiang, Y.J.; Schmuth, M. Pathogenesis of permeability barrier abnormalities in the ichthyoses: Inherited disorders of lipid metabolism. *J. Lipid Res.* **2008**, *49*, 697–714. [CrossRef]

16. Elias, P.M.; Crumrine, D.; Paller, A.; Rodriguez-Martin, M.; Williams, M.L. Pathogenesis of the cutaneous phenotype in inherited disorders of cholesterol metabolism: Therapeutic implications for topical treatment of these disorders. *Dermatoendocrinology* **2011**, *3*, 100–106. [CrossRef]

17. Seeger, M.A.; Paller, A.S. The role of abnormalities in the distal pathway of cholesterol synthesis in the Congenital Hemidysplasia with Ichthyosiform erythroderma and Limb Defects (CHILD) syndrome. *Biochim. Biophys. Acta Mol. Cell Biol. Lipids* **2014**, *1841*, 345–352. [CrossRef] [PubMed]

18. Alexopoulos, A.; Kakourou, T. CHILD syndrome: Successful treatment of skin lesions with topical simvastatin/cholesterol ointment—A case report. *Pediatr. Dermatol.* **2015**, *32*, e145–e147. [CrossRef]

19. Cho, S.K.; Ashworth, L.D.; Goldman, S. Topical cholesterol/simvastatin gel for the treatment of CHILD syndrome in an adolescent. *Int. J. Pharm. Compd.* **2020**, *24*, 367–369. [PubMed]

20. Jagannathan, V.; Drögemüller, C.; Leeb, T.; Aguirre, G.; André, C.; Bannasch, D.; Becker, D.; Davis, B.; Ekenstedt, K.; Faller, K.; et al. A comprehensive biomedical variant catalogue based on whole genome sequences of 582 dogs and eight wolves. *Anim. Genet.* **2019**, *50*, 695–704. [CrossRef] [PubMed]

21. Richards, S.; Aziz, N.; Bale, S.; Bick, D.; Das, S.; Gastier-Foster, J.; Grody, W.W.; Hegde, M.; Lyon, E.; Spector, E.; et al. Standards and guidelines for the interpretation of sequence variants: A joint consensus recommendation of the American College of Medical Genetics and Genomics and the Association for Molecular Pathology. *Genet. Med.* **2015**, *17*, 405–424. [CrossRef] [PubMed]

A *CNTNAP1* Missense Variant is Associated with Canine Laryngeal Paralysis and Polyneuropathy

Anna Letko [1,*,†], **Katie M. Minor** [2,†], **Steven G. Friedenberg** [3], **G. Diane Shelton** [4], **Jill Pesayco Salvador** [4], **Paul J. J. Mandigers** [5], **Peter A. J. Leegwater** [5], **Paige A. Winkler** [6], **Simon M. Petersen-Jones** [6], **Bryden J. Stanley** [6], **Kari J. Ekenstedt** [7], **Gary S. Johnson** [8], **Liz Hansen** [8], **Vidhya Jagannathan** [1], **James R. Mickelson** [2,‡] **and Cord Drögemüller** [1,‡]

[1] Institute of Genetics, Vetsuisse Faculty, University of Bern, 3012 Bern, Switzerland; vidhya.jagannathan@vetsuisse.unibe.ch (V.J.); cord.droegemueller@vetsuisse.unibe.ch (C.D.)

[2] Department of Veterinary and Biomedical Sciences, College of Veterinary Medicine, University of Minnesota, Saint Paul, MN 55108, USA; minork@umn.edu (K.M.M.); micke001@umn.edu (J.R.M.)

[3] Department of Veterinary Clinical Sciences, College of Veterinary Medicine, University of Minnesota, Saint Paul, MN 55108, USA; fried255@umn.edu

[4] Department of Pathology, School of Medicine, University of California San Diego, La Jolla, CA 92093-0709, USA; gshelton@ucsd.edu (G.D.S.); jpesayco@ucsd.edu (J.P.S.)

[5] Department of Clinical Sciences, Utrecht University, 3584 CM Utrecht, The Netherlands; p.j.j.mandigers@veterinair-neuroloog.nl (P.J.J.M.); P.A.J.Leegwater@uu.nl (P.A.J.L.)

[6] Department of Small Animal Clinical Sciences, College of Veterinary Medicine, Michigan State University, East Lansing, MI 48824, USA; winkler.paige@gmail.com (P.A.W.); peter315@msu.edu (S.M.P.-J.); stanle32@msu.edu (B.J.S.)

[7] Department of Basic Medical Sciences, College of Veterinary Medicine, Purdue University, West Lafayette, IN 47907, USA; kje0003@purdue.edu

[8] Department of Veterinary Pathobiology, University of Missouri, Columbia, MO 65211, USA; JohnsonGS@missouri.edu (G.S.J.); HansenL@missouri.edu (L.H.)

* Correspondence: anna.letko@vetsuisse.unibe.ch;

† These authors contributed equally to the work.

‡ James R. Mickelson and Cord Drögemüller shared last author.

Abstract: Laryngeal paralysis associated with a generalized polyneuropathy (LPPN) most commonly exists in geriatric dogs from a variety of large and giant breeds. The purpose of this study was to discover the underlying genetic and molecular mechanisms in a younger-onset form of this neurodegenerative disease seen in two closely related giant dog breeds, the Leonberger and Saint Bernard. Neuropathology of an affected dog from each breed showed variable nerve fiber loss and scattered inappropriately thin myelinated fibers. Using across-breed genome-wide association, haplotype analysis, and whole-genome sequencing, we identified a missense variant in the *CNTNAP1* gene (c.2810G>A; p.Gly937Glu) in which homozygotes in both studied breeds are affected. *CNTNAP1* encodes a contactin-associated protein important for organization of myelinated axons. The herein described likely pathogenic *CNTNAP1* variant occurs in unrelated breeds at variable frequencies. Individual homozygous mutant LPPN-affected Labrador retrievers that were on average four years younger than dogs affected by geriatric onset laryngeal paralysis polyneuropathy could be explained by this variant. Pathologic changes in a Labrador retriever nerve biopsy from a homozygous mutant dog were similar to those of the Leonberger and Saint Bernard. The impact of this variant on health in English bulldogs and Irish terriers, two breeds with higher *CNTNAP1* variant allele frequencies, remains unclear. Pathogenic variants in *CNTNAP1* have previously been reported in human patients with lethal congenital contracture syndrome and hypomyelinating neuropathy, including vocal cord palsy and severe respiratory distress. This is the first report of contactin-associated LPPN in dogs characterized by a deleterious variant that most likely predates modern breed establishment.

Keywords: *Canis familiaris*; whole-genome sequencing; rare disease; contactin; neurological disorder; Leonberger; Saint Bernard; Labrador retriever

1. Introduction

Laryngeal paralysis (LP) can result from trauma or neoplasia involving the recurrent laryngeal nerves, peripheral nerve disease, or a primary or secondary disease affecting the muscle or neuromuscular junction. Loss of normal function of the larynx leads to breathing difficulties, reduced exercise and heat tolerance, as well as an increased risk of aspiration pneumonia [1]. Laryngeal nerve disease results in degeneration and atrophy of intrinsic laryngeal muscles followed by decreased or absent movement of the attendant laryngeal cartilages. During breathing, these cartilages control airflow into and out of the trachea. Affected dogs have stridor, may have a change in vocalization, and difficulty breathing due to the flaccid laryngeal vocal folds and corniculate processes of the arytenoid obstructing the lumen of the airway [1]. Normal laryngeal function protects the airway by closing off the lumen to prevent aspiration of food or water. In LP-affected dogs, the vocal folds remain in a paramedian position, causing airway resistance and turbulence, instead of abducting, as they normally would, to open the airway during inspiration. Frequently, affected dogs suffering from LP are treated by crico- or thyro-arytenoid laryngoplasty surgery, to improve breathing and, therefore, quality of life [2]. As the recurrent laryngeal nerve axons are some of the longest in the body [3], LP is often reported as part of a more generalized length-dependent polyneuropathy (PN) complex, which manifests with additional signs including proprioceptive and motor abnormalities, slowly progressing pelvic limb weakness, and loss of limb muscle mass [4].

Various mostly breed-specific canine inherited neuropathies form a heterogeneous group of degenerative diseases affecting motor and/or sensory and autonomic peripheral nerves. This group includes mixed forms of LP and PN [5], i.e., the laryngeal paralysis and polyneuropathy complex (LPPN), which has variable ages of onset among and across several dog breeds (OMIA 001206-9615, OMIA 001292-9615). Late-onset forms, e.g., geriatric onset laryngeal paralysis polyneuropathy (GOLPP), are also observed in various breeds including Labrador retrievers [6]. Leonberger dogs are known to be susceptible to LPPN; recently, a short list of potentially pathogenic variants for neurological disorders in this breed derived from whole-genome sequencing has been presented [7]. To date, variants in *ARHGEF10* [8] and *GJA9* [9] have already been associated with certain forms of the disorder and designated with breed-specific names Leonberger polyneuropathy type 1 (LPN1; OMIA 001917-9615) and Leonberger polyneuropathy type 2 (LPN2; OMIA 002119-9615), respectively. These two variants, however, do not explain all the phenotypically described cases in Leonbergers [7]. The *ARHGEF10* variant has also been reported in the related Saint Bernard breed, but again it did not explain all LPPN cases [8]. Alaskan huskies, black Russian terriers, and Rottweilers with PN including LP and respiratory distress are known to have deleterious variants in the *RAB3GAP1* gene, a member of the RAB3 protein family implicated in regulated exocytosis of neurotransmitters and hormones (OMIA 001970-9615) [10–12]. Another major risk factor for canine LP recently described in miniature bull terriers and bull terriers is a variant in the *RAPGEF6* gene encoding a widely expressed nucleotide exchange factor whose function is not well understood (OMIA 002222-9615) [13].

In general, there are limits to precisely diagnosing neurological diseases in dogs in the clinic. For example, in a previous study [14], we noticed Leonbergers that were initially clinically diagnosed as polyneuropathy-affected, although, in fact, they were suffering from leukoencephalomyelopathy, a juvenile-onset neurodegenerative disorder of the CNS white matter with distinctive pathological features, caused by a recessive variant in the *NAPEPLD* gene (OMIA 001788-9615).

Our aim in this study was to identify additional causative genetic variants associated with younger-onset laryngeal paralysis and polyneuropathy (LPPN), by focusing on two closely related giant dog breeds [15], namely the Leonberger and Saint Bernard.

2. Materials and Methods

2.1. Ethics Statement

All animal experiments were performed according to local regulations, and all animals in this study were examined with the consent of their owners. The study was approved under IACUC protocol 1903-36865A at the University of Minnesota, the Michigan State University Institutional Animal Care and Use Committee (AUF number 01/11-009-00), and by the Cantonal Committee for Animal Experiments (Canton of Bern; permit 71/19) at the University of Bern.

2.2. Animal Selection

Data on 15,378 dogs from 243 breeds, 321 dogs of mixed or unknown heritage, and 62 wild canids were collected in three different sets for this study (Table 1 and Supplementary Table S1). The discovery cohort included 426 Leonbergers either showing signs of LPPN with an age of onset ≤5 years or healthy control dogs at ≥8 years of age, and 91 Saint Bernards either showing signs of LPPN with an age of onset ≤5 years or population control dogs with genome-wide association study (GWAS) data available from unrelated studies [15,16]. All 517 Leonbergers and Saint Bernards were genotyped for the ARHGEF10 variant [8], and the Leonbergers were also genotyped for the GJA9 variant [9], in order to include only dogs homozygous wild type for these loci. In addition, the Leonbergers were genotyped for a previously reported leukoencephalopathy-associated NAPEPLD variant [14], in order to rule out another known underlying neurological disease with similar clinical phenotype.

Table 1. Number of canids in each studied cohort.

Cohort [1]	Dog Breed/Species	Total	Phenotype		
			LPPN-Affected [2]	LPPN Non-Affected [3]	Unknown
Discovery (n = 517)	Leonberger	426	126	300	0
	Saint Bernard	91	18	14	59
Validation (n = 1070)	Leonberger	859	500	359	0
	Saint Bernard	11	11	0	0
	Labrador retriever [4]	200	150	50	0
Population (n = 14,174)	243 dog breeds	13,798	0	0	13,798
	Unknown/mixed heritage	314	0	0	314
	Wolf	58	0	0	58
	Golden jackal	2	0	0	2
	Andean fox	1	0	0	1
	Dhole	1	0	0	1

[1] Additional details including the source of all data are available in Supplementary Materials Table S1. [2] Includes affected dogs with previously described laryngeal paralysis and polyneuropathy (LPPN)-associated variants in ARHGEF10 [8] and GJA9 [9]. [3] Includes dogs homozygous for the previously described leukoencephalomyelopathy-associated variant in NAPEPLD [14]. [4] Includes seven mixed-breed dogs enrolled in the Michigan State University's GOLPP study [6].

A validation cohort used for targeted genotyping of the newly discovered variant consisted of 1070 dogs with known LPPN phenotypes (Table 1 and Supplementary Table S1). There was no age of onset restriction for the cases in the validation cohort. Included in the validation cohort were 193 Labrador retrievers and seven mixed-breed dogs from an ongoing geriatric onset laryngeal paralysis polyneuropathy (GOLPP) study; these were used as an independent validation group (Table 1).

Finally, a population cohort consisting of 14,112 dogs, 58 wolves, two golden jackals, one Andean fox, and one dhole (Table 1 and Supplementary Table S1), with no available information about their health status, was used to determine the absence/presence and frequency of the described variant-associated haplotype across canids.

The information about age of onset of clinical signs in the LPPN-affected dogs was available for a subset of 770 dogs from the discovery and validation cohorts with detailed health information from three breeds (596 Leonbergers, 28 Saint Bernards, and 146 Labrador retrievers) The statistical significance of the differences between groups was evaluated with Student's *t*-test and $p < 0.05$ was considered as significant.

2.3. Sample Preparation

Genomic DNA was isolated from EDTA blood samples, buccal swabs, or archived muscle biopsies by using either the Gentra PureGene kit (Qiagen, Hilden, Germany) or the Maxwell RSC Whole Blood DNA kit (Promega, Dübendorf, Switzerland).

Clinical cases of polyneuropathy and laryngeal paralysis were evaluated in three dogs homozygous for the studied *CNTNAP1* variant with available nerve biopsies; these included a 3-year-old Saint Bernard, a 3-year-old Leonberger, and a 9-year-old Labrador retriever (Supplementary Table S1). Three normal adult dog samples from Labrador retrievers were used as controls. The ages for the control dogs were 8–10 years of age. All the archived nerve specimens were obtained years prior to the identification of the *CNTNAP1* variant. Peroneal nerve specimens, pinned on cork discs to maintain length and orientation, were immersion-fixed in 2.5% glutaraldehyde in 0.1 M phosphate buffer before shipment. Upon receipt, the nerves were postfixed in 1% aqueous osmium tetroxide for 3 to 4 h before dehydration in a graded alcohol series and propylene oxide. After infiltration with a 1:1 mixture of propylene oxide and araldite resin for 4 h, nerves were placed in 100% araldite resin overnight before embedding in fresh araldite resin. Thick sections (1 μm) were cut with glass knives and either stained with toluidine blue prior to light microscopic examination, or stained with paraphenylenediamine prior to morphometry.

2.4. Axonal Size Frequency Distributions and G-Ratios

Axonal size-frequency distributions of myelinated fibers were performed on transverse sections of selected peroneal nerve biopsies determined to be adequately fixed, free from artifact, and with an intact perineurium. Images were obtained from a single section of each nerve biopsy using the Photoshop image analysis system. Profiles containing paranodal regions or Schmidt–Lanterman clefts were not included. Using a ×60 objective, the final magnification of the digitized image was equivalent to 1 pixel = 0.091 μm. Myelinated fibers were individually identified and selected prior to being sorted with an automated process into bins based on axonal area. G-ratios were calculated as the ratio between the diameter of the axon itself and the outer diameter of the myelinated fiber.

2.5. Single Nucleotide Polymorphism Array Genotyping and Imputation

The discovery cohort (426 Leonbergers and 91 Saint Bernards) was genotyped by using either the Axiom Canine Set A or HD arrays (Thermo Fisher Scientific, Waltham, MA, USA) or the Illumina CanineHD BeadChip array (Illumina, San Diego, CA, USA). Samples genotyped on lower single nucleotide polymorphism (SNP) density arrays were imputed with Beagle 4.1 [17,18], using a diverse reference dataset containing 526,045 variants in 49 wolves and 2871 dogs (including 65 Leonbergers and 23 Saint Bernards; Supplementary Table S1). The data were filtered to include only biallelic SNPs with a minor allele frequency ≥0.02, a per-SNP genotyping rate ≥95%, and a per-individual genotyping rate ≥95%. The reference dataset was phased on a per-chromosome basis, using Beagle 4.1 with default parameters of 10 iterations and an effective population size of 200. Next, a target dataset containing approximately 174,000 variants in 402 Leonbergers and 66 Saint Bernards (Supplementary Table S1) was filtered to include only biallelic SNPs with a minor allele frequency ≥0.02, and then checked for concordance with the filtered and phased reference dataset, using the Beagle 4 utility conform-gt [19]. Conforming sites of the target dataset were imputed to the reference dataset on a per-chromosome basis, using Beagle 4.1 with the following settings: window size 50 kb, overlap 3 kb, effective population size 200, and 10 iterations. The per-chromosome imputed data were concatenated and sorted, using VCFtools 0.1.13 [20]; variants with a Beagle 4.1 dosage R-squared (DR2) ≥0.7 were retained for downstream analysis. In total, we used imputed SNP data for 468 Leonberger and Saint Bernard dogs in this study.

To evaluate haplotypes across breeds, approximately 126,000 SNPs common across genotyping platforms were extracted from non-imputed SNP genotype data for 12,931 canids, which were either generated during this study or publicly available (Supplementary Table S1) and phased with Beagle 4.1 as described above.

2.6. Genome-Wide Association Study and Fine-Mapping

The discovery cohort from the two breeds combined contained 517 dogs (144 LPPN-cases and 373 controls). Quality control filtering steps of the imputed SNP array genotyping data were carried out by using PLINK v1.9 [21]. The dataset was pruned for low minor allele frequency (0.05) and failure to meet Hardy–Weinberg equilibrium (0.0001) and consisted of 289,553 markers. An across-breed genome-wide association study (GWAS) was performed with GEMMA v0.98 [22], using a linear mixed model including an estimated kinship matrix from centered genotypes to correct for the genomic inflation. The significance threshold was estimated by Bonferroni correction. Manhattan and Q–Q plots of the corrected p-values were generated in R environment v3.6.0 [23], using the qqman package [24]. Haplotypes around the significantly associated locus obtained from GWAS were constructed by using Beagle 4.1 for all canids with available SNP genotype data (n = 13,399) (Supplementary Table S1). All genome positions refer to the CanFam3.1 reference assembly.

2.7. Whole-Genome Sequencing

Whole-genome sequence (WGS) data of 716 publicly available dogs of 131 different breeds, and nine wolves [25] (Supplementary Table S2) were studied in order to identify the causative variant in the disease-associated region obtained by the GWAS. This set included 34 Leonbergers and two Saint Bernards diagnosed with a form of LPPN unexplained by the previously known variants in *ARHGEF10* [8], *GJA9* [9], *RAB3GAP1* [10–12] and *RAPGEF6* [13], as well as seven Leonbergers and one Saint Bernard used as controls. The sequence data analysis and calling of single nucleotide variants and small indels (SNVs), including the prediction of functional effects, were described previously [25]. The Integrative genomics viewer (IGV) software 2.8.2 [26] was used for visual inspection and screening for structural variants in the region of interest in the affected dogs' WGS.

2.8. Targeted Genotyping

Polymerase chain reaction (PCR) and Sanger sequencing were used to validate and genotype the variant identified from WGS. PCR products from genomic DNA were amplified by using AmpliTaqGold360 MasterMix (Thermo Fisher Scientific), and the purified PCR amplicons were directly sequenced on an ABI3730 capillary sequencer (Thermo Fisher Scientific). The *CNTNAP1* missense variant (XM_548083.6:c.2810G>A) was genotyped, using the following primers: TCCCTTGCCCTCCCTATATC (forward) and AGTCCTAATGCCCTCTGCTG (reverse). The sequence data were analyzed by using Sequencher 5.1 software (GeneCodes, Ann Arbor, MI, USA).

2.9. Protein Predictions

The MutPred2 [27], PROVEAN [28] and PON-P2 [29] in silico prediction tools were used to predict biological consequences of the discovered variant on the encoded protein. All references to the canine *CNTNAP1* gene correspond to the accessions NC_006591.3 (NCBI accession), XM_548083.6 (mRNA), and XP_548083.3 (protein). The Genome Aggregation Database (gnomAD) [30] was searched for the corresponding variant in the human *CNTNAP1* gene (NP_003623.1).

2.10. Availability of Data and Material

The WGS are freely available at the European Nucleotide Archive (ENA). All accession numbers of the used genomes are available in the Supplementary Table S2. The sources of SNP array genotyping data published before are detailed in the Supplementary Table S1, and the dataset generated for this study is available from the corresponding author on reasonable request. All genome positions are reported with respect to the dog reference genome assembly CanFam3.1 and NCBI annotation release 105.

3. Results

3.1. Phenotype

The herein studied affected dogs showed generic signs of LPPN (Supplementary Table S1) with the key feature across breeds being breathing difficulty, often described as noisy or raspy breathing (Supplementary Video S1). Due to LP, 247 dogs (121 Leonbergers, 10 Saint Bernards, 114 Labrador retrievers, and 2 mixed-breed dogs) underwent an arytenoid lateralization surgery, 25 of which (ten Leonbergers, seven Saint Bernards, six Labrador retrievers, and two mixed-breed dogs) tested homozygous for the studied *CNTNAP1* variant (Supplementary Table S1). Additional clinical signs, which were noted variably among the dogs, included difficulty swallowing, changes in barking frequency and quality, high-stepping and uncoordinated gait, stumbling and tripping, exercise intolerance, and limb muscle atrophy.

3.2. Neuropathological and Morphometric Findings

Peroneal nerve biopsies were evaluated from three archived normal adult Labrador retriever (8–10 years) samples (representative image in Figure 1a), and three LPPN-affected dog samples: a nine-year-old male Labrador retriever (Figure 1b), a three-year-old male Leonberger (Figure 1c), and a three-year-old male Saint Bernard (Figure 1d), all of which tested homozygous for the studied *CNTNAP1* variant. Compared to control nerve, pathological changes were similar among affected dogs of all three breeds and included a subjective decrease in the number of myelinated nerve fibers compared to control nerve (Figure 1b–d) with scattered inappropriately thin myelin sheaths for the axon diameter (best demonstrated in Figure 1b,c). The inappropriately thin myelinated fibers were not found in the nerves of control dogs. Myelin splitting and ballooning, onion-bulb formations, and axonal degeneration were not observed in any of the biopsies.

A histogram of axonal size-frequency distribution of the relative percentage of small (<5 μm) and large (>5 μm) myelinated nerve fibers is shown for the three control Labrador retrievers, the LPPN-affected Leonberger, and the LPPN-affected Labrador retriever (Supplementary Figure S1) described above. As only a partial nerve fascicle was available for the LPPN-affected Saint Bernard, those data were not included. The large and small nerve fibers are determined by the axon diameters and this does not refer to the thickness of the myelin sheath. Compared to the average values for the control Labrador retrievers, the affected Labrador retriever showed an increased population of small caliber nerve fibers and a decreased population of large caliber nerve fibers. In contrast, the affected Leonberger showed a decreased population of small fibers and an increased population of larger fibers. Calculated G-ratio, a quantitative measure of myelin thickness, was 0.586 ± 0.031 (range 0.552–0.609) for the control Labrador retrievers, 0.543 for the affected Leonberger, and 0.575 for the affected Labrador retriever.

3.3. Genome-Wide Association Study and Fine-Mapping

The across-breed GWAS using the discovery cohort of *ARHGEF10*- and *GJA9*-negative Leonbergers and Saint Bernards (144 cases vs. 373 controls) revealed a single genome-wide significantly associated region for LPPN (Figure 2a). The 15 best-associated markers were used to define a 4.6 Mb region of interest between 19.1 and 23.7 Mb on chromosome 9 (Supplementary Table S3). Fine-mapping of this region, using the available haplotypes from non-imputed SNP array genotyping data, included 87 markers centered on the best associated SNP (chr9:20,271,681). This revealed one homozygous haplotype present most frequently in LPPN-affected dogs ($n = 21$) of both breeds and not present in homozygosity in any of the controls (Supplementary Table S4). Therefore, the disease-associated region was narrowed to ~0.98 Mb (bp position 19,393,936 to 20,371,611), by a combination of sharing in the 21 homozygous cases from the discovery cohort (14 Leonbergers and 7 Saint Bernards), coupled with recombination events. Based on this analysis, we hypothesized that the causative variant explaining the GWAS hit was localized on this specific haplotype occurring in both breeds from the discovery cohort. Subsequent haplotype analysis of all 13,399 canids with available SNP genotype data provided evidence for the presence of this haplotype in total of 25 dog breeds (Supplementary Table S4).

3.4. Identification of the Candidate Causative Variant

In total, 38 protein coding genes and five lncRNAs were annotated within the disease-associated ~0.98 Mb critical interval on chromosome 9 (Figure 2b). Visual inspection of this region in the WGS of five LPPN-affected dogs homozygous for the associated haplotype (four Leonbergers and one Saint Bernard) revealed no evidence for the presence of structural variants. Filtering variants for homozygous alternative genotypes shared in these five dogs within the critical interval yielded 872 intronic or intergenic, 12 synonymous, and 18 protein-changing variants (Supplementary Table S5). In addition, WGS data were available for three Leonbergers out of the 55 dogs from the discovery cohort (Supplementary Table S1) carrying a single copy of the identified disease-associated haplotype (Supplementary Table S4). Filtering for heterozygous variants in complete linkage disequilibrium with this haplotype in three dogs reduced the number of putative variants to 93 intronic or intergenic, one synonymous, and one protein-changing variant (Supplementary Table S5).

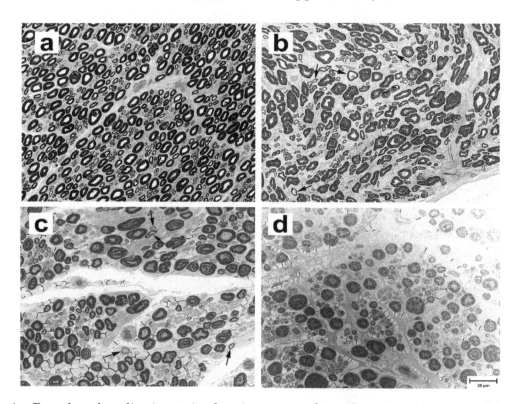

Figure 1. Paraphenylenediamine-stained resin sections from the peroneal nerves of four dogs. (**a**) An adult normal control Labrador retriever, (**b**) a nine-year-old LPPN-affected Labrador retriever, (**c**) a three-year-old LPPN-affected Leonberger, and (**d**) a three-year-old LPPN-affected Saint Bernard. All three LPPN-affected dogs were homozygous for the *CNTNAP1* variant. Arrows in (**b**) and (**c**) point to nerve fibers that are inappropriately thin for the axon diameters. Bar in lower right image indicates 25 μm and is valid for all images.

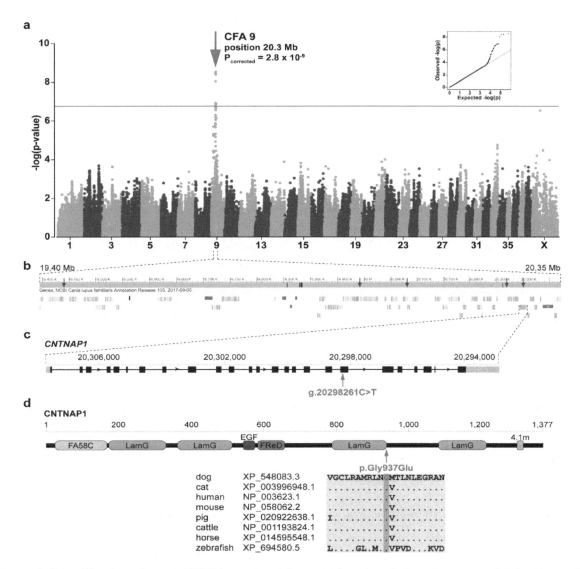

Figure 2. Identification of a new LPPN-associated locus and variant in Leonbergers and Saint Bernards. (**a**) Manhattan plot for the two-breed genome-wide association study (GWAS) using 144 LPPN-affected dogs and 373 normal control dogs indicates a signal with multiple associated single nucleotide polymorphisms (SNPs) on chromosome 9. The -log p-values for each SNP are plotted on the y-axis versus each canine chromosome on the x-axis. The red line represents the Bonferroni corrected significance threshold ($-\log(p\text{-value}) = 6.76$). Inset: Corrected Q–Q plot confirms that the observed p-values of the best-associated markers have stronger association with the trait than expected by chance (null hypothesis, red line). (**b**) Gene content in the ~0.98 Mb region of interest. Blue arrows show the best-associated markers from GWAS. Green bars represent the different genes and violet bars represent lncRNAs. (**c**) Schematic representation of the *CNTNAP1* gene showing the variant (XM_548083.6:c.2810G>A) location in exon 18. (**d**) Schematic representation of the CNTNAP1 protein with its domains: coagulation factor 5/8 C-terminal domain (FA58C), laminin G domains (LamG), calcium-binding EGF-like domain (EGF), fibrinogen-related domain (FReD), and putative band 4.1 homologues' binding motif (4.1m). The CNTNAP1 amino acid substitution (XP_548083.3:p.Gly937Glu) position is shown together with the amino acid multiple alignment indicating the residue is highly conserved across species.

CNTNAP1 represents a functional candidate gene due to its involvement in human congenital hypomyelination, where vocal cord palsy is a common clinical finding [31], so we pursued the lone remaining missense variant in the *CNTNAP1* gene (CFA9:g.20298261C>T; c.2810G>A; p.Gly937Glu) further. This *CNTNAP1* variant was predicted to be deleterious by several prediction tools (MutPred2 score: 0.884, PROVEAN score: −7.667, PON-P2 probability for pathogenicity: 0.848). It is located in exon 18 of the *CNTNAP1* gene (Figure 2c) and affects a highly conserved amino acid residue at the end of the third laminin G domain of the CNTNAP1 protein (Figure 2d). Two missense variants (rs905697967:p.Gly938Arg and rs763033339:p.Gly938Glu) in the human *CNTNAP1* coding region at the corresponding position were found in the gnomAD [30]. Both variants were reported with allele frequency 7.95×10^{-4} and no homozygous individuals were detected [30]. The canine missense variant in *CNTNAP1* was present in 5 of the 688 control canid WGS with a frequency of 0.004 (Supplementary Table S5), including one homozygous (English bulldog) and four heterozygous dogs (golden retriever, Labrador retriever, English bulldog, and Kerry blue terrier).

3.5. The CNTNAP1 Variant Occurs in Several Breeds

Available SNP array genotype data of 13,337 dogs and 62 wild canids (Supplementary Table S1) were inspected for the identified *CNTNAP1*-associated haplotype (Supplementary Table S4). Out of this group, targeted genotyping by PCR and Sanger sequencing was performed in 2469 canids and demonstrated perfect concordance between the *CNTNAP1*-associated haplotype and the *CNTNAP1*:c.2810G>A genotype (Supplementary Table S4). In addition, 2362 dogs without SNP array data were directly genotyped for the variant (Supplementary Table S1); this included 557 dogs from the validation cohort and 1805 from the population cohort.

In total, the variant was found in 25 different breeds and no wild canids. Homozygotes for the missense allele in breeds other than the Leonberger, Saint Bernard, and Labrador retriever were identified in 46 English bulldogs, six Irish terriers, two boxers, one bullmastiff, one Peruvian hairless dog, one Yorkshire terrier, and one golden retriever (Supplementary Table S1), all with unknown precise health history. Additionally, two LPPN-affected mixed-breed dogs enrolled in the Michigan State University's GOLPP study [6] were also homozygous for the missense allele (Supplementary Table S1).

Analysis of the validation cohort that included the three breeds with available health information (Leonberger, Saint Bernard, and Labrador retriever) demonstrated that the *CNTNAP1* variant is not present in a homozygous state in any dog apparently non-affected with LPPN (Table 2). The 18 homozygous LPPN-affected Leonbergers represent 4.1% of all as yet unexplained cases with any age of onset that were not carrying the previously identified disease-causing variants in *ARHGEF10* and *GJA9*. For the Saint Bernard, 10 out of 24 (41.6%) diagnosed dogs were homozygous mutant, whereas only 4.7% of GOLPP-affected Labrador retrievers carried two copies of the *CNTNAP1* variant. The homozygous A/A *CNTNAP1* genotype also occurred rarely in single dogs of the population controls from each of the three studied breeds (Table 2). Altogether, the mutant allele frequency was estimated as 6.6% in the studied Leonbergers ($n = 2738$ dogs), 13.9% in Saint Bernards ($n = 305$ dogs), and 5.2% in Labrador retrievers ($n = 1524$ dogs). Among the 22 other breeds segregating for this variant, the allele frequency was highest in the English bulldogs ($n = 193$ dogs) and Irish terriers ($n = 184$ dogs), estimated at 46.6% and 17.1%, respectively (Supplementary Table S1).

Mean age of onset in the LPPN-affected dogs was investigated for a subset of 770 dogs with detailed health information from three breeds (596 Leonbergers, 28 Saint Bernards, and 146 Labrador retrievers) and showed a marked difference between the cases depending on the different underlying genetic causes (Figure 3). The average age of onset of clinical signs in the limited number of dogs homozygous for the herein described *CNTNAP1* variant was 3.4, 2.1, and 7.5 years in Leonbergers, Saint Bernards, and Labrador retrievers, respectively. In comparison, the age of onset of clinical signs in the previously characterized *ARHGEF10*-associated polyneuropathy [8] was seen in Leonbergers and Saint Bernards with average ages of 2.2 and 1.6 years, respectively. Additionally, affected Leonbergers with the *GJA9* frameshift variant [9] had average age of onset of their clinical signs of 6.2 years. Interestingly, the LPPN-affected Labrador retrievers that do not carry the herein identified *CNTNAP1* variant and come from the GOLPP study [6] showed a higher average age of onset of 11.5 years (Figure 3). The difference in age of disease onset between the dogs with the identified *CNTNAP1* variant and the cases without known disease-causing mutation was statistically significant in all three breeds (Leonberger p-value = 0.000001002, Saint Bernard p-value = 0.01681, Labrador retriever p-value = 0.002662). The difference between dogs with the *CNTNAP1* variant and the *ARHGEF10* variant was significant in Leonbergers (p-value = 0.002538) but not significant in Saint Bernards (p-value = 0.3095). The difference between Leonbergers with the *CNTNAP1* variant and the *GJA9* variant was statistically significant (p-value = 0.00000001797).

Table 2. Segregation of the *CNTNAP1*:c.2810G>A genotypes with laryngeal paralysis and polyneuropathy (LPPN) in three breeds with available health information.

| Breed | LPPN Status | CNTNAP1 Genotypes | | |
		G/G	G/A	A/A [1]
Leonberger (n = 2738)	Affected (n = 434) [2]	358	58	18
	LPN1/LPN2 (n = 192) [3]	180	11	1
	Non-affected (n = 659) [4]	605	54	0
	Population controls (n = 1453)	1258	192	3
Saint Bernard (n = 305)	Affected (n = 24) [2]	9	5	10
	LPN1 (n = 5) [3]	2	3	0
	Non-affected (n = 14)	9	5	0
	Population controls (n = 262)	213	46	3
Labrador retriever (n = 1524)	Affected (n = 148)	132	9	7
	Non-affected (n = 45)	42	3	0
	Population controls (n = 1331)	1200	128	3

[1] Includes the three herein described histopathologically confirmed cases. [2] LPPN-affected dogs that tested negative for *ARHGEF10* [8] and *GJA9* [9] mutations. [3] LPPN-affected dogs homozygous for the previously described polyneuropathy-associated variant in *ARHGEF10* (LPN1) [8], and homozygous or heterozygous for the variant in *GJA9* (LPN2) [9]. [4] Includes cases homozygous for the previously described leukoencephalomyelopathy-associated variant in *NAPEPLD* [14].

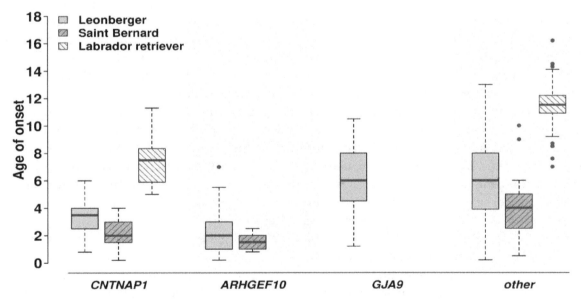

Figure 3. Age of onset of clinical signs for laryngeal paralysis and polyneuropathy (LPPN) differs depending on underlying genetic variants and across the three breeds. Comparison of the age of onset of clinical signs in the LPPN-affected dogs (n = 770), which were genotyped homozygous for the polyneuropathy-associated variants in *CNTNAP1*:c.2810G>A, or *ARHGEF10*:c.1955_1958+6delCACGGTGAGC [8], and homozygous or heterozygous for the variant in *GJA9*:c.1107_1108delAG [9], as well as the age of onset in the yet unexplained cases (other), is shown for Leonbergers (gold bars; n = 596), Saint Bernards (pink bars; n = 28), and Labrador retrievers (yellow bars; n = 146). Note that the *ARHGEF10* variant is only present in Leonbergers and Saint Bernards, and the *GJA9* variant only in Leonbergers.

4. Discussion

This study has revealed strong evidence for a new potentially pathogenic variant associated with laryngeal paralysis and polyneuropathy (LPPN) initially observed in two closely related giant dog breeds, the Leonberger and Saint Bernard. Interestingly, the variant also explains some cases of GOLPP in Labrador retrievers and segregates at different frequencies in 22 other unrelated dog breeds, including English bulldogs and Irish terriers, suggesting that the derived allele predates modern breed formation. Apparently, the variant was not purged by either selection or drift.

The affected *contactin-associated protein 1* (*CNTNAP1*) gene has been previously implicated in human autosomal recessive neurological diseases with a broad spectrum of clinical phenotypes and neonatal and childhood onsets: congenital hypomyelinating neuropathy type 3 (OMIM 618186), lethal congenital contracture syndrome 7 (OMIM 616286), and childhood-onset Charcot–Marie–Tooth disease [32]. *CNTNAP1* is essential in the formation of paranodal axoglial junctions in myelinated axons and is also involved in regulating neural progenitor cells and the development of the cerebral cortex [33]. Pathological variants in the *CNTNAP1* gene may lead to defective or absent proteins critical to development of central or peripheral nervous systems. Even though, based on the current gnomAD [30] database, the corresponding glycine to glutamic acid exchange occurs very rarely in humans, so far, there is no evidence reported for disease association. Human patients with other *CNTNAP1* homozygous frameshift or nonsense variants show a more severe disorder with early-onset neurological disease, including severe respiratory compromise and early lethality, while those carrying missense variants can survive beyond infancy [34]. This suggests that the missense alleles affecting the myelination and development of paranodal junctions may be hypomorphic and have some residual function. Although the precise role of the protein domains in ligand binding is not fully understood, several missense variants were predicted to impact the domain structure and protein folding [34].

Pathological changes in semi-thin transverse resin sections of the peroneal nerves of three affected dogs had similarities to those in published human cases, including reduced myelinated nerves and inappropriately thin myelin sheaths for the axon diameters [35]; however, in the affected dogs, thinly myelinated fibers were scattered and fewer in number. This may reflect the severity of disease in neonatal onset human cases and milder disease with an adult onset in dogs. The increased population of small fibers in the affected Labrador retriever, as compared to the affected Leonberger, may reflect attempts at regeneration in the Labrador retriever or genetic differences in other modifying genes. There are several limitations to the pathological studies in these dogs: The number of affected dogs with available peripheral nerve biopsies was small; detailed study of the paranodal areas of the peroneal nerves was limited by the retrospective nature of the study, the use of archived nerve specimens obtained many years prior to the identification of the variant, and the necessity of preparation of the nerves at the time of original processing for teased fibers and for longitudinal evaluation; and the standard processing for diagnostic specimens in the laboratory of one of the authors (GDS) is in transverse section. Future in-depth prospective studies of the peripheral nerves, including laryngeal nerves in more cases of confirmed LPPN with the *CNTNAP1* gene variant in each breed, are necessary to fully evaluate the observed pathological changes.

The neurological diseases identified in humans associated with variants in *CNTNAP1* support our recent speculation, based on the enrichment of this allele in Leonbergers [7], that the herein-described missense variant predicted in silico to be deleterious represents a promising candidate causative mutation for inherited neurological disorders in dogs. The striking genetic association data implicate that this mutation affects the function of the encoded protein, although we have not studied this further. Homozygosity for the missense variant in the *CNTNAP1* gene is significantly associated with the development of LPPN in large and giant-sized dogs, indicating recessive inheritance in all three studied breeds (Leonberger, Saint Bernard, and Labrador retriever). As yet we do not have convincing evidence for causality in smaller dog breeds segregating for this variant, such as the English bulldog or Irish terrier, and further study with reliably phenotyped populations is needed. However, we hypothesize that the apparently higher allele frequency in English bulldogs may be a result of underdiagnosed LP due to breathing difficulties related to brachycephalic airway syndrome, including laryngeal collapse [36] obscuring a neurodegenerative LP. The observed higher allele frequency in Irish terriers, although without available health information, suggests that the association between the variant and LPPN phenotype is breed-specific and may not be pathogenic in some breeds although this needs to be evaluated. We also hypothesize that the observed later age of onset in the Labrador retriever group, compared to the Leonbergers and Saint Bernards, might be either due to the different genetic breed background and/or their smaller stature and correspondingly shorter laryngeal nerve length; the latter was previously suggested by correlation between growth (specifically height) and laryngeal neuropathy in horses [37].

5. Conclusions

In conclusion, we identified a potentially causative genetic variant in *CNTNAP1* associated with autosomal recessive younger-onset LPPN in large and giant dogs, specifically Leonbergers, Saint Bernards, and Labrador retrievers. Our results represent the first large animal model for a *CNTNAP1*-related neurodegenerative disease. The developed genetic test enables veterinary diagnostics and selective breeding against this deleterious variant across breeds to reduce the occurrence of LPPN. Therefore, selecting based on this additional disease-associated variant, which we have designated LPPN3, will enable dog breeders to make even greater strides in controlling the propagation of this devastating disorder and maintaining the health of Leonberger, Saint Bernard, and Labrador retriever populations. However, the fact that not all LPPN cases from the three intensively studied breeds carried the described variant, together with the broad range in age of onset of the clinical signs for the as yet unexplained cases, indicates that still unknown genetic heterogeneity of different forms of canine LPPN need to be studied in future.

Supplementary Materials:
Figure S1: Histogram showing the axonal size-frequency distribution of myelinated nerve fibers in peroneal nerve sections from control Labrador retrievers (average of three archived adult control dog samples), an LPPN-affected Labrador retriever, and an LPPN-affected Leonberger. Both affected dogs were homozygous for the *CNTNAP1* variant. Axons are distributed into bins determined by axonal diameter based on perimeter. Table S1: Sample designations and detailed information of all dogs used in the study. Table S2: Sample designations and affection status of all whole-genome sequences used for filtering variants. Table S3: The 10,000 most significant markers sorted by *p*-value obtained from the across-breed genome-wide association study. Table S4: Haplotype diversity for the LPPN-associated genome region on chromosome 9. Table S5: Variants in the region of interest obtained from GWAS on chromosome 9. Video S1: Video illustrating the clinical phenotype of two LPPN-affected dogs: a Leonberger and a Saint Bernard.

Author Contributions: Conceptualization, J.R.M. and C.D.; data curation, B.J.S. and V.J.; formal analysis, A.L. and K.M.M.; funding acquisition, J.R.M. and C.D.; investigation, A.L., K.M.M., G.D.S., and J.P.S.; methodology, A.L. and K.M.M.; resources, P.J.J.M., P.A.J.L., P.A.W., S.M.P.-J., K.J.E., G.S.J., and L.H.; software, S.G.F. and V.J.; supervision, J.R.M. and C.D.; visualization, A.L., K.M.M., and G.D.S.; writing—original draft, A.L., K.M.M., G.D.S., J.R.M., and C.D.; writing—review and editing, A.L., K.M.M., S.G.F., G.D.S., K.J.E., J.R.M., and C.D. All authors have read and agreed to the published version of the manuscript.

Acknowledgments: The authors are grateful to the breeders and owners of all dogs who provided samples and shared valuable information about their dogs. We thank Nathalie Besuchet Schmutz for expert technical assistance. The Next Generation Sequencing Platform and the Interfaculty Bioinformatics Unit of the University of Bern are acknowledged for performing the WGS and providing high-performance computational infrastructure.

References

1. Kitshoff, A.M.; Van Goethem, B.; Stegen, L.; Vandekerckhov, P.; De Rooster, H. Laryngeal paralysis in dogs: An update on recent knowledge. *J. S. Afr. Vet. Assoc.* **2013**, *84*, 1–9. [CrossRef]

2. Monnet, E. Surgical Treatment of Laryngeal Paralysis. *Vet. Clin. N. Am. Small Anim. Pract.* **2016**, *46*, 709–717. [CrossRef]

3. Mackin, G.A. Diagnosis of patients with peripheral nerve disease. *Clin. Podiatr. Med. Surg.* **1994**, *11*, 545–569. [PubMed]

4.   Gabriel, A.; Poncelet, L.; Van Ham, L.; Clercx, C.; Braund, K.G.; Bhatti, S.; Detilleux, J.; Peeters, D. Laryngeal paralysis-polyneuropathy complex in young related Pyrenean mountain dogs. *J. Small Anim. Pract.* **2006**, *47*, 144–149. [CrossRef] [PubMed]

5.   Granger, N. Canine inherited motor and sensory neuropathies: An updated classification in 22 breeds and comparison to Charcot-Marie-Tooth disease. *Vet. J.* **2011**, *188*, 274–285. [CrossRef] [PubMed]

6.   GOLPP|College of Veterinary Medicine at MSU. Available online: https://cvm.msu.edu/scs/research-initiatives/golpp (accessed on 7 September 2020).

7.   Letko, A.; Minor, K.M.; Jagannathan, V.; Seefried, F.R.; Mickelson, J.R.; Oliehoek, P.; Drögemüller, C. Genomic diversity and population structure of the Leonberger dog breed. *Genet. Sel. Evol.* **2020**, *52*, 61. [CrossRef]

8.   Ekenstedt, K.J.; Becker, D.; Minor, K.M.; Shelton, G.D.; Patterson, E.E.; Bley, T.; Oevermann, A.; Bilzer, T.; Leeb, T.; Drögemüller, C.; et al. An ARHGEF10 Deletion Is Highly Associated with a Juvenile-Onset Inherited Polyneuropathy in Leonberger and Saint Bernard Dogs. *PLoS Genet.* **2014**, *10*, e1004635. [CrossRef]

9.   Becker, D.; Minor, K.M.; Letko, A.; Ekenstedt, K.J.; Jagannathan, V.; Leeb, T.; Shelton, G.D.; Mickelson, J.R.; Drögemüller, C. A GJA9 frameshift variant is associated with polyneuropathy in Leonberger dogs. *BMC Genom.* **2017**, *18*, 662. [CrossRef]

10. Wiedmer, M.; Oevermann, A.; Borer-Germann, S.E.; Gorgas, D.; Shelton, G.D.; Drögemüller, M.; Jagannathan, V.; Henke, D.; Leeb, T. A RAB3GAP1 SINE Insertion in Alaskan Huskies with Polyneuropathy, Ocular Abnormalities, and Neuronal Vacuolation (POANV) Resembling Human Warburg Micro Syndrome 1 (WARBM1). *G3 Genes Genomes Genet.* **2016**, *6*, 255–262. [CrossRef]

11. Mhlanga-Mutangadura, T.; Johnson, G.S.; Schnabel, R.D.; Taylor, J.F.; Johnson, G.C.; Katz, M.L.; Shelton, G.D.; Lever, T.E.; Giuliano, E.; Granger, N.; et al. A mutation in the Warburg syndrome gene, RAB3GAP1, causes a similar syndrome with polyneuropathy and neuronal vacuolation in Black Russian Terrier dogs. *Neurobiol. Dis.* **2016**, *86*, 75–85. [CrossRef]

12. Mhlanga-Mutangadura, T.; Johnson, G.S.; Ashwini, A.; Shelton, G.D.; Wennogle, S.A.; Johnson, G.C.; Kuroki, K.; O'Brien, D.P. A Homozygous RAB3GAP1:c.743delC Mutation in Rottweilers with Neuronal Vacuolation and Spinocerebellar Degeneration. *J. Vet. Intern. Med.* **2016**, *30*, 813–818. [CrossRef] [PubMed]

13. Rasouliha, S.H.; Barrientos, L.; Anderegg, L.; Klesty, C.; Lorenz, J.; Chevallier, L.; Jagannathan, V.; Rösch, S.; Leeb, T. A RAPGEF6 variant constitutes a major risk factor for laryngeal paralysis in dogs. *PLoS Genet.* **2019**, *15*, 1–17. [CrossRef] [PubMed]

14. Minor, K.M.; Letko, A.; Becker, D.; Drögemüller, M.; Mandigers, P.J.J.; Bellekom, S.R.; Leegwater, P.A.J.; Stassen, Q.E.M.; Putschbach, K.; Fischer, A.; et al. Canine NAPEPLD-associated models of human myelin disorders. *Sci. Rep.* **2018**, *8*, 5818. [CrossRef] [PubMed]

15. Parker, H.G.; Dreger, D.L.; Rimbault, M.; Davis, B.W.; Mullen, A.B.; Carpintero-Ramirez, G.; Ostrander, E.A. Genomic Analyses Reveal the Influence of Geographic Origin, Migration, and Hybridization on Modern Dog Breed Development. *Cell Rep.* **2017**, *19*, 697–708. [CrossRef]

16. Huang, M.; Hayward, J.J.; Corey, E.; Garrison, S.J.; Wagner, G.R.; Krotscheck, U.; Hayashi, K.; Schweitzer, P.A.; Lust, G.; Boyko, A.R.; et al. A novel iterative mixed model to remap three complex orthopedic traits in dogs. *PLoS ONE* **2017**, *12*, e0176932. [CrossRef]

17. Browning, S.R.; Browning, B.L. Rapid and Accurate Haplotype Phasing and Missing-Data Inference for Whole-Genome Association Studies by Use of Localized Haplotype Clustering. *Am. J. Hum. Genet.* **2007**, *81*, 1084–1097. [CrossRef]

18. Browning, B.L.; Browning, S.R. Genotype Imputation with Millions of Reference Samples. *Am. J. Hum. Genet.* **2016**, *98*, 116–126. [CrossRef]

19. Browning, B. Conform-gt Program. Available online: https://faculty.washington.edu/browning/conform-gt.html (accessed on 22 September 2020).

20. Danecek, P.; Auton, A.; Abecasis, G.; Albers, C.A.; Banks, E.; DePristo, M.A.; Handsaker, R.E.; Lunter, G.; Marth, G.T.; Sherry, S.T.; et al. The variant call format and VCFtools. *Bioinformatics* **2011**, *27*, 2156–2158. [CrossRef]

21. Chang, C.C.; Chow, C.C.; Tellier, L.C.A.M.; Vattikuti, S.; Purcell, S.M.; Lee, J.J. Second-generation PLINK: Rising to the challenge of larger and richer datasets. *Gigascience* **2015**, *4*, 7. [CrossRef]

22. Zhou, X.; Stephens, M. Genome-wide efficient mixed-model analysis for association studies. *Nat. Genet.* **2012**, *44*, 821–824. [CrossRef]

23. R Core Team. *R: A Language and Environment for Statistical Computing*; R Foundation for Statistical Computing: Vienna, Austria, 2019.

24. Turner, S.D.; Turner, D.S. qqman: An R package for visualizing GWAS results using Q-Q and manhattan plots. *bioRxiv* **2014**, *81*, 559–575. [CrossRef]

25. Jagannathan, V.; Drögemüller, C.; Leeb, T. Dog Biomedical Variant Database Consortium, (DBVDC) A comprehensive biomedical variant catalogue based on whole genome sequences of 582 dogs and eight wolves. *Anim. Genet.* **2019**, *50*, 695–704. [CrossRef] [PubMed]

26. Thorvaldsdóttir, H.; Robinson, J.T.; Mesirov, J.P. Integrative Genomics Viewer (IGV): High-performance genomics data visualization and exploration. *Brief. Bioinform.* **2013**, *14*, 178–192. [CrossRef] [PubMed]

27. Pejaver, V.; Urresti, J.; Lugo-Martinez, J.; Pagel, K.A.; Lin, G.N.; Nam, H.-J.; Mort, M.; Cooper, D.N.; Sebat, J.; Iakoucheva, L.M.; et al. MutPred2: Inferring the molecular and phenotypic impact of amino acid variants. *bioRxiv* **2017**, 134981. [CrossRef]

28. Choi, Y.; Chan, A.P. PROVEAN web server: A tool to predict the functional effect of amino acid substitutions and indels. *Bioinformatics* **2015**, *31*, 2745–2747. [CrossRef]

29. Niroula, A.; Urolagin, S.; Vihinen, M. PON-P2: Prediction method for fast and reliable identification of harmful variants. *PLoS ONE* **2015**, *10*, e117380. [CrossRef]

30. Karczewski, K.J.; Francioli, L.C.; Tiao, G.; Cummings, B.B.; Alföldi, J.; Wang, Q.; Collins, R.L.; Laricchia, K.M.; Ganna, A.; Birnbaum, D.P.; et al. The mutational constraint spectrum quantified from variation in 141,456 humans. *Nature* **2020**, *581*, 434–443. [CrossRef]

31. Low, K.; Stals, K.; Caswell, R.; Clayton-Smith, J.; Donaldson, A.; Foulds, N.; Splitt, M.; Norman, A.; Urankar, K.; Vijayakumar, K.; et al. CNTNAP1: Extending the phenotype of congenital hypomyelinating neuropathy in 6 further patients. *Neuromuscul. Disord.* **2017**, *27*, S148. [CrossRef]

32. Freed, A.S.; Weiss, M.D.; Malouf, E.A.; Hisama, F.M. CNTNAP1 mutations in an adult with Charcot Marie Tooth disease. *Muscle Nerve* **2019**, *60*, E28–E30. [CrossRef]

33. Sabbagh, S.; Antoun, S.; Mégarbané, A. CNTNAP1 Mutations and Their Clinical Presentations: New Case Report and Systematic Review. *Case Rep. Med.* **2020**, *2020*. [CrossRef]

34. Low, K.; Stals, K.; Caswell, R.; Wakeling, M.; Clayton-Smith, J.; Donaldson, A.; Foulds, N.; Norman, A.; Splitt, M.; Urankar, K.; et al. Phenotype of CNTNAP1: A study of patients demonstrating a specific severe congenital hypomyelinating neuropathy with survival beyond infancy. *Eur. J. Hum. Genet.* **2018**, *26*, 796–807. [CrossRef] [PubMed]

35. Vallat, J.-M.; Nizon, M.; Magee, A.; Isidor, B.; Magy, L.; Péréon, Y.; Richard, L.; Ouvrier, R.; Cogné, B.; Devaux, J.; et al. Contactin-Associated Protein 1 (CNTNAP1) Mutations Induce Characteristic Lesions of the Paranodal Region. *J. Neuropathol. Exp. Neurol.* **2016**, *75*, 1155–1159. [CrossRef] [PubMed]

36. Meola, S.D. Brachycephalic Airway Syndrome. *Top. Companion Anim. Med.* **2013**. [CrossRef] [PubMed]

37. Boyko, A.R.; Brooks, S.A.; Behan-Braman, A.; Castelhano, M.; Corey, E.; Oliveira, K.C.; Swinburne, J.E.; Todhunter, R.J.; Zhang, Z.; Ainsworth, D.M.; et al. Genomic analysis establishes correlation between growth and laryngeal neuropathy in Thoroughbreds. *BMC Genom.* **2014**, *15*, 259. [CrossRef] [PubMed]

A Missense Variant Affecting the C-Terminal Tail of UNC93B1 in Dogs with Exfoliative Cutaneous Lupus Erythematosus (ECLE)

Tosso Leeb [1,2,*], Fabienne Leuthard [1,2], Vidhya Jagannathan [1,2], Sarah Kiener [1,2], Anna Letko [1,2], Petra Roosje [2,3], Monika M. Welle [2,4], Katherine L. Gailbreath [5], Andrea Cannon [6], Monika Linek [7], Frane Banovic [8], Thierry Olivry [9], Stephen D. White [10], Kevin Batcher [11], Danika Bannasch [11], Katie M. Minor [12], James R. Mickelson [12], Marjo K. Hytönen [13,14,15], Hannes Lohi [13,14,15], Elizabeth A. Mauldin [16] and Margret L. Casal [16]

[1] Institute of Genetics, Vetsuisse Faculty, University of Bern, 3001 Bern, Switzerland; fabileuthard@gmail.com (F.L.); vidhya.jagannathan@vetsuisse.unibe.ch (V.J.); sarah.kiener@vetsuisse.unibe.ch (S.K.); anna.letko@vetsuisse.unibe.ch (A.L.)

[2] Dermfocus, University of Bern, 3001 Bern, Switzerland; petra.roosje@vetsuisse.unibe.ch (P.R.); monika.welle@vetsuisse.unibe.ch (M.M.W.)

[3] Division of Clinical Dermatology, Department of Clinical Veterinary Medicine, Vetsuisse Faculty, University of Bern, 3001 Bern, Switzerland

[4] Institute of Animal Pathology, Vetsuisse Faculty, University of Bern, 3001 Bern, Switzerland

[5] ZNLabs Veterinary Diagnostics, Garden City, ID 83714, USA; katherine@znlabs.com

[6] Westvet, Garden City, ID 83714, USA; cannonderm@sbcglobal.net

[7] AniCura Tierärztliche Spezialisten, 22043 Hamburg, Germany; monikalinek@gmail.com

[8] Department of Small Animal Medicine and Surgery, College of Veterinary Medicine, University of Georgia, Athens, GA 30602, USA; fbànovic@uga.edu

[9] Department of Clinical Sciences, College of Veterinary Medicine, North Carolina State University, Raleigh, NC 27607, USA; tolivry@ncsu.edu

[10] Department of Medicine and Epidemiology, School of Veterinary Medicine, University of California Davis, Davis, CA 95616, USA; sdwhite@ucdavis.edu

[11] Department of Population Health and Reproduction, School of Veterinary Medicine, University of California, Davis, CA 95616, USA; klbatcher@ucdavis.edu (K.B.); dlbannasch@ucdavis.edu (D.B.)

[12] Department of Veterinary and Biomedical Sciences, University of Minnesota, Saint Paul, MN 55108, USA; minork@umn.edu (K.M.M.); micke001@umn.edu (J.R.M.)

[13] Department of Veterinary Biosciences, University of Helsinki, 00014 Helsinki, Finland; marjo.hytonen@helsinki.fi (M.K.H.); hannes.lohi@helsinki.fi (H.L.)

[14] Department of Medical and Clinical Genetics, University of Helsinki, 00014 Helsinki, Finland

[15] Folkhälsan Research Center, 00290 Helsinki, Finland

[16] School of Veterinary Medicine, University of Pennsylvania, Philadelphia, PA 19104, USA; emauldin@vet.upenn.edu (E.A.M.); casalml@vet.upenn.edu (M.L.C.)

* Correspondence: tosso.leeb@vetsuisse.unibe.ch;

Abstract: Cutaneous lupus erythematosus (CLE) in humans encompasses multiple subtypes that exhibit a wide array of skin lesions and, in some cases, are associated with the development of systemic lupus erythematosus (SLE). We investigated dogs with exfoliative cutaneous lupus erythematosus (ECLE), a dog-specific form of chronic CLE that is inherited as a monogenic autosomal recessive trait. A genome-wide association study (GWAS) with 14 cases and 29 controls confirmed a previously published result that the causative variant maps to chromosome 18. Autozygosity mapping refined the ECLE locus to a 493 kb critical interval. Filtering of whole genome sequence data from two cases against 654 controls revealed a single private protein-changing variant in this critical interval, *UNC93B1*:c.1438C>A or p.Pro480Thr. The homozygous mutant genotype was exclusively observed in 23 ECLE affected German Shorthaired Pointers and an ECLE affected Vizsla, but absent from 845 controls. UNC93B1 is a transmembrane protein located in the endoplasmic reticulum and endolysosomes, which is required for correct trafficking of several Toll-like receptors (TLRs). The p.Pro480Thr variant is predicted to affect the C-terminal tail of the UNC93B1 that has recently been shown to restrict TLR7 mediated autoimmunity via an interaction with syndecan binding protein (SDCBP). The functional knowledge on UNC93B1 strongly suggests that p.Pro480Thr is causing ECLE in dogs. These dogs therefore represent an interesting spontaneous model for human lupus erythematosus. Our results warrant further investigations of whether genetic variants affecting the C-terminus of UNC93B1 might be involved in specific subsets of CLE or SLE cases in humans and other species.

Keywords: *Canis familiaris*; dermatology; immunology; animal model; skin; TLR7; toll-like receptor; syndecan binding protein; syntenin-1; systemic lupus erythematosus; SLE; CLE

---

1. Introduction

In humans, cutaneous lupus erythematosus (CLE) represents a group of lupus erythematosus (LE)-associated autoimmune skin diseases exhibiting a cell-rich interface dermatitis leading to erosions and ulcerations with subsequent scarring, disfiguration and decreased quality of life [1–4]. CLE can affect only the skin or be present as part of a diverse range of potentially life-threatening and debilitating symptoms in patients with systemic lupus erythematosus (SLE) [1–4].

The incidence of CLE has been reported at ~4 cases per 100,000 persons per year [5–8]; 10% to 30% of human patients with CLE exhibit a transition from cutaneous into SLE forms, suggesting shared pathways and genetic background relevant to both cutaneous and systemic manifestations [5,6,9].

It has been proposed that some CLE forms, similarly to SLE, have an underlying genetic predisposition that combines with environmental factors to elicit an abnormal immune response with a continuous activation of the innate immune system. Several genetic associations have been identified in human CLE, with the majority of them involving type I interferon pathways, cell death and clearance of cell debris, antigen presentation and immune cell regulation [10,11]. To date, a single monogenic form of CLE caused by heterozygous variants in the *TREX1* gene encoding the three prime repair exonuclease has been identified in human patients with familial chilblain lupus erythematosus [12]. The pathogenic *TREX1* variants lead to chronic hyperactivation of the type I interferon system via cytosolic DNA recognition pathways [11,13]. A rare monogenic form of SLE in humans is caused by variants in the *DNASE1* gene encoding deoxyribonuclease 1 [14]. Mice deficient for Dnase I also develop an SLE-like autoimmune disease [15].

Dogs may also suffer from various forms of CLE, some of which resemble or are identical to their human homologs [4]. The so-called exfoliative cutaneous lupus erythematosus (ECLE) is a dog-specific variant of chronic CLE that has a very strong hereditary component and appears to be inherited as a monogenic autosomal trait [16–18]. Despite its current designation, signs of ECLE are not restricted to the skin. In most patients, ECLE starts with characteristic skin lesions in juvenile or young adult dogs (Figure 1). In later stages, ECLE often additionally affects the joints with severe pain, but a progression to classic antinuclear antibody-positive SLE is usually not seen [4,16–18]. The treatment of ECLE-affected dogs with immunomodulatory drugs often is insufficient to achieve long-lasting control of the disease, leading to a guarded prognosis [18,19]. Dogs affected with ECLE often are euthanized due to the severity of their disease. ECLE has been observed in several closely related hunting dog breeds, German Shorthaired Pointers, Braques du Bourbonnais, and Vizslas.

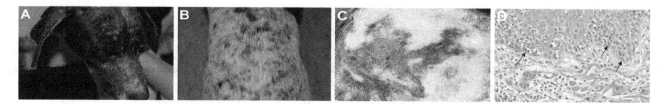

Figure 1. Exfoliative Cutaneous Lupus Erythematosus (ECLE) phenotype. (**A**) Scarring alopecia, generalized hair loss and adherent crusts on the face of a 2-year-old male dog. (**B**) Erythematous lesions on the back of a 1.5-year old male dog. (**C**) Close up of patchy lesions on the abdomen. (**D**) Haired skin from an ECLE affected dog with typical histological changes that include a cell-rich interface inflammation with frequent basal keratinocyte apoptosis (arrows). Hematoxylin and eosin stain.

A previously reported genome-wide association study (GWAS) mapped the causative genetic defect for ECLE to chromosome 18, but the causative variant has not yet been identified [20]. The best-associated marker was located at position 53,913,829 (CanFam 2) [20], which corresponds to 50,888,317 in the current CanFam 3.1 assembly.

In the present study, we performed a new GWAS followed by a whole genome sequencing approach with the goal to identify the causative genetic variant for ECLE in dogs.

2. Materials and Methods

2.1. Ethics Statement

All the dogs in this study were privately owned and samples were collected with the consent of their owners. The collection of blood samples was approved by the "Cantonal Committee for Animal Experiments" (Canton of Bern; permit 75/16).

2.2. Animal Selection

This study included 877 dogs. They consisted of 552 German Shorthaired Pointers (26 ECLE cases/526 controls), 52 unaffected German Longhaired Pointers, 210 unaffected German Wirehaired Pointers, 7 unaffected Braques du Bourbonnais, and 56 Vizslas (1 ECLE case/55 controls). The 27 ECLE cases were diagnosed by licensed veterinarians. The 850 dogs classified as unaffected represented population controls without reports of severe immunological or skin-related health issues. Peripheral blood samples were collected in EDTA vacutainers and stored at −20°C. Additional details on samples are given in Table S1.

2.3. DNA Extraction and SNV Genotyping

Genomic DNA was either available from a previous study [20], isolated from EDTA blood with the Maxwell RSC Whole Blood Kit using a Maxwell RSC instrument (Promega, Dübendorf, Switzerland), or from formalin-fixed paraffin-embedded (FFPE) tissue samples using the Maxwell RSC DNA FFPE kit according to the manufacturer's instructions. DNA from 14 ECLE cases and 29 controls was genotyped on illumina_HD canine BeadChips containing 220,853 markers (Neogen, Lincoln, NE, USA). The raw SNV genotypes are available in File S1. We did not have complete pedigree information on all 43 dogs that were genotyped on the SNV arrays. Some of the dogs were closely related, including, for example, 5 cases that were full siblings. Table S2 lists the pairwise IBD between all dogs and gives an objective measure of the relatedness between the genotyped dogs. A multiple dimension scaling (MDS) plot is shown in Figure S1.

The previously published GWAS [20] had been done with Affymetrix v2 127 k SNV genotyping arrays. A total of 6 cases and 2 controls were shared between the two analyses. The other 35 samples herein were from dogs different from those of the previous study.

For some dogs from the previous study [20] only very little DNA was left. The remaining DNA of 8 German Shorthaired Pointers was used up for SNV genotyping on the illumina_HD canine BeadChips. In these dogs, no specific targeted genotyping could be performed (see Section 2.8 below).

2.4. GWAS and Autozygosity Mapping

We used PLINK v.1.9 for basic file manipulation of the SNV genotypes [21]. We removed markers and individuals with less than 90% call rates. We further removed markers with minor allele frequency of less than 10% and markers deviating from the Hardy–Weinberg equilibrium in controls with a p-value of less than 10^{-5}. An allelic GWAS was then performed with the GEMMA 0.98 software using a linear mixed model including an estimated kinship matrix as covariable to correct for the genomic inflation [22]. Manhattan and QQ plots of the corrected p-values were generated in R [23].

For autozygosity mapping, the genotype data of 14 ECLE cases were used. A tped-file containing the markers on chromosome 18 was visually inspected in an Excel spreadsheet to find a homozygous shared haplotype in the cases (Table S3).

2.5. Whole Genome Sequencing of Two Affected German Shorthaired Pointers

Illumina TruSeq PCR-free DNA libraries with ~450 bp insert size of two affected German Shorthaired Pointers without known relationships were prepared. We collected 277 and 160 million 2×150 bp paired-end reads on a NovaSeq 6000 instrument corresponding to 29.3× and 17.9× coverage, respectively. Mapping and alignment were performed as described previously [24]. The sequence data were deposited under study accession PRJEB16012 and sample accessions SAMEA5657398 and SAMEA6249504 at the European Nucleotide Archive.

2.6. Variant Calling

Variant calling was performed using GATK HaplotypeCaller [25] in gVCF mode as described [24]. To predict the functional effects of the called variants, SnpEff [26] software together with NCBI annotation release 105 for the CanFam 3.1 genome reference assembly was used. For variant filtering we used 654 control genomes, which were either publicly available [27,28] or produced during other projects of our group [24] (Table S4).

2.7. Gene Analysis

We used the CanFam 3.1 dog reference genome assembly and NCBI annotation release 105. Numbering within the canine *UNC93B1* gene corresponds to the NCBI RefSeq accession numbers XM_540813.6 (mRNA) and XP_540813.3 (protein).

2.8. Sanger Sequencing

The *UNC93B1*:c.1438C>A variant was genotyped by direct Sanger sequencing of PCR amplicons. On high-quality genomic DNA samples, a 399 bp PCR product was amplified from genomic DNA using AmpliTaqGold360Mastermix (Thermo Fisher Scientific, Waltham, MA, USA) together with primers 5'-ATC CGT GTC TGT GCC CTC A-3' (Primer F) and 5'-CGA CCT GAG ACG CGG TAA A-3' (Primer R). For FFPE-derived DNA samples, a smaller amplicon of 124 bp was amplified with the primers 5'-CCT CGT ACC TGT GGA TGG AG-3' (Primer F2) and 5'-CTC TCG TCG GAG TTG TCC TC-3' (Primer R2). After treatment with exonuclease I and alkaline phosphatase, amplicons were sequenced on an ABI 3730 DNA Analyzer (Thermo Fisher Scientific). Sanger sequences were analyzed using the Sequencher 5.1 software (GeneCodes, Ann Arbor, MI, USA).

3. Results

3.1. Mapping of the ECLE Locus

We performed a GWAS with genotypes from 43 German Shorthaired Pointers. After quality control, the pruned dataset consisted of 14 ECLE cases, 29 controls and 116,891 markers. We obtained a single association signal with 35 markers exceeding a suggestive significance threshold of $p = 5 \times 10^{-5}$ after adjustment for genomic inflation. All associated markers were located on chromosome 18 within an interval spanning from 49.0 Mb–53.9 Mb. The top-associated marker at Chr18:49,835,345 had a p-value of 1.5×10^{-6} (Figure 2).

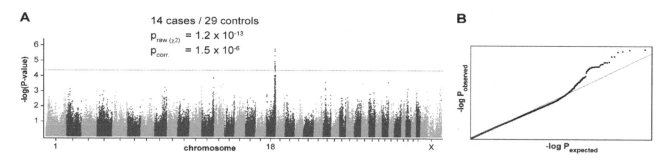

Figure 2. Mapping of the ECLE locus by genome-wide association. (**A**) Manhattan plot illustrating a single signal on chromosome 18. The dashed red line indicates the threshold for suggestive significance at $p = 5 \times 10^{-5}$ according to [29]. The best associated marker did not reach the stringent Bonferroni significance threshold ($p_{Bonf.} = 4.3 \times 10^{-7}$) due to several close relationships and extreme genomic inflation in the dataset. The genomic inflation factor was 1.90 before and 0.99 after the correction. (**B**) The quantile–quantile (QQ) plot shows the observed versus expected –log(p) values. The straight red line in the QQ plot indicates the distribution of p-values under the null hypothesis. The deviation of p-values at the right side indicates that these markers are stronger associated with the trait than would be expected by chance. This supports the biological significance of the association.

To narrow down the identified region, we visually inspected the genotypes of the cases and performed an autozygosity mapping. We searched for homozygous regions with allele sharing and found one region of ~493 kb which was shared between all 14 cases. The critical interval for the causative ECLE variant corresponded to the interval between the first flanking heterozygous markers on either side of the homozygous segment or Chr18:49,545,431-50,038,225 (CanFam 3.1 assembly).

3.2. Identification of a Candidate Causative Variant

We sequenced the genome of two affected dogs at $29.3 \times$ and $17.9 \times$ coverage and called SNVs and small indel variants with respect to the reference genome. We then compared these variants to whole genome sequence data of 8 wolves and 646 control dogs from genetically diverse breeds. This analysis identified two private homozygous variants in the critical interval in the affected dogs (Table 1). A visual inspection of the short read alignments ruled out any additional structural variants affecting protein-coding sequences in the critical interval in the two sequenced cases.

Table 1. Variants detected by whole genome re-sequencing of two ECLE-affected dogs.

Filtering Step	Variants
Shared homozygous variants in whole genome	1,420,602
Private homozygous variants (absent from 654 control genomes) in whole genome	25
Shared homozygous variants in 493 kb critical interval	851
Private variants (absent from 654 control genomes) in critical interval	2
Protein changing private variants in critical interval	1

One of the two private variants in the critical interval, Chr18:49,733,311C>T, was located in an intron of the *CHKA* gene and thus not investigated further. The other variant, Chr18:49,834,825C>A was a missense variant in the last exon of the *UNC93B1* gene. The formal designation of this variant is XM_540813.6:c.1438C>A or XP_540813.3:p.(Pro480Thr). It is predicted to change a highly conserved amino acid in the C-terminal tail of the UNC93B1 protein. We confirmed the variant by Sanger sequencing (Figure 3).

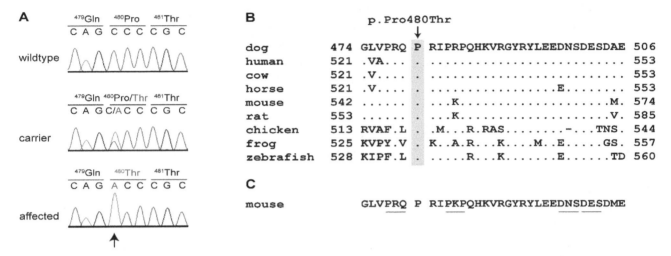

Figure 3. Details of the *UNC93B1* missense variant. (**A**) Representative Sanger electropherograms from dogs with the three different genotypes at c.1438C>A are shown. The amino acid translation is indicated. (**B**) Evolutionary conservation of the SDCBP binding domain [30]. The proline at position 480 of the canine UNC93B1 protein is strictly conserved across all vertebrates. The sequences were derived from the following database accessions: dog XP_540813.3, human NP_112192.2, cow XP_540813.3, horse XP_023510352.1, mouse NP_062322.2, rat NP_001101983.1, chicken XP_004941322.1, frog NP_001093723.1, zebrafish XP_0026660582.1. (**C**) Scanning-alanine mutagenesis in mouse macrophages identified four mutants that disrupt SDCBP binding and lead to upregulated TLR7 signaling [30]. The altered residues in these mutants are underlined.

3.3. Genotype Phenotype Association of the UNC93B1:p.Pro480Thr Variant

We genotyped 544 German Shorthaired Pointers for the p.Pro480Thr variant and found a near perfect association of the genotypes at this variant with ECLE ($p_{Fisher} = 1.2 \times 10^{-39}$). None of the 520 genotyped controls were homozygous for the mutant A/A genotype. However, one of the 24 genotyped cases was not homozygous A/A. We speculate that this single discordant dog is likely due to a phenotyping error as it had an atypically late age of onset and was not clinically confirmed as having ECLE by a board certified veterinary dermatologist (Table S1). The analysis of additional animals from related hunting dog breeds revealed the presence of the mutant allele in German Longhaired Pointers and Vizslas. A single ECLE-affected Vizsla also had the homozygous mutant A/A genotype (Table 2).

Table 2. Association of the genotypes at *UNC93B1*:c.1438C>A with ECLE.

ECLE Phenotype	Breed	C/C	C/A	A/A
Affected	German Shorthaired Pointer ($n = 24$)	1	–	23
Control	German Shorthaired Pointer ($n = 520$)	457	63	–
Control	German Longhaired Pointer ($n = 52$)	50	2	–
Control	German Wirehaired Pointer ($n = 210$)	210	–	–
Control	Braque du Bourbonnais ($n = 7$)	7	–	–
Affected	Vizsla ($n = 1$)			1
Control	Vizsla ($n = 56$)	51	5	–

4. Discussion

In this study, we identified UNC93B1:pPro480Thr as a candidate causative variant for ECLE in dogs. We performed a new GWAS and obtained the strongest association signal on the same chromosome, but approximately 1 Mb more proximal than the location in the previously reported GWAS [20]. Given that linkage disequilibrium within breeds can span several Mb, we consider our new result a confirmation and refinement of the previously reported association. Compared to the previous study [20], we detected a different ~500 kb homozygous haplotype block harboring the 7 top markers of our GWAS that was shared among all 14 investigated ECLE cases.

Whole genome sequencing data of two cases and 654 controls revealed a single private protein changing variant in the critical interval, UNC93B1:pPro480Thr. All but one of the designated ECLE cases were homozygous for the mutant allele with the single discordant dog believed to represent a phenotype mismatch. Conversely, the mutant allele was not found in a homozygous state in more than 1000 control dogs.

The mutant allele was also detected in heterozygous status in controls of two related breeds, German Longhaired Pointers and Vizslas. These breeds share a common ancestry with German Shorthaired Pointers. This provides indirect support for the previous observation that ECLE also can affect dogs from breeds related to the German Shorthaired Pointer. The hypothesis of a common genetic defect in these breeds was confirmed by our finding of an ECLE affected Vizsla that was also homozygous mutant at the *UNC93B1* variant.

The *UNC93B1* gene encodes a protein named "unc-93 homolog B1, TLR signaling regulator". The human UNC93B1 consists of 597 amino acids and is a 12 transmembrane domain containing protein located in endosomal membranes [31]. It acts as a trafficking chaperone of the intracellular nucleic acid-sensing Toll-like receptors (TLRs) 3, 7 and 9 [32–35]. These TLRs are essential components of the innate immune system and activated when pathogen derived nucleic acids appear in endolysosomes. *UNC93B1* mediates the correct trafficking and localization of these TLRs to endolysosomes [32]. Complete loss-of-function of UNC93B1 results in a severe immune deficiency in human patients [36] and the *3d* mouse mutant [37].

Recently, the molecular mechanisms of the interaction of UNC93B1 with TLRs were studied in great detail. A 33 amino acid sequence motif in the cytoplasmic C-terminal domain of UNC93B1 binds to syndecan binding protein (SDCBP), also called syntenin-1. SDCBP interacts with both UNC93B1 and TLR7 [30]. This interaction dampens TLR7 signaling and prevents autoimmune activation of TLR7 by endogenous nucleic acids [30,35]. Gene-edited mice expressing a mutant Unc93b1 in which three critical amino acids of this C-terminal domain were altered (530-PKP/AAA-532) developed hallmarks of systemic inflammation and autoimmunity [30], similar to what has been observed in Tlr7 overexpressing mice [38–40]. In summary, the available literature suggests that complete loss of function of UNC93B1 leads to an immune deficiency, while UNC93B1 variants that only affect the C-terminal tail containing the SDCBP binding domain lead to upregulation of TLR7 signaling with subsequent development of systemic autoimmune disease.

The detailed functional knowledge on the role of the C-terminal tail of UNC93B1 for the regulation of TLR7 signaling strongly suggests that ECLE in dogs is due to dysregulated TLR7 signaling caused by the canine UNC93B1:p.Pro480Thr variant.

To the best of our knowledge, ECLE affected dogs represent the first spontaneous *UNC93B1* mutant that develops an autoimmune disease of the lupus group. Therefore, these dogs represent an interesting model for human CLE and/or SLE. As already suggested by [30], it seems possible that lupus erythematosus or other related autoimmune diseases in some human patients might be due to comparable genetic variants in *UNC93B1*.

5. Conclusions

We identified the spontaneously arisen UNC93B1:p.Pro480Thr variant as likely causative for ECLE in dogs. Knowledge of this variant will facilitate genetic testing of dogs to prevent the non-intentional breeding of ECLE-affected dogs. This unique canine form of CLE in dogs represents an interesting model for lupus erythematosus and potentially other autoimmune diseases in humans.

Author Contributions: Conceptualization, T.L.; Data curation, V.J.; Investigation, T.L., F.L., S.K., A.L., K.B., K.M.M., M.K.H.; M.L.C.; Methodology, V.J., A.L.; Resources, K.L.G., A.C., M.L., F.B., T.O., S.D.W., D.B., J.R.M., H.L., E.A.M., M.L.C.; Supervision, T.L.; Visualization, T.L.; Writing—original draft, T.L.; Writing—review and editing, T.L. F.L., V.J., S.K., A.L., P.R., M.M.W., K.L.G., A.C., M.L., F.B., T.O., S.D.W., K.B., D.B., K.M.M., J.R.M., M.K.H., H.L., E.A.M., and M.L.C. All authors have read and agreed to the published version of the manuscript.

Acknowledgments: The authors are grateful to all dog owners who donated samples and shared health and pedigree data of their dogs. We thank Eva Andrist, Nathalie Besuchet Schmutz, Sini Karjalainen, Sabrina Schenk, and Daniela Steiner for expert technical assistance, the Next Generation Sequencing Platform of the University of Bern for performing the high-throughput sequencing experiments, and the Interfaculty Bioinformatics Unit of the University of Bern for providing high performance computing infrastructure. We thank the Dog Biomedical Variant Database Consortium (Gus Aguirre, Catherine André, Danika Bannasch, Doreen Becker, Brian Davis, Cord Drögemüller, Kari Ekenstedt, Kiterie Faller, Oliver Forman, Steve Friedenberg, Eva Furrow, Urs Giger, Christophe Hitte, Marjo Hytönen, Vidhya Jagannathan, Tosso Leeb, Hannes Lohi, Cathryn Mellersh, Jim Mickelson, Leonardo Murgiano, Anita Oberbauer, Sheila Schmutz, Jeffrey Schoenebeck, Kim Summers, Frank van Steenbeek, Claire Wade) for sharing whole genome sequencing data from control dogs. We also acknowledge all researchers who deposited dog or wolf whole genome sequencing data into public databases.

References

1. Sontheimer, R.D. The lexicon of cutaneous lupus erythematosus—A review and personal perspective on the nomenclature and classification of the cutaneous manifestations of lupus erythematosus. *Lupus* **1997**, *6*, 84–95. [CrossRef] [PubMed]

2. Rothfield, N.; Sontheimer, R.D.; Bernstein, M. Lupus erythematosus: Systemic and cutaneous manifestations. *Clin. Dermatol.* **2006**, *24*, 348–362. [CrossRef] [PubMed]

3. Kuhn, A.; Landmann, A. The classification and diagnosis of cutaneous lupus erythematosus. *J. Autoimmun.* **2014**, *48–49*, 14–19. [CrossRef]

4. Olivry, T.; Linder, K.E.; Banovic, F. Cutaneous lupus erythematosus in dogs: A comprehensive review. *BMC Vet. Res.* **2018**, *14*, 132. [CrossRef] [PubMed]

5. Durosaro, O.; Davis, M.D.; Reed, K.B.; Rohlinger, A.L. Incidence of cutaneous lupus erythematosus, 1965-2005: A population-based study. *Arch. Dermatol.* **2009**, *145*, 249–253. [CrossRef] [PubMed]

6. Grönhagen, C.M.; Fored, C.M.; Granath, F.; Nyberg, F. Cutaneous lupus erythematosus and the association with systemic lupus erythematosus: A population-based cohort of 1088 patients in Sweden. *Br. J. Dermatol.* **2011**, *164*, 1335–1341. [CrossRef] [PubMed]

7. Biazar, C.; Sigges, J.; Patsinakidis, N.; Ruland, V.; Amler, S.; Bonsmann, G.; Kuhn, A.; EUSCLE co-authors. Cutaneous lupus erythematosus: First multicenter database analysis of 1002 patients from the European Society of Cutaneous Lupus Erythematosus (EUSCLE). *Autoimmun. Rev.* **2013**, *12*, 444–454. [CrossRef]

8. Jarukitsopa, S.; Hoganson, D.D.; Crowson, C.S.; Sokumbi, O.; Davis, M.D.; Michet, C.J., Jr.; Matteson, E.L.; Maradit Kremers, H.; Chowdhary, V.R. Epidemiology of systemic lupus erythematosus and cutaneous lupus erythematosus in a predominantly white population in the United States. *Arthritis Care Res. (Hoboken)* **2015**, *67*, 817–828. [CrossRef]

9. Chong, B.F.; Song, J.; Olsen, N.J. Determining risk factors for developing systemic lupus erythematosus in patients with discoid lupus erythematosus. *Br. J. Dermatol.* **2012**, *166*, 29–35. [CrossRef]

10. Hersh, A.O.; Arkin, L.M.; Prahalad, S. Immunogenetics of cutaneous lupus erythematosus. *Curr. Opin. Pediatr.* **2016**, *28*, 470–475. [CrossRef]

11. Wenzel, J. Cutaneous lupus erythematosus: New insights into pathogenesis and therapeutic strategies. *Nat. Rev. Rheumatol.* **2019**, *15*, 519–532. [CrossRef] [PubMed]

12. Rice, G.; Newman, W.G.; Dean, J.; Patrick, T.; Parmar, R.; Flintoff, K.; Robins, P.; Harvey, S.; Hollis, T.; O'Hara, A.; et al. Heterozygous mutations in TREX1 cause familial chilblain lupus and dominant Aicardi-Goutieres syndrome. *Am. J. Hum. Genet.* **2007**, *80*, 811–815. [CrossRef] [PubMed]

13. Peschke, K.; Friebe, F.; Zimmermann, N.; Wahlicht, T.; Schumann, T.; Achleitner, M.; Berndt, N.; Luksch, H.; Behrendt, R.; Lee-Kirsch, M.A.; et al. Deregulated type I IFN response in TREX1-associated familial chilblain lupus. *J. Investig. Dermatol.* **2014**, *134*, 1456–1459. [CrossRef] [PubMed]

14. Yasutomo, K.; Horiuchi, T.; Kagami, S.; Tsukamoto, H.; Hashimura, C.; Urushihara, M.; Kuroda, Y. Mutation of DNASE1 in people with systemic lupus erythematosus. *Nat. Genet.* **2001**, *28*, 313–314. [CrossRef] [PubMed]

15. Napirei, M.; Karsunky, H.; Zevnik, B.; Stephan, H.; Mannherz, H.G.; Möröy, T. Features of systemic lupus erythematosus in Dnase1-deficient mice. *Nat. Genet.* **2000**, *25*, 177–181. [CrossRef] [PubMed]

16. Vroom, M.W.; Theaker, A.J.; Rest, J.R.; White, S.D. Case report: Lupoid dermatosis in 5 German short-hair pointer. *Vet. Dermatol.* **1995**, *6*, 93–98. [CrossRef]

17. Bryden, S.L.; White, S.D.; Dunston, S.M.; Burrows, A.K.; Olivry, T. Clinical, histopathological and immunological characteristics of exfoliative cutaneous lupus erythematosus in 25 German short-haired pointers. *Vet. Dermatol.* **2005**, *16*, 239–252. [CrossRef]

18. Mauldin, E.A.; Morris, D.O.; Brown, D.C.; Casal, M.L. Exfoliative cutaneous lupus erythematosus in German shorthaired pointer dogs: Disease development, progression and evaluation of three immunomodulatory drugs (ciclosporin, hydroxychloroquine, and adalimumab) in a controlled environment. *Vet. Dermatol.* **2010**, *21*, 373–382. [CrossRef]

19. Ferrigno, A.; Hoover, K.; Blubaugh, A.; Rissi, D.; Banovic, F. Treatment of exfoliative cutaneous lupus erythematosus in a German shorthaired pointer dog with mycophenolate mofetil. *Vet. Dermatol.* **2019**, *30*, 350. [CrossRef]

20. Wang, P.; Zangerl, B.; Werner, P.; Mauldin, E.A.; Casal, M.L. Familial cutaneous lupus erythematosus (CLE) in the German shorthaired pointer maps to CFA18, a canine orthologue to human CLE. *Immunogenetics* **2010**, *63*, 197–207. [CrossRef]

21. Purcell, S.; Neale, B.; Todd-Brown, K.; Thomas, L.; Ferreira, M.A.; Bender, D.; Maller, J.; Sklar, P.; de Bakker, P.I.; Daly, M.J.; et al. PLINK: A tool set for whole-genome association and population-based linkage analyses. *Am. J. Hum. Genet.* **2007**, *81*, 559–575. [CrossRef]

22. Zhou, X.; Stephens, M. Genome-wide efficient mixed-model analysis for association studies. *Nat. Genet.* **2012**, *44*, 821–824. [CrossRef]

23. Qqman: Q-Q and Manhattan Plots for GWAS Data. R Package Version 0.1.4. Available online: https://CRAN.R-project.org/package=qqman (accessed on 5 December 2019).

24. Jagannathan, V.; Drögemüller, C.; Leeb, T.; Dog Biomedical Variant Database Consortium (DBVDC). A comprehensive biomedical variant catalogue based on whole genome sequences of 582 dogs and eight wolves. *Anim. Genet.* **2019**, *50*, 695–704. [CrossRef]

25. McKenna, A.; Hanna, M.; Banks, E.; Sivachenko, A.; Cibulskis, K.; Kernytsky, A.; Garimella, K.; Altshuler, D.; Gabriel, S.; Daly, M.; et al. The Genome Analysis Toolkit: A MapReduce framework for analyzing next-generation DNA sequencing data. *Genome Res.* **2010**, *20*, 1297–1303. [CrossRef]

26. Cingolani, P.; Platts, A.; Wang, L.L.; Coon, M.; Nguyen, T.; Wang, L.; Land, S.J.; Lu, X.; Ruden, D.M. A program for annotating and predicting the effects of single nucleotide polymorphisms, SnpEff: SNPs in the genome of Drosophila melanogaster strain w1118; iso-2; iso-3. *Fly* **2012**, *6*, 80–92. [CrossRef]

27. Bai, B.; Zhao, W.M.; Tang, B.X.; Wang, Y.Q.; Wang, L.; Zhang, Z.; Yang, H.C.; Liu, Y.H.; Zhu, J.W.; Irwin, D.M.; et al. DoGSD: The dog and wolf genome SNP database. *Nucleic Acids Res.* **2015**, *43*, 777–783. [CrossRef]

28. Plassais, J.; Kim, J.; Davis, B.W.; Karyadi, D.M.; Hogan, A.N.; Harris, A.C.; Decker, B.; Parker, H.G.; Ostrander, E.A. Whole genome sequencing of canids reveals genomic regions under selection and variants influencing morphology. *Nat. Commun.* **2019**, *10*, 1489. [CrossRef]

29. The Welcome Trust Case Control Consortium. Genome-wide association study of 14,000 cases of seven common diseases and 3,000 shared controls. *Nature* **2007**, *447*, 661–678. [CrossRef]

30. Majer, O.; Liu, B.; Kreuk, L.S.M.; Krogan, N.; Barton, G.M. UNC93B1 recruits syntenin-1 to dampen TLR7 signaling and prevent autoimmunity. *Nature* **2019**, *575*, 366–370. [CrossRef]

31. Kashuba, V.I.; Protopopov, A.I.; Kvasha, S.M.; Gizatullin, R.Z.; Wahlestedt, C.; Kisselev, L.L.; Klein, G.; Zabarovsky, E.R. hUNC93B1: A novel human gene representing a new gene family and encoding an unc-93-like protein. *Gene* **2002**, *283*, 209–217. [CrossRef]

32. Kim, Y.-M.; Brinkmann, M.M.; Paquet, M.-E.; Ploegh, H.L. UNC93B1 delivers nucleotide-sensing toll-like receptors to endolysosomes. *Nature* **2008**, *452*, 234–238. [CrossRef]

33. Saitoh, S.; Miyake, K. Regulatory molecules required for nucleotide-sensing Toll-like receptors. *Immunol. Rev.* **2009**, *227*, 32–43. [CrossRef]

34. Majer, O.; Liu, B.; Woo, B.J.; Kreuk, L.S.M.; Van Dis, E.; Barton, G.M. Release from UNC93B1 reinforces the compartmentalized activation of select TLRs. *Nature* **2019**, *575*, 371–374. [CrossRef]

35. Fukui, R.; Saitoh, S.; Kanno, A.; Onji, M.; Shibata, T.; Ito, A.; Onji, M.; Matsumoto, M.; Akira, S.; Yoshida, N.; et al. Unc93B1 restricts systemic lethal inflammation by orchestrating Toll-like receptor 7 and 9 trafficking. *Immunity* **2011**, *35*, 69–81. [CrossRef]

36. Casrouge, A.; Zhang, S.Y.; Eidenschenk, C.; Jouanguy, E.; Puel, A.; Yang, K.; Alcais, A.; Picard, C.; Mahfoufi, N.; Nicolas, N.; et al. Herpes simplex virus encephalitis in human UNC-93B deficiency. *Science* **2006**, *314*, 308–312. [CrossRef]

37. Tabeta, K.; Hoebe, K.; Janssen, E.M.; Du, X.; Georgel, P.; Crozat, K.; Mudd, S.; Mann, N.; Sovath, S.; Goode, J.; et al. The Unc93b1 mutation 3d disrupts exogenous antigen presentation and signaling via Toll-like receptors 3, 7 and 9. *Nat. Immunol.* **2006**, *7*, 156–164. [CrossRef]

38. Deane, J.A.; Pisitkun, P.; Barrett, R.S.; Feigenbaum, L.; Town, T.; Ward, J.M.; Flavell, R.A.; Bolland, S. Control of toll-like receptor 7 expression is essential to restrict autoimmunity and dendritic cell proliferation. *Immunity* **2007**, *27*, 801–810. [CrossRef]

39. Pisitkun, P.; Deane, J.A.; Difilippantonio, M.J.; Tarasenko, T.; Satterthwaite, A.B.; Bolland, S. Autoreactive B cell responses to RNA-related antigens due to TLR7 gene duplication. *Science* **2006**, *312*, 1669–1672. [CrossRef]

40. Subramanian, S.; Tus, K.; Li, Q.Z.; Wang, A.; Tian, X.H.; Zhou, J.; Liang, C.; Bartov, G.; McDaniel, L.D.; Zhou, X.J.; et al. A Tlr7 translocation accelerates systemic autoimmunity in murine lupus. *Proc. Natl. Acad. Sci. USA* **2006**, *103*, 9970–9975. [CrossRef]

Deletion in the Bardet–Biedl Syndrome Gene *TTC8* Results in a Syndromic Retinal Degeneration in Dogs

Suvi Mäkeläinen [1], Minas Hellsand [2], Anna Darlene van der Heiden [1], Elina Andersson [3], Elina Thorsson [3], Bodil S. Holst [4], Jens Häggström [4], Ingrid Ljungvall [4], Cathryn Mellersh [5], Finn Hallböök [2], Göran Andersson [1], Björn Ekesten [4] and Tomas F. Bergström [1,*]

[1] Department of Animal Breeding and Genetics, Swedish University of Agricultural Sciences (SLU), Box 7023, SE-750 07 Uppsala, Sweden; suvi.makelainen@slu.se (S.M.); anna.darlene.heiden@slu.se (A.D.v.d.H.); goran.andersson@slu.se (G.A.)

[2] Department of Neuroscience, Uppsala University, Box 593, SE-751 24 Uppsala, Sweden; minas.hellsand@neuro.uu.se (M.H.); finn.hallbook@neuro.uu.se (F.H.)

[3] Section of Pathology, Department of Biomedical Sciences and Veterinary Public Health, Faculty of Veterinary Medicine and Animal Science, Swedish University of Agricultural Sciences (SLU), Box 7028, SE-750 07 Uppsala, Sweden; elina.andersson@slu.se (E.A.); elina.thorsson@slu.se (E.T.)

[4] Department of Clinical Sciences, Swedish University of Agricultural Sciences, Box 7054, SE-750 07 Uppsala, Sweden; Bodil.Strom-Holst@slu.se (B.S.H.); jens.haggstrom@slu.se (J.H.); ingrid.ljungvall@slu.se (I.L.); bjorn.ekesten@slu.se (B.E.)

[5] Canine Genetics Research Group, Kennel Club Genetics Centre, Animal Health Trust, Lanwades Park, Kentford, Newmarket, CB8 7UU Suffolk, UK; cathrynmellersh@yahoo.co.uk

* Correspondence: tomas.bergstrom@slu.se;

Abstract: In golden retriever dogs, a 1 bp deletion in the canine *TTC8* gene has been shown to cause progressive retinal atrophy (PRA), the canine equivalent of retinitis pigmentosa. In humans, *TTC8* is also implicated in Bardet–Biedl syndrome (BBS). To investigate if the affected dogs only exhibit a non-syndromic PRA or develop a syndromic ciliopathy similar to human BBS, we recruited 10 affected dogs to the study. The progression of PRA for two of the dogs was followed for 2 years, and a rigorous clinical characterization allowed a careful comparison with primary and secondary characteristics of human BBS. In addition to PRA, the dogs showed a spectrum of clinical and morphological signs similar to primary and secondary characteristics of human BBS patients, such as obesity, renal anomalies, sperm defects, and anosmia. We used Oxford Nanopore long-read cDNA sequencing to characterize retinal full-length *TTC8* transcripts in affected and non-affected dogs, the results of which suggest that three isoforms are transcribed in the retina, and the 1 bp deletion is a loss-of-function mutation, resulting in a canine form of Bardet–Biedl syndrome with heterogeneous clinical signs.

Keywords: Bardet–Biedl syndrome (BBS); primary cilia; ciliopathy; BBS8; progressive retinal atrophy (PRA); retinitis pigmentosa

1. Introduction

Inherited retinal degenerations (IRDs) are a diverse group of retinopathies leading to visual impairment and blindness in humans and other species. Most of the IRDs, such as retinitis pigmentosa (RP) in humans (OMIM # 268000) and the canine equivalent, termed progressive retinal atrophy (PRA), are non-syndromic and only affect vision. Syndromic IRDs are less common and besides visual impairment, other organs are also affected. In golden retriever (GR) dogs with PRA, a 1 bp deletion in exon 7 of the Tetratricopeptide repeat domain 8 (*TTC8*) gene was identified in 2014 (CanFam3.1 Chr8:60,090,185delA, rs852355138, OMIA 001984-9615, here denoted as *TTC8*^{delA}) [1]. This form of

PRA is generally referred to as GR-PRA2. The deletion was predicted to cause a frameshift of the open reading frame leading to a premature stop codon in exon 8, 15 codons downstream of the deletion. If translated, the truncated protein would lack most of the tetratricopeptide repeat motifs. In humans, mutations in the *TTC8* gene cause Bardet–Biedl syndrome (BBS; OMIM # 615985), a clinically and genetically heterogeneous autosomal recessive ciliopathy and the second most common human syndromic IRD after Usher syndrome [2,3].

BBS was first described by Georges Bardet and Artur Biedl in the early 1920s [4,5]. The symptoms are highly variable, even between patients from the same family, and are divided into primary and secondary characteristics [6,7]. Primary symptoms include retinal degeneration, obesity, polydactyly, kidney abnormalities, learning disabilities or cognitive impairment, hypogonadism in males, and genital abnormalities in females. Secondary features include speech delay, developmental delay, behavioral abnormalities, eye abnormalities, brachydactyly/syndactyly, ataxia/poor coordination/imbalance, short stature, mild hypertonia, diabetes mellitus, orodental abnormalities, cardiovascular anomalies, situs inversus, hepatic involvement, craniofacial dysmorphism, Hirschsprung disease, and anosmia [2,7,8]. For clinical diagnosis of BBS, it has been suggested that four of the primary characteristics or alternatively three primary and two secondary characteristics should be observed [8].

With 24 genes associated with BBS (OMIM # 209900) to date [9], the syndrome shows large non-allelic heterogeneity [10–13]. The most common cause of the disorder in humans are mutations in the *BBS1* and *BBS10* genes, each accounting for approximately 20% of human cases [14–16]. *TTC8* mutations account for approximately 2% of the cases, being amongst the less frequent causes for BBS [17]. In 2003, Ansley et al. discovered that the *TTC8* gene is associated with BBS and identified the syndrome as a basal body dysfunction of the ciliated cells [2]. The *TTC8* gene, also referred to as *BBS8*, is one of the eight *BBS* genes (*BBS1, BBS2, BBS4, BBS5, BBS7, TTC8, BBS9,* and *BBIP1*), encoding proteins that assemble into a stable octameric protein complex termed the BBSome [18,19]. The BBSome forms a membrane coat that sorts membrane receptors to the primary cilium and its dysfunction leads to the failure of cell-specific signal transduction affecting multiple cell-types and organs [20].

In addition to pleiotropic disorder, there are also reports of non-syndromic retinal degeneration caused by mutations in the BBS genes *BBS1, BBS2, ARL6/BBS3,* and *TTC8* [21–24], disrupting the normal function of photoreceptor cilia. At the time of the discovery of the canine *TTC8* deletion in 2014, there were indications that dogs homozygous for the deletion might exhibit clinical signs other than retinal degeneration [1]. However, only ophthalmic examinations of the affected dogs were performed and other BBS-associated characteristics could not be clinically investigated. In addition, it was not possible to analyze tissues from affected individuals. Here, we describe a detailed examination of two golden retrievers, homozygous for the *TTC8* variant (*TTC8*[delA]) that were followed from the time of the PRA-diagnosis until they were euthanized and a full necropsy was performed. This allowed for a rigorous clinical characterization of this canine form of a *TTC8*-mediated disease, and to investigate the effect of the canine *TTC8* mutation on the transcriptional and protein level in the canine retina.

2. Materials and Methods

2.1. Animals and Samples

A golden retriever sib-pair, a male (GR01) and a female (GR02), was followed from the time of their PRA-diagnosis until euthanasia, after which a necropsy was conducted and tissue samples were collected. The male dog was 6 years and 1 month old, and the female was 3 months older at the time of euthanization. Both dogs tested homozygous for the *TTC8*[delA] allele. Tissue samples were also collected from five unaffected dogs (RW01, BE02, LR02, GS01, and GSP01) euthanized for reasons unrelated to this study (Table S1). In addition, two unaffected dogs (BE01 and LR01; Table S1) were included in the clinical ophthalmic examination (see below). Interviews were conducted with owners of the sib-pair, as well as the owners of eight additional affected golden retrievers, all tested homozygous for the $TTC8^{delA}$ allele (Table S2). All samples were obtained with informed consent from the dog owners. Ethical approval was granted by the regional animal ethics committee (Uppsala ethics committee on animal experiments/Uppsala djurförsöksetiska nämnd; Dnr C12/15, Dnr 5.8.18-15533/2018, and Dnr 5.8.18-04682/2020).

2.2. Ophthalmic Examination, Confocal Scanning Ophthalmoscopy (cSLO), Optical Coherence Tomography (OCT) and Electroretinography (ERG)

Ophthalmic examination of GR01 and GR02, as well as an unaffected beagle (BE01) and an unaffected Labrador retriever (LR01) included reflex testing, testing of vision with falling cotton balls under dim and daylight conditions, and tonometry (Tonovet, Icare Finland Oy, Vantaa, Finland), as well as indirect ophthalmoscopy (Heine 500, Heine Optotechnik GmbH, Herrsching, Germany) and slit-lamp biomicroscopy (Kowa SL-17, Kowa Company Ltd., Tokyo, Japan) after dilation of pupils with tropicamide (Mydriacyl 0.5%, Alcon Nordic AS, København, Denmark).

cSLO- and OCT-imaging (Spectralis HRT + OCT, Heidelberg Engineering, Heidelberg, Germany) were performed after dilation of pupils with tropicamide and under light sedation with 5 µg/kg medetomidine (Sedator, Dechra Veterinary Products AB, Upplands Väsby, Sweden) and 50 µg/kg butorphanol (Dolorex, Intervet AB, Stockholm, Sweden). The cornea was kept moist using artificial tears throughout the procedure. Total retinal thickness in GR02 was measured as previously described [25], and compared to data from an unaffected 5-year-old female Labrador retriever (LR01) and a 7-year-old female beagle (BE01).

We recorded a bilateral, full-field ERG in GR02 under general anesthesia and compared to data from the unaffected LR01. Sedation with intramuscular acepromazine 0.03 mg/kg (Plegicil vet., Pharmaxim Sweden AB, Helsingborg, Sweden) was followed by induction with propofol 10 mg/kg, intravenously (Propovet, Orion Pharma Animal Health AB, Danderyd, Sweden). After intubation, inhalation anesthesia was maintained with isoflurane (Isoflo vet., Orion Pharma Animal Health AB). Corneal electrodes (ERG-JET, Cephalon A/S, Aalborg, Denmark) were used with isotonic eye drops (Comfort Shield, i.com medical GmbH, Munich, Germany) as a coupling agent. Gold-plated, cutaneous electrodes served as ground and reference electrodes (Grass, Natus Neurology Inc. Middleton, WI, USA) at the vertex and approximately 3 cm caudal to the lateral canthi, respectively. Light stimulation, calibration of lights, and processing of signals were performed as previously described [26] and the ECVO protocol for canine clinical ERGs was followed [27].

2.3. Clinical Andrological Examination and Semen Analysis

Semen from the affected male (GR01, age 6 years and 1 month), was collected using digital manipulation with a bitch in estrus present. The sperm concentration was measured using a Bürker chamber. Sperm morphology was evaluated using standard procedures in wet preparations of semen fixed in buffered formalin and in air-dried smears stained with carbolfuchsin–eosin. Due to a very low sperm concentration and volume, only 50 spermatozoa were examined in the wet preparation, under a phase-contrast microscope at 1000× magnification. All abnormalities on any given spermatozoon were counted and the overall frequencies were classified according to a system developed by Bane (1961) [28]. For a more detailed examination of the sperm heads, 100 spermatozoa were evaluated in a smear under a light microscope at 1000× magnification. Presence of spermatogenic cells was recorded in smears stained in accordance with standard well-established methodology. The head morphologies were classified as pear-shaped, narrow at the base, abnormal contour, undeveloped, loose and abnormal, narrow, and variable size.

2.4. Echocardiography and Electrocardiographic (ECG) Examinations

For the echocardiographic examinations of the sib-pair (GR01 and GR02, at an age of 6 years and 1 month), the dogs were placed in right and then left lateral recumbency on an ultrasound examination table. The echocardiographic evaluation was conducted by use of an ultrasonographic unit (EPIQ 7G, Philips Ultrasound, Bothell, WA, USA) equipped with a 5-1 matrix transducer and ECG monitoring. The heart was examined and subjectively assessed in standard right- and left-sided views [29]. Blood flow over heart valves was interrogated using color mode Doppler echocardiography and measured using spectral Doppler echocardiography. Left ventricular dimensions were measured using M-mode echocardiography in the right parasternal short axis view at the level of the papillary muscles. The left atrial diameter was measured in the right parasternal short axis view at the level of the aortic valve. Left ventricular dimensions were compared to published weight-based normal reference ranges [30] and left atrial diameter was indexed to the aortic diameter as previously described [31].

2.5. Histopathological Examinations

Tissue samples from the affected siblings GR01 and GR02 (Table S3), as well as a retinal sample from an unaffected 3-year-old Rottweiler (RW01), were fixed in 10% neutral buffered formalin for >24 h, paraffin wax embedded, sectioned at 4 μm and stained with hematoxylin and eosin (HE). In addition, kidney sections were also stained with periodic acid-Schiff (PAS). All sections were evaluated using light microscopy.

2.6. Total RNA Extraction

The retinal tissue sample from the affected female GR02 was collected directly in TRIzol Reagent (Invitrogen™, Carlsbad, CA, USA) for immediate RNA extraction. Retinal samples from three unaffected dogs—a beagle (BE02), a Labrador retriever (LR02), and a German shepherd (GS01)—were preserved in RNAlater (SigmaAldrich, Saint Louis, MO, USA) directly after euthanasia. The samples were then washed with 1 × PBS and between 50 to 100 mg of tissue was used for extraction. The samples from GR02, BE02, and GS01 were then homogenized in TRIzol Reagent with Precellys homogenizer (Bertin Instruments, Montigny-le-Bretonneux, France) and total RNA was extracted following the manufacturer's instructions (Pub. No. MAN0001271, Rev. B.0.). Total RNA from LR02 was extracted with RNeasy mini kit (Qiagen, Hilden, Germany) according to the manufacturer's instructions. RNA concentration was measured using Qubit RNA BR Assay kit (Invitrogen™, Waltham, MA, USA). RNA integrity and quality were inspected with Agilent TapeStation 4150 with an Agilent RNA ScreenTape (Agilent Technologies, Santa Clara, CA, USA). PolyA-selection was carried out utilizing Dynabeads mRNA Purification Kit (Invitrogen™, Waltham, MA, USA), applying the manufacturer-provided protocol.

2.7. Long-Read cDNA Sequencing with Oxford Nanopore Sequencing Technology (ONT)

Oxford Nanopore long-read cDNA sequencing libraries for the polyA-selected RNA of the canine retina from the affected GR02 as well as unaffected BE02 and GS01 were prepared using the Direct cDNA Sequencing kit (SQK-DCS109, Oxford Nanopore Technologies Ltd., Oxford, UK) following the manufacturer's instructions (Protocol version DCS_9090_v109_revC_04Feb2019; updated 02 May 2019). The input material for each library was 100 ng of polyA-selected RNA. The prepared libraries were sequenced on a MinION sequencer using R9.4.1 flow-cells and MinKNOW (v.19.06.7) software. The resulting raw fast5 files were basecalled using Guppy version 3.1.5+781ed57 with the –trim_strategy DNA flag. The quality control for each run was performed using an R markdown script developed by ONT (Nanopore_SumStatQC_Tutorial.Rmd). To characterize the retinal *TTC8* transcripts, quality passed reads (quality score > 7) were mapped to the canine reference genome sequence CanFam3.1 using MiniMap2 (v.2.16) with -ax splice parameter (Li, 2018) [32]. A reference-guided assembly of the transcriptome was produced using StringTie2 (v.2.1.1) with default settings for long-reads (-L) [33], with Ensembl anotation build 100 (CanFam3.1). The assembled transcripts were compared to the raw sequnce data using The Integrative Genomics Viewer (IGV) [34,35]. Transcripts with less then 20× coverage were discared. To quantify the expression levels, quality passed reads (quality score > 7) were mapped to the canine reference transcriptome consisting of protein coding gene sequences and non-coding RNA sequences from Ensembl build 100 (CanFam3.1) using Minimap2 (v2.16) with the settings -ax map-ont -N 100 [32]. The transcript counts were produced using Salmon (v.1.1.0) in aligned based mode and –libType A for automatic detection of library type [36]. The results for each transcript expressed as transcripts per million (TPM) were summarized to produce gene level TPM values. We then analyzed the expression levels of genes considered to be expressed in a cell-specific manner (retinal marker genes) [37–57]. The complete list of marker genes and their respective references can be found in Table S4.

2.8. Quantitative RT-qPCR

cDNA was synthesized using RNA prepared from retinal samples of the affected female (GR02) and three unaffected dogs (BE02, LR02, and GS01) using RT^2 First Strand kit (Qiagen, Hilden, Germany) with random hexamers provided in the kit. cDNA concentration was measured using Qubit ssDNA Assay kit (Invitrogen™, Waltham, MA, USA). To amplify the target and the reference genes, custom primers were designed using the software Primer3 [58,59] (Table S5). The cDNA fragments encoding regions of interest were amplified using RT^2 SYBR Green ROX qPCR Mastermix (Qiagen, Hilden, Germany) on a StepOnePlus Real-Time PCR system (Applied Biosystems™, Waltham, MA, USA), according to the manufacturer's instructions. Target gene expression was normalized to expression of *GAPDH* as well as *ACTB* reference genes, and shown relative to a control sample (BE02) (△△CT method). The results were confirmed in two independent experiments.

2.9. Fluorescence Histochemistry

Retina from the affected female (GR02) and an unaffected 10-year-old male German spaniel (GSP01) were analyzed by means of fluorescence histochemistry. The lens and anterior segment were removed and the vitreous punctured before the eye cups were fixed in 4% PFA in 1 × PBS for 15 min on ice, washed in 1 × PBS for 10 min on ice, and cryoprotected in 30% sucrose in 1 × PBS at 4 °C until saturated. The eye cups were embedded in Neg-50™ frozen section medium (Thermo Scientific, Waltham, MA, USA) and 10 μm sections were collected on Superfrost Plus slides (J1800AMNZ, Menzel-Gläser, Thermo Fisher Scientific, Waltham, MA, USA). Sections were re-hydrated in 1 × PBS for 10 min, incubated in blocking solution (1% donkey serum, 0.02% thimerosal, and 0.1% Triton X-100 in 1 × PBS) for 30 min at room temperature, and incubated in blocking solution containing Alexa Fluor™ 488-conjugated PNA (1:400, L21409, Invitrogen™, Waltham, MA, USA) and a rhodopsin primary antibody (1:5000, NBP2-25160, Novus Biologicals, Abingdon, UK) overnight at 4 °C. The sections were then washed in 1 × PBS, 3 × 5 min, incubated in Alexa 568 secondary antibody (1:2000, A10037, Invitrogen™, Waltham, MA, USA) for at least 2 h at room temperature, washed in 1 × PBS, 3 × 5 min, and the slides mounted using ProLong™ Gold Antifade Mountant with DAPI (P36931, Molecular Probes, Waltham, MA, USA). Images were captured using a Zeiss Imager.Z2 microscope equipped with an Axiocam 512 mono camera (Carl Zeiss Microscopy GmbH, Jena, Germany).

3. Results

3.1. Desciption of Primary and Secondary Bardet-Biedl Syndrome Characteristics

To investigate if the dogs exhibit other BBS-related problems, we interviewed the owners of 10 affected dogs. Two of the dogs were also part of the 2014 study [1], and we based the interviews on the questionnaire developed by Downs et al. (2014) [1]. Among the 10 affected dogs, 4 were reported to exhibit a minimum of four characteristics matching human primary BBS-signs (Table S2). The remaining dogs displayed three (two dogs) and two (three dogs) primary signs, respectively, and for one dog, PRA was the only reported primary characteristic. All of the dogs had been diagnosed with PRA, and the average age of diagnosis was 4 years and 8 months. None of the dogs were reported to have polydactyly or any other malformations of the paws, but obesity or polyphagia, renal problems, cognitive dysfunction, irregular estrous cycles, and decreased libido in males were among the reported primary signs. As for secondary BBS signs, many dogs were described to have a short stature relative to the standard for the breed. Partial or complete loss of the sense of smell (anosmia), worsening with age, was noticed by most of the owners (Table S2). Half of the individuals were also diagnosed with cataracts. At the time of this study, seven of these dogs were no longer alive. The oldest dog was reported to have died in his sleep at 10 years of age, while the other dogs had been euthanized at an average age of 7.5 years. Among the dogs in the questionnaires was the BBS-affected sib-pair (GR01 and GR02), which were further investigated in this study.

3.2. Ophthalmic Examinations of the Affected Sib-Pair

The male dog GR01 was initially diagnosed with PRA at the age of 4 years and 3 months, after which he and his female littermate GR02 were genotyped and found to be homozygous for the $TTC8^{delA}$ allele and subsequently recruited for this study. The two dogs were then examined ophthalmologically on three occasions: at the age of 4.5 and 5.5 years, and finally at the age of 6 years and 1 month. At the first examination, both dogs had mildly dilated pupils in room light. Pupillary light reflexes and menace responses were considered normal, but the dazzle reflex was mildly impaired in both eyes (oculi uterque, OU). The results of the cotton ball test in room light were unremarkable for both dogs, whereas the female detected approximately 50% and the male only between 10–20% of the cotton balls under dim light conditions. On indirect ophthalmoscopy, generalized abnormal tapetal reflection going from hypo- via normo- to hyperreflection (in the male) was seen when the indirect ophthalmoscopy lens was tilted back and forth. Furthermore, retinal vascular attenuation and pigment clumping in the non-tapetal fundus were observed. Compared to the female dog, the male showed signs of more advanced retinal degeneration. Findings were symmetrical between eyes. In addition to the abnormal retinal appearance, equatorial and anterior cortical cataracts were seen in the eyes of both individuals. The male had multiple, pigmented iridociliary cysts mainly emerging through the nasal portion of the pupils (OU), but free-floating and collapsed cysts were also seen in the anterior chambers. Intraocular pressures (IOP) were normal (OU) in both dogs.

To further investigate the retinal phenotype, we performed cSLO and OCT on the affected female (GR02). Reduced fundus autofluorescence (FAF) in the entire tapetal fundus was seen on cSLO (Figure 1a), whereas the non-tapetal fundus appeared slightly hyperreflective indicating accumulation of lipofuscin in the degenerating retina. Retinal vascular attenuation in the affected fundus was evident, as well as islets with bright tapetal hyperreflection (Figure 1b), compared to the unaffected dog (Figure 1c,d).

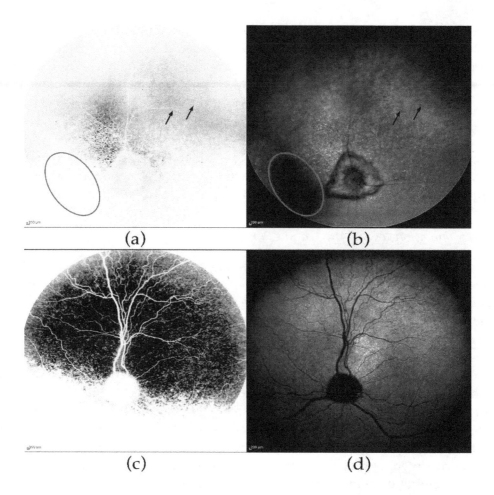

Figure 1. Fundus autofluorescence (FAF) and infrared confocal scanning laser ophthalmoscopy (IR-cSLO). cSLO FAF- and IR-cSLOs of the left eye of GR02 (panels (**a**,**b**), respectively) and age-matched, unaffected Labrador retriever LR01 (panels (**c**,**d**), respectively). Both FAF-images are inverted and hence, the tapetal reflection in GR02 (**a**) is remarkably faint. Detection of FAF in the tapetal fundus is difficult because of the normal, bright reflection from the tapetum lucidum. Black arrows indicate areas with bright reflection in the tapetal fundus on FAF (**a**), but hyporeflection on IR (**b**), which is suggestive of lipofuscin accumulation. The slight hyperreflection (the grey shade below the optic nerve head in the inverted image) (**a**) in the non-tapetal area autofluorescence indicates storage of lipofuscin. The IR-image (**b**) shows the large, myelinated optic nerve head often seen in the golden retriever breed, but very attenuated retinal vessels (red arrows) and islets of hyperreflectivity. Cast shadows in the cSLOs from GR02 were caused by the cataracts present in this dog (one shadowed area indicated by the blue oval).

OCT showed considerable retinal thinning (Figure 2a) compared to two unaffected dogs (LR01 and BE01). Mainly the outer retinal layers were reduced in thickness and outer retinal landmarks, such as the external limiting membrane (ELM), ellipsoid zone (EZ), and interdigitation zone (IZ), could not easily be identified in the affected dog (Figure 2b). The inner nuclear layer (INL) was thin and often fragmented, making the segmentation of the outer plexiform layer (OPL) and inner plexiform layer (IPL) difficult. In the ventral (inferior) non-tapetal fundus, retinal thickness was also reduced, but more irregularly, giving a patchier appearance. Again, segmentation of the outer retinal layer on the OCT image was difficult and a distinct outer nuclear layer ONL occasionally missing. Both fragmentation and thickening of the retinal pigment epithelium (RPE)was observed (Figure 2c). The cataracts in the male (GR01) hindered the cSLO and OCT examinations.

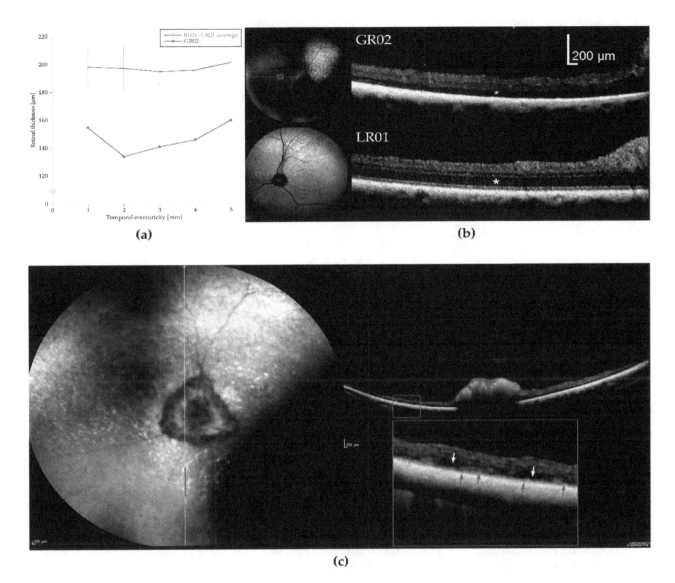

Figure 2. Retinal thickness and optical coherence tomography (OCT). (**a**) Total retinal thickness temporally from the optic nerve head (ONH) towards the periphery of the retina is reduced in the affected dog (GR02) compared to the thickness observed in an unaffected Labrador retriever (LR01) and a Beagle (BE01). (**b**) OCTs from the nasal part of the fundus (red rectangles) from the affected dog (GR02, top) and the unaffected dog (LR01, bottom) showing both the marked thinning of the outer nuclear layer (ONL) (asterisk) and less distinct segmentation of retinal layers in the affected dog. (**c**) Appearance of the retina in the non-tapetal, ventral fundus of GR02. The vertical red bar in the cSLO-image shows the area outlined by the red rectangle on the OCT photograph, which is then magnified below (the area inside the large red rectangle). Cast shadows on the cSLO-image were caused by cataracts. The thinned retina is more variable in thickness than in the tapetal fundus dorsal to the ONH. The retinal pigment epithelium (RPE) is occasionally fragmented (red arrows) or appears thickened (blue arrows). The segmentation of the outer retina is difficult and dark areas probably representing clusters of nuclei in the ONL are seen occasionally (white arrows).

Flash-electroretinography (FERG) was performed in the female, but not in the male, because of the ophthalmoscopic signs of more advanced retinal degeneration. In the female, rod responses were non-detectable throughout the 20 min dark adaptation. Neither was the a-wave of the mixed, dark-adapted rod-cone response discernible and the b-wave had profoundly subnormal amplitude and was dominated by the early, mainly cone-driven part. The light-adapted cone-driven transient b-wave was relatively better preserved, but biphasic with a late, second peak, whereas the a-wave was essentially missing. The cone flicker response was more abnormal, as the cone-driven responses were unable to follow the 30 Hz stimuli (Figure 3).

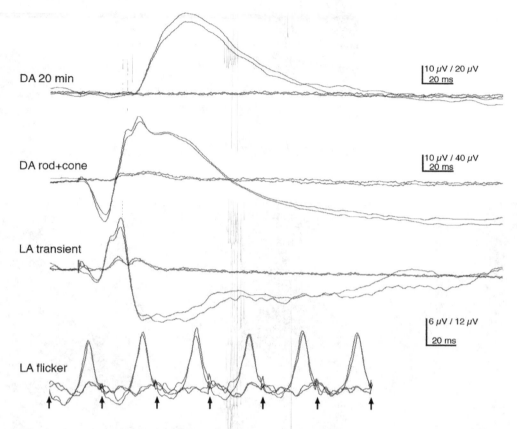

Figure 3. Flash-electroretinographs (FERGs). Both dark-adapted (DA) and light-adapted (LA) responses of the FERG had subnormal amplitudes in the affected golden retriever (GR02; red tracings) compared to the unaffected Labrador retriever (LR01) (blue tracings). Rod responses were essentially non-detectable and even the dark-adapted responses to the bright rod-cone stimulus seem to be mainly cone-driven. Light-adapted cone transients lacked a-wave and had a biphasic waveform. When a 30 Hz stimulus was employed, the cone responses of GR02 came out of sync and were not time-locked to the individual stimuli. Calibrations show the time base and the different amplitude scales for GR02 and LR01.

The siblings were re-examined 11 months later at the age of 5.5 years. Pupils were now moderately to widely dilated in both dogs, pupillary light reflexes sluggish and incomplete, and dazzle reflexes impaired. The male dog showed poor menace responses and did not respond to falling cotton balls regardless of lighting, but did occasionally follow hand movements at 30 cm in bright light. Vision was less impaired in the female; menace responses were retained and approximately 50% of the falling cotton balls were perceived in room light, whereas no cotton balls were detected in dim light. Ophthalmoscopy showed generalized tapetal hyperreflection in both dogs with a brighter hyperreflection in the male than in the female. Retinal vascular attenuation was now moderate to advanced and the optic nerve heads appeared pale. In the non-tapetal area, pigment clumping was observed, as on the previous examination. Cataractous changes had progressed in both dogs and were seen in both the anterior and posterior cortices of both eyes, as well as in the equatorial region. Iridociliary cysts were still present in the male and his eyes were normotensive.

Both dogs were examined a third time at the age of 6 years and 1 month. At this time, the male was severely visually impaired both under daylight and dim light conditions, and had developed bilateral mature-hypermature total cataracts. In addition, the dog showed both intact and ruptured iridociliary cysts bilaterally (Figure 4a) and had normal IOP. However, the ocular fundi could not be examined in vivo because of the cataracts. Postmortem gross examination of the fundi revealed bright hyperreflection in the tapetal area (Figure 4b). The network of retinal blood vessels was severely attenuated (even for a postmortem specimen) and difficult to follow towards the periphery (Figure 4b). The pupils of the female dog (GR02) were dilated in room light conditions, the pupillary light reflexes (PLRs) were sluggish and incomplete, dazzle reflexes were poor, and menace responses were present in room light, but not in dim light conditions. The female was unable to detect falling cotton balls regardless of lighting. The cataractous changes had progressed (OU), particularly in the posterior than in the anterior cortex, and the tapetal hyperreflectivity and retinal vascular attenuation could now only be seen like through a haze.

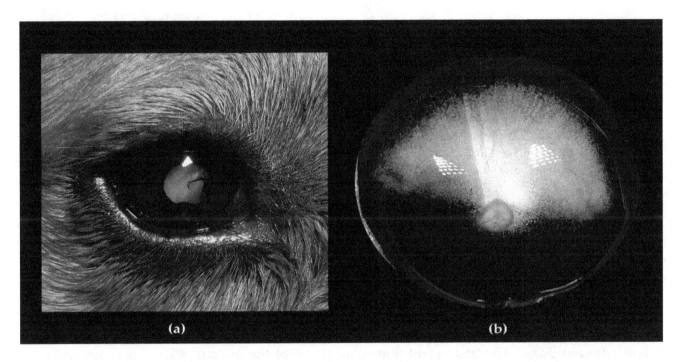

Figure 4. Iridociliary cysts and fundus imaging of the affected male (GR01). (**a**) Iridociliary cysts both at the posterior side of the iris and free-floating in the anterior chamber were seen in both eyes of the affected male (GR01). Pigment and remnants of ruptured cysts were seen on the anterior capsules of the cataractous lenses. (**b**) The eyecup of the affected male (GR01), *postmortem*. Bright tapetal hyperreflection is seen close to the optic nerve head (ONH), whereas the rest of the tapetum is faintly colored. The retinal vessels, including the larger venules, are almost impossible to follow.

3.3. Andrological Examination

The testes of the affected male dog GR01 were both palpable in the scrotum and found to be smaller than normal for the age and breed. An ejaculate of a very small volume (<0.5 mL), and light grey in color, was obtained. The sperm concentration was 15×10^6/mL and motility was <5%. The total sperm count could not be calculated exactly, but was estimated to be $<7 \times 10^6$/mL. There was a high proportion of spermatozoa with abnormalities, and less than 1% were considered morphologically normal. Midpiece defects were predominant (82% of spermatozoa), consisting of "Dag defect" [60], with strong folding, coiling, and fracture of the distal part of the midpiece, and "tail stump defect", where, in place of normal tails, short "stumps" were found. Other defects were coiled tails (12%), and double bent tails (6%), as well as proximal droplets (12%), acrosome defects (4%), and nuclear pouches (20%). Head defects were detected in 36% of the spermatozoa, the most common being pear shaped (11%), variable size (10%), and loose abnormal heads (7%). In addition, a large number of spermatogenic cells, inflammatory cells, and epithelial cells, as well as necrotic cells of varying sizes, were present (Figure 5a).

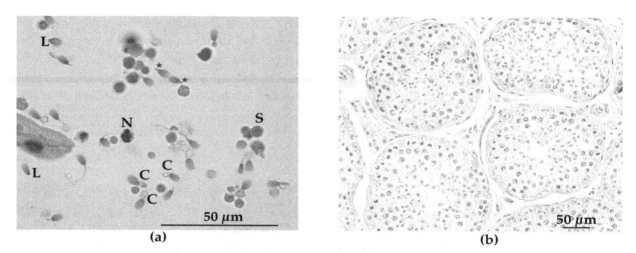

Figure 5. Light microscopy of sperm and seminiferous tubules from the affected male (GR01). (a) Papanicolaou staining of semen showing several abnormal spermatozoa. Different tail defects are evident, including coiled tails (C), tail stumps (*) and loose heads (L). S: spermatogenic cell, N: neutrophil leukocyte. (b) Tubuli seminiferi in testis stained with hematoxylin and eosin, showing mainly early stages of spermatogenesis and few elongated spermatids (ES).

3.4. Cardiac Examination

Both dogs (GR01 and GR02) presented normal respiratory sinus arrhythmia at a normal heart rate (between 80–90 BPM). Echocardiography showed normal cardiac morphology, dimensions, and motion in both dogs. Minimal regurgitation over the mitral valve was detected in both dogs, but valve morphology appeared normal. None of the dogs manifested *situs inversus*.

3.5. Necropsy Findings

To further investigate clinical features associated with BBS, a thorough necropsy was conducted on both affected dogs. The body condition score (BCS) of the male (GR01) was estimated to be 9/9, consistent with obesity [61]. In gross examination of the male, an abnormal head shape with a broadened muzzle and flat forehead was perceived, as was a low withers height. Furthermore, there was gingival hyperplasia and moderately increased interdental spaces (diastema) in both lower and upper jaw. The testicles were also seemingly small for the dog's breed and age. Gross examination of the kidneys revealed suspected chronic infarcts bilaterally, with the most marked changes in the right kidney (Table S3). Mild myxomatous valvular degeneration was seen in the heart of the affected male. The body condition score (BCS) of the female (GR02) was assessed to be 7/9, consistent with heavy [61]. The interdental spaces were also moderately increased. The kidneys showed signs of mild chronic glomerulonephritis bilaterally (Table S3).

3.6. Histopathology Findings

Next, we examined the histopathology of tissue samples collected during the necropsy. Abnormal changes were observed in the retina, kidney, and testis. The majority of the retina from the male (GR01) exhibited severe retinal thinning with complete loss of normal architecture with most pronounced degenerative changes in the non-tapetal fundus. Compared to a normal retina (Figure S1a), the ONL of the affected male GR01 was severely affected in the tapetal fundus and completely missing in the non-tapetal fundus (Figure S1b,c).

Histopathological examination of the testicles revealed only few (or no) late spermatids in the tubuli seminiferi (Figure 5b). A reduced number of spermatocytes was also observed. Microscopically, sections from the lesions in the right kidney of the male (GR01) corresponded to segmental areas of fibrosis, infiltrated by a moderate number of lymphocytes and plasma cells, extending from cortex to medulla (Figure 6a,b). In the fibrotic tissue, there were some degenerated glomeruli and lack of tubular structures. Furthermore, a disarray of occasional small glomeruli with peripheral nuclei and inapparent capillaries (fetal glomeruli), as well as atypical tubular structures outlined by pseudostratified cuboidal epithelium with large, basophilic, plump cells, were seen. No cellular atypia or mitotic activity were evident. Occasional dilated tubular structures were seen (Figure 6b). No chronic infarcts were confirmed histologically in the left kidney. On microscopic examination of the kidneys from the female (GR02), changes consistent with mild chronic glomerulonephritis was evident.

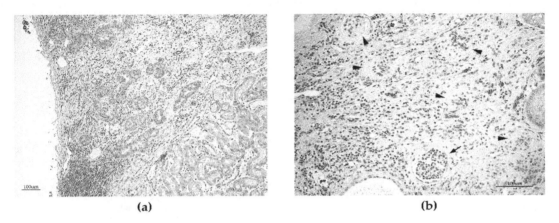

(a)   (b)

Figure 6. Renal histopathology of the affected male dog (GR01). Light microscopy of the right kidney stained with hematoxylin and eosin, showing a segmental area of fibrosis, (**a**) infiltrated by lymphocytes and plasma cells, extending from cortex, with the presence of a disarray of atypical tubular structures, and (**b**) with occasional small glomeruli with peripheral nuclei and inapparent capillaries (fetal glomeruli, marked with an arrow). Furthermore, multiple degenerated glomeruli are seen (arrowheads).

3.7. Characterization of Canine TTC8 Transcripts in the Retina

To comprehensively characterize the different *TTC8* transcripts expressed in the canine retina and to investigate the effect of the 1 bp deletion (*TTC8*^{delA}) in an affected dog, we performed full-length cDNA sequencing of the neural retina from the female (GR02), as well as of two 12-year-old unaffected female dogs, a beagle (BE02) and a German shepherd (GS01), using Oxford Nanopore Technologies (ONT) for long-read sequencing. This produced 3.6 M reads and 5.86 Gb of quality passed DNA sequence for GR02, 7.8 M reads and 10.68 Gb for BE02, as well as 7.6 M reads and 7.06 Gb for GS01 (Table 1).

Table 1. Full-length cDNA sequencing (ONT).

Dog	Reads Produced	Bases Called *	Quality Passed Reads	Quality Passed Bases *	Mean Read Length (bp)	N50 (bp)	Mean Read Quality
GR02	4,895,849	6.78	3,577,000 (73.1%)	5.86 (86.3%)	1637	2277	10.1
BE02	10,284,735	12.36	7,819,514 (76%)	10.68 (86.4%)	1365	1756	10.6
GS01	11,717,598	9.01	7,629,750 (65.1%)	7.06 (78.4%)	926	1135	9.5

* Gb of DNA sequence.

The cDNA sequence data was assembled into transcripts using reference-guided assembly. The predicted transcripts of the *TTC8* gene were then manually curated with the raw sequence data. We could not assemble any full-length *TTC8* transcripts from the sample of the affected dog (GR02) due to lack of read coverage over the *TTC8* locus. In contrast, sequence data from the unaffected dogs (BE02 and GS01) suggested transcription of three different retinal isoforms at the *TTC8* gene, here denoted tr1, tr2, and tr3 (Figure 7a). Fourteen exons were detected in tr1, 15 in tr2, and 16 in tr3, comprising 6.5%, 76.1%, and 17.4% of the *TTC8* transcripts, respectively. In tr1, exons 1b and the retinal specific exon 2a were missing. In tr2, exon 1b was absent, whereas tr3 featured both exons 1b and 2a. The comparison of the identified transcripts to existing annotations showed that the exon-intron boundaries and sequence between the first and the last exon of tr1 corresponds to the curated NCBI RefSeq transcript NM_001284469.1, tr2 corresponds to the predicted NCBI RefSeq transcript XM_003639207.4, as well as Ensembl transcript ENSCAFT00000027700.5, and tr3 corresponds to the predicted NCBI RefSeq transcript XM_014115661.2. The exon-intron boundaries of the identified transcripts show similarity to human *TTC8* transcripts (Figure 7b). In all three transcripts, a putative translation initiation site (TIS) was identified in exon 1 (Chr8:60,061,732) containing an AUG start codon with an adjacent optimal (GCCRCCAUGG) Kozak consensus sequence (Figure 7a) [62,63]. Using the TIS, tr1 and tr2 have an open reading frame extending to the last exon, encoding for 505 and 515 aa protein products, respectively. However, in tr3, the TIS would lead to a termination codon two exons downstream of exon 1, producing a 49 aa protein product and would lack the tetratricopeptide repeat (TPR) motifs. An alternative TIS is found at position Chr8:60,077,223 of exon 2 and, although the adjacent Kozak consensus is not optimal, it is classified as strong (NNNRNNAUGG) [63]. This alternative TIS is in-frame with the original coding sequence, and its open reading frame would produce a 455 aa protein product for all three transcripts, including the TPR motifs (Figure 7a). We did not observe any transcripts skipping exon 7, where the deletion Chr8:60,090,185[delA] is located, nor any exons downstream the deletion.

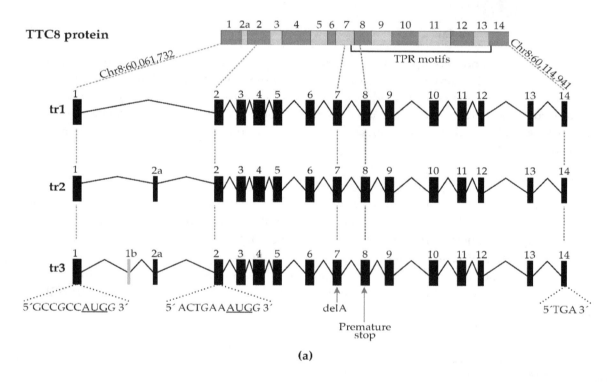

(a)

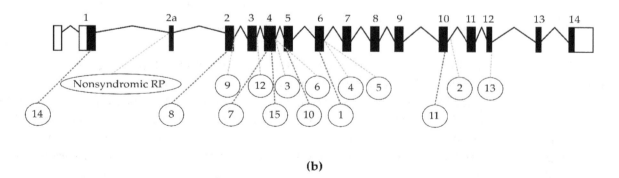

(b)

Figure 7. Retinal isoforms of canine the *TTC8* gene and human variants associated with Bardet-Biedl syndrome (BBS). (a) On top, a schematic representation of the TTC8 protein including the approximate location of the TPR motifs, and below, the three identified canine retinal transcripts. The black dashed lines indicate the two alternative TIS including the Kozak consensus sequence, and the translation termination site in exon 14. The red dashed lines indicate the 1 bp deletion of adenine in exon 7 and the premature stop codon in exon 8. (**b**) An overview of identified human *TTC8* coding variants (red dashed line) and splice-site variants (blue dashed line), see Table S6. The positions of the human mutations are based on the reported positions in the original publications, and the exon numbering may therefore differ from the positions in the presented transcript (ENST00000345383.9). tr1: transcript 1, tr2: transcript 2, tr3: transcript 3, TPR: tetratricopeptide repeat, TIS: translation initiation site.

Next, we compared *TTC8* gene expression levels of the unaffected BE02 and GS01 with the *TTC8* levels of the affected GR02 with 1 bp deletion in the exon 7 (Figure 8). We first estimated the transcript abundance for each annotated gene with Salmon (v.1.1.0) [36] using canine transcriptome from Ensembl build 100 and then summarized the level of transcript expression of each gene in the annotation. In BE02, the *TTC8* gene was expressed at a level of 99.8 transcripts per million (TPM) (856th most highly expressed gene), and in GS01 at a level of 60.6 TPM (859th most highly expressed gene). As suggested by the low read coverage of GR02 of *TTC8* transcripts, the expression levels were low in the affected dog, with 16.8 TPM (3625th most highly expressed gene). We then summarized the expression levels of known marker genes for different cell types in the retina (Table S4, Figure 8). The expression of genes transcribed in the rod photoreceptor cells (*PDE6A*, *PDE6B*, *CNGB1*, *CNGA1*, and *GNAT1*) [39,43,64–66] accounted for 25–27% of the total marker gene expression (TPM) in both the unaffected dogs (Figure 8a,b). For the affected GR02, the expression was estimated to 0.2%, indicating that the sample only included a small fraction of rod cells compared to the unaffected dogs (Figure 8c). The rhodopsin gene (*RHO*), encoding for a specialized G protein-coupled receptor known to be expressed exclusively in rod photoreceptors, was not included in the most recent Ensembl annotation release (build 100) used in the analysis, and therefore not included in the rod marker gene list. Similarly, the POU Class 4 Homeobox 1 (*POU4F1*), marker for retinal ganglion cells [67], was not among the genes annotated in Ensembl build 100. Both *RHO* and *POU4F1* were instead included in the quantification using reverse transcription quantitative real-time PCR (see below). The expression levels of cone photoreceptor cell markers (*ARR3*, *GUCA1C*, *PDE6C*, *PDE6H*, and *OPN1LW*) [37–43] were also lower in GR02, whereas the expression levels of macroglial cell (MG) marker genes (*RLBP1*, *SLC1A3*, *GLUL*, *CLU*, and *GFAP*) [43–46] were elevated (Figure 8a–c). The marker gene expression levels of the horizontal cells (HC) [47,48], retinal ganglion cells (RGC) [49–54], RPE cells [50,55], amacrine cells (AC) [47,56], or bipolar cells (BC) [57] did not differ drastically between the three dogs, although the proportional expression of BC and RPE markers was higher in the affected female. The complete list of marker genes and their expression values in each sample can be found in Table S4.

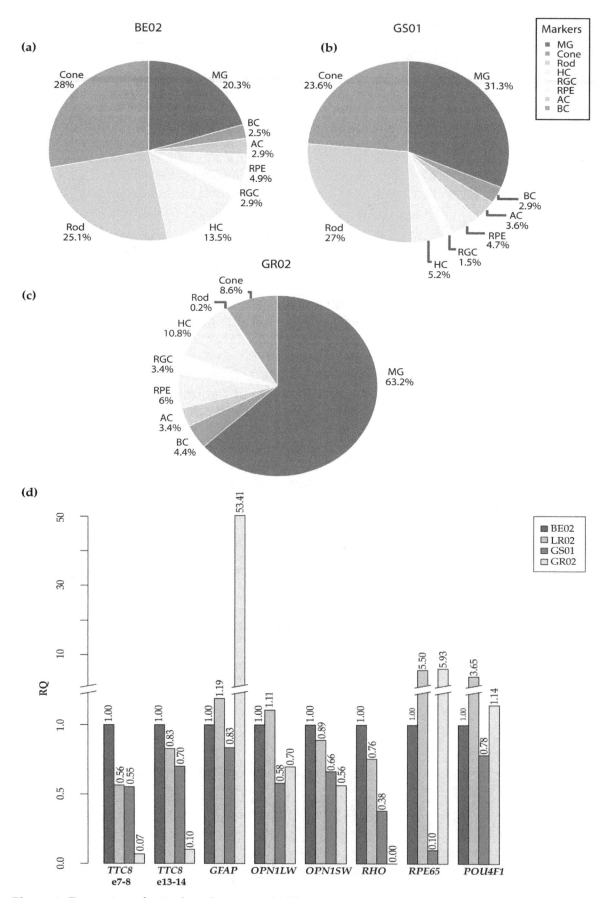

Figure 8. Expression of retinal marker genes. (**a**) The average expression of marker genes for each retinal cell type in the unaffected BE02 (**a**) and GS01 (**b**) dogs as well as the affected GR02 (**c**), based on cDNA sequencing. (**d**) Relative mRNA expression levels by quantitative RT-qPCR in two different regions

(exons 7–8 and exons 13–14) of the *TTC8* gene, as well as the retinal marker genes *GFAP* (macroglial cells), *OPN1LW* and *OPN1SW* (cone photoreceptors), *RHO* (rod photoreceptors), *RPE65* (RPE cells), and *POU4F1* (retinal ganglion cells) expression in three unaffected dogs (BE02, LR02, GS01) and the affected GR02, normalized to *GAPDH* and *ACTB* gene expression. Rod: rod photoreceptors, cone: cone photoreceptors, RGC: retinal ganglion cells, AC: amacrine cells, HC: horizontal cells, BC: bipolar cells, MG: macroglial cells, RPE: retinal pigment epithelium, BE02: unaffected beagle, GS01: unaffected German shepherd, GR02: affected golden retriever, LR02: unaffected Labrador retriever.

To verify the relative differences in the expression levels of *TTC8* and retinal marker genes in the affected GR02 and unaffected BE02 and GS01, as well as in an unaffected Labrador retriever (LR02, not used in the cDNA sequencing), we performed reverse transcription quantitative real-time PCR (RT-qPCR). We amplified two separate regions of the *TTC8* gene over the exons 7 to 8 and 13 to 14 (Figure 8d). In addition, we amplified canine long-wave (*OPN1LW*), and short-wave (*OPN1SW*) opsins expressed in cone photoreceptors, as well as, retinoid isomerohydrolase RPE65 (*RPE65*) and glial fibrillary acidic protein (*GFAP*) genes (markers for RPE cells and macroglia, respectively) to compare their cDNA sequencing levels to RT-qPCR. We also used *RHO* to evaluate relative rod photoreceptor levels and POU Class 4 Homeobox 1 (*POU4F1*) to evaluate retinal ganglion cells in these retinal samples. With the exception of *RPE65* expression, the RT-qPCR results reflected the cDNA sequencing quantification showing that the expression of both *TTC8* amplicons, as well as *RHO* expression, were lower in the GR02 compared to the three unaffected dogs and *GFAP* expression was higher than in the unaffected dogs (Figure 8d).

3.8. Fluorescence Histochemical Analysis of the TTC8^{delA} Retina

RT-qPCR analysis revealed low expression of markers of rod and, to a lesser extent, cone photoreceptors in the affected female (GR02; Figure 8), and the histopathology analysis for the affected male (GR01; Figure S1) and OCT analysis for the affected female (GR02; Figure 2) showed that both the ONL and photoreceptor layer were thinner compared to control retinas. To investigate the presence of photoreceptors in the TTC8^{delA} retina, we performed fluorescence histochemistry using an antibody directed against rhodopsin and fluorophore-conjugated peanut agglutinin (PNA), which binds selectively to cone photoreceptors in the retina [68]. Retinal sections from an unaffected, 10-year-old German spaniel (GSP01) and the affected, 6-year-old female golden retriever (GR02) were analyzed (Figure 9). We found that the ONL and the photoreceptor layer were thinner in the GR02 retina compared to control. In the unaffected retina, both rhodopsin and PNA staining were found in the photoreceptor layer (Figure 9a), whilst in the affected GR02 retina, rhodopsin staining was absent and PNA labeled what appeared to be truncated cone outer segments in the photoreceptor layer (Figure 9b). The fluorescence data corroborate the histopathology and OCT findings.

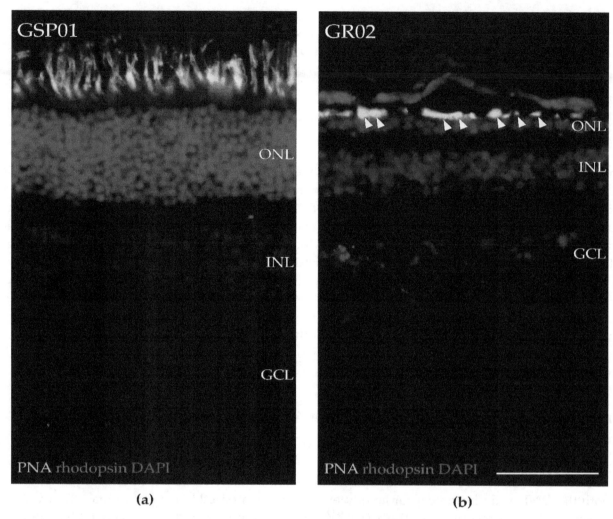

Figure 9. Fluorescence histochemistry of dog retinas for rhodopsin and cone photoreceptors. Fluorescence micrograph showing rhodopsin expression (red), Alexa™ 488-conjugated PNA (green), and DAPI (blue) in (**a**) a male, unaffected, 10-year-old German spaniel (GSP01) and (**b**) a female, affected, 6-year-old golden retriever (GR02). Note the thin ONL, lack of rhodopsin staining, and the truncated cone outer segments (exemplified with arrowheads) in the retina of the affected compared that of the unaffected dog. PNA: peanut agglutinin, ONL: outer nuclear layer, INL: inner nuclear layer, GCL: ganglion cell layer. Scale bar: 50 μm and applies to both images.

4. Discussion

When the deletion at the *TTC8* locus (*TTC8*^{delA}) in golden retrievers was discovered in 2014, there were indications that the mutation did not only lead to progressive retinal degeneration in the affected dogs, but could also cause additional clinical signs, suggesting a syndromic type of disease [1]. However, at the time, no cases were available for a thorough clinical examination apart from ophthalmoscopy, and no tissue samples could be collected. With the increasing number of genetically affected dogs detected by DNA-testing, we were able to continue the questionnaires and interviews initiated by Downs et al. The results strengthened the view that the disease in golden retrievers (generally referred to as GR_PRA2) may indeed be similar to Bardet–Biedl syndrome (BBS) in humans. To diagnose BBS patients correctly is often challenging due to the heterogeneity of the disease with symptoms that vary even between individuals within families carrying identical mutations. In addition, the symptoms overlap with other diseases, such as Laurence–Moon syndrome, which may in fact, to some extent be considered a variation of the same condition [69]. Polydactyly or similar congenital digit abnormalities can be cues in the search for a correct diagnosis. In the absence of digit malformations, the relatively early onset of retinal degeneration [6,7], can guide clinicians towards a BBS diagnosis. Both polydactyly and retinal degeneration are primary characteristics of BBS, as well as obesity, kidney abnormalities, cognitive impairment, hypogonadism in males, and genital abnormalities in females [7]. To date, 15 mutations in the human *TTC8* gene have been reported to cause BBS [2,17,70–76] (Table S6; Figure 7b). These mutations include six intronic splice-site variants, as well as three exonic splice-site variants (one missense, one nonsense, and one silent mutation). In addition, the identified mutations include three frameshift insertions/deletions, one complex variant, one nonsense variant, and one non-frameshift deletion in the coding sequence. Moreover, one *TTC8* splice-site variant has been associated with non-syndromic RP in humans [24]. Interestingly, one of the exonic splice-site variants (NM_144596.3: c.1347G>C; p.Gln449His) has been reported to cause both non-syndromic RP [77] and BBS [70], suggesting that the genetic background of each patient may play a significant role in the development of BBS symptoms in humans. Similar to humans, the genetic background is also likely to result in the heterogeneous clinical signs in dogs (Table S2).

All the dogs in this study were diagnosed with PRA initially causing visual problems in dim light, later also under daylight conditions and eventually causing blindness. This is consistent with BBS, where rod-cone dystrophy is the most frequently observed clinical sign, diagnosed in about 93% of the patients with approximately three out of four becoming legally blind by the second to third decade of life [6,7]. FERGs from the middle-aged female dog (GR02) showed bilateral loss of rod function, as well as profoundly subnormal and delayed cone-amplitudes, supporting a diffuse rod-cone degeneration (Figure 3). This is similar to human patients with *TTC8* mutations, where loss of rod and cone function has been reported [24,72,77]. Early in the course of the disease, human BBS patients may have cone flicker responses with marked delays and near normal amplitudes that deteriorate over time [78]. *Ttc8*-knockout mouse models show both reduced rod and cone ERGs at an early age [79]. Interestingly, the mouse models also demonstrate that cone structure, function, and viability depend on the normal expression of *Ttc8*. Loss of the TTC8 protein results in shortened and disorganized photoreceptor outer segments already before retinal maturation, as early as post-natal day 10 in *Ttc8*-knockout mice [79]. The lack of rhodopsin staining, and the appearance of truncated cone outer segments observed in the retina of the affected female using fluorescence histochemistry (Figure 9), suggests that the deletion at the *TTC8* gene (*TTC8*^{delA}) eventually results in a photoreceptor phenotype similar to the *Ttc8*-knockout mice. Taken together, the progressive reduction of cone photoreceptors and concomitant decline of cone ERGs may not only be secondary to degeneration of rods, as the TTC8 protein appears to be essential for normal cone function.

We were able to investigate the retina of the affected female using OCT, and considerable outer retinal thinning was observed (Figure 2), corroborating the results from ERG and postmortem findings. The abnormal appearance and thinning of the INL was judged as secondary to the photoreceptor degeneration. OCT-scans from the ventral (inferior) retina showed a more patchy degeneration with irregular RPE lining, also reported in some human patients with BBS [80], and clusters of nuclei in the ONL. Accumulation of lipofuscin, most clearly seen as increased autofluorescence in the non-tapetal fundus (Figure 1) has also been reported in human patients with BBS. However, the precise distribution of lipofuscin in the canine fundus is difficult to determine on cSLO because of the tapetal reflection in this species.

In addition to retinal degeneration, both the clinically investigated siblings, as well as three other affected dogs, were diagnosed with cataracts, a common secondary characteristic in human BBS [78]. In contrast to the posterior polar cataracts typically seen in human patients, both the affected male and the female developed cataracts that rather rapidly spread in the posterior, equatorial, and anterior cortices. The cataracts contributed to the dogs' visual impairment. The prevalence of posterior polar cataracts in human BBS has been reported to be similar in patients with different genotypes, although none of the patients studied was homozygous for pathogenic mutations in the *TTC8* gene [81]. We cannot exclude that the cataracts of the affected dogs were secondary to the retinal degeneration, because secondary cataracts are frequently seen in late-stage hereditary photoreceptor degenerations

(PRA) in dogs [82]. Toxic dialdehydes from decaying photoreceptors have been proposed to induce cataract formation [83] and the location of the cataractous changes in GR01 and GR02 in the more metabolically active equatorial and cortical regions of the lenses may also suggest a toxic effect on the lens. However, the cataracts in the golden retriever sib-pair were observed already at the initial examination when the degeneration of the retinae was judged as moderately advanced.

The affected male was also diagnosed with iridociliary cysts (Figure 4a). Iridociliary cysts have previously been reported in golden retrievers with glaucoma [84] and retinal detachments, but have not been associated with progressive retinal degenerations. Our observation of iridociliary cysts in the affected male is most likely a coincidental finding, but could possibly be a result of the deletion at the TTC8 gene and a consequence of abnormal ciliary trafficking.

When Ansley et al. identified TTC8 as a novel BBS gene in 2003 [2], situs inversus was observed in one of the patients with a TTC8 splice-site mutation. This led to the important conclusion that BBS is a disease caused by ciliary dysfunction. The TTC8 protein is part of the BBSome, an octameric protein complex which functions in the exit of activated G protein–coupled receptors (GPCRs) from cilia [19,85,86]. Thus, the underlying cause of the syndrome is malfunction of primary cilia, an organelle emanating from the cell surface of most mammalian cell types during growth arrest [87]. Primary cilia function in cell signaling during development and in homeostasis, thus explaining the multitude of organs affected in each BBS patient and the repertoire of different symptoms experienced. Nodal cilia, a type of motile primary cilia transiently present during embryonal development, are crucial for breaking the left-right symmetry during the embryogenesis, and defects in this process may cause different forms of heterotaxy such as partial or total situs inversus, as well as congenital heart defects [88,89]. Manifestation of situs inversus and other forms of heterotaxy is rare in the general population (1/10,000). However, in a study of 368 participants in the Clinical Registry Investigating Bardet–Biedl Syndrome (CRIBBS), six patients (1.6%) were found to have disorders of asymmetry, suggesting a 170-fold increase compared to the general population [90]. Cardiovascular diseases and congenital heart defects have also been reported for human BBS patients [7,91]. Of the 19 patients with TTC8 mutations (Table S6), 3 were diagnosed with hypertension or haemophilia [2,72,76]. We therefore investigated the cardiac status of the two affected golden retrievers. Both dogs showed normal cardiac morphology, dimensions and motion, and a normal left-right body axis. In the postmortem gross examination, a mild myxomatous valvular degeneration was seen in the heart tissue of the affected male. While the finding is common in dogs [92], it has recently been shown that defects of the primary cilia in the extra-cellular matrix can lead to myxomatous mitral valve disease in humans and mice [93].

Hypogonadism in males and genital abnormalities in females are considered primary characteristics of human BBS [6,7]. Hypogonadism was also common for the male patients with TTC8 mutations (Table S6). The affected the males had a low total sperm count and a high number of abnormal sperm cells, mainly lacking flagellum or having other tail-defects, indicating infertility (Figure 5a). He did not display any interest in the female dog in heat at the time of sampling. The histopathological examination of the testes revealed only a few elongated spermatids (Figure 5b). Severe sperm defects, including tail abnormalities as well as a low total sperm count, have previously been reported in Hungarian Puli dogs with a loss-of-function mutation in the Bardet–Biedl syndrome 4 (BBS4) gene [94]. The importance of BBS-genes for the normal formation of flagella in spermatogenesis has further been shown in mouse models. Genetically modified mice for any of the genes Bbs1 [95], Bbs2 [96], Bbs3 (Arl6) [97], Bbs4 [98], Bbs6 (Mkks) [99], or Bbs7 [100], result in failure to form normal flagella. In a Bbs8-knockout mouse model, the sperm defects were not described, but the males were found to be infertile [79].

Interestingly, many of these mouse models, including the Ttc8 knockout mouse [101], also showed partial or complete anosmia. This is a secondary characteristic experienced by many BBS patients in general [102], but it was not reported for the 19 human patients with TTC8 mutations. This is in contrast with the present study, where most of the owners of the affected dogs (8/10) reported their dogs having poor or gradually worsening sense of smell (Table S2). This appear to be a characteristic that is shared between dogs and mice, but not with humans. Moreover, as was the case for the dogs, none of the mouse models exhibited polydactyly, and the phenotype of dogs may therefore resemble the mouse phenotype more closely than that of human patients with *TTC8* mutations.

Obesity was reported for 16 of the 19 human patients. Although we did not formally investigate the body condition score for more than two dogs, the majority of them appeared overweight or heavy according to the owners (Table S2). It should, however, be noted that we have not compared this to the general golden retriever population. Similar to the two golden retriever siblings in this study, dental anomalies were reported for one human patient with a *TTC8* splice-site mutation [76] and for 27% of the BBS patients in general [7].

The histopathological changes in the right kidney of the affected male were most similar to a renal dysplasia-like lesion (Figure 6). The female sibling had mild chronic bilateral glomerulonephritis, but such mild chronic inflammatory changes are an unspecific finding, which probably did not affect the animal clinically. In total, 4 of the 10 dogs included in this study had renal problems (Table S2), suggesting that, as in humans, mutations in the *TTC8* gene may result in variable renal phenotypes. Among the 10 golden retrievers included in this study (Table S2), 1 dog was reported to be euthanized due to kidney failure. Other reasons for euthanasia included gastrointestinal problems (2 dogs), as well as problems related to sensory deprivation (visual and olfactory impairments: 2 dogs) and neoplastic disease (1 dog). Interviews indicated a rather low average lifespan of the affected golden retrievers: 7 years and 8 months for the nine dogs in the questionnaires (one of the ten dogs is still alive as of preparing this manuscript, 5 years of age). Data from 1995–2002 show that almost 90% of golden retrievers survive to 8 years of age and more than 80% to the age of 10 [103]. The 1 bp deletion in the canine *TTC8* gene had detrimental effects on the dogs' health and longevity. In human BBS patients, kidney failure is a frequent cause of death and the average survival of the patients overall is substantially reduced [104]. Taken together, the deletion in the canine *TTC8* gene is associated with additional clinical features apart from PRA in the affected dogs, such as obesity, renal and genital anomalies, anosmia, short stature, and dental anomalies that are similar to human BBS.

The major isoforms of the TTC8 protein are predicted to consist of approximately 500 amino acid residues, and the exon-intron structure is well conserved between human, dog, and mouse. Two canine retinal transcripts were previously predicted to exist based on Sanger sequencing of cDNA by Downs et al (2014) [1], one with and one without the retinal specific exon termed 2a. The transcript with the retinal specific exon was originally reported in humans [24]. It was shown that an in-frame splice-site mutation leading to the skipping of exon 2a is sufficient to cause a non-syndromic retinal degeneration in humans. In mice, the retinal specific exon 2a was found to be exclusively expressed in the ocular tissue, having the highest expression in the outer segments (OS) of both rod and cone photoreceptor cells [24,105]. In addition to retinal photoreceptor cells, exon 2a has also been found expressed in pinealocytes of rat pineal gland, and it has been suggested that these two cell types have evolved from a common precursor photodetector cell [106]. In our study, we used Oxford Nanopore Sequencing Technology for long-read sequencing, capable of reading through full-length transcripts and therefore enhancing the detection of different splice sites. Notably, the data only gave support for three different transcripts expressed in the retinal tissue (Figure 7), while the Ensembl annotation (release 100) predicts the existence of seven canine transcripts, of which only one (ENSCAFT00000027700.5 corresponding to tr2) was identified in this study. The six additional Ensembl canine transcripts are either skipping exon(s): E5 (ENSCAFT00000043691.2), E6 (ENSCAFT00000050179.3), E5-6 (ENSCAFT00000093101.1), E2a-10 (ENSCAFT00000070341.1), E1-2a (ENSCAFT00000086744.1), or E1-5 (ENSCAFT00000087482.1). We found no evidence for the presence of these other transcripts in our data from the canine retina.

As expected, the tr2 transcript, which includes the retinal specific exon 2a, was found to be the most highly expressed of the three identified transcripts. We also identified a short transcript (tr1) without the retinal specific exon 2a, with low expression in the dog retina. In mice, despite having a lower expression than the retinal specific transcript, the short transcript lacking the exon 2a is expressed throughout the retinal cell layers and shows the highest expression in the RPE [24]. The retinal samples investigated in this study did not exclusively include photoreceptor cells, but also consisted of other neural cells and RPE cells (Figure 8), which likely express the short transcript tr1. In addition to these two previously identified canine retinal transcripts, we also found evidence for a third transcript (tr3) including both exon 2a as well as a short exon with 22 nucleotides, here denoted 1b. A transcript similar to tr3 is also reported in GenBank (XM_014115661.2), likely annotated by an ab initio prediction detecting an open reading frame of sufficient length, but likely without supporting alignment (The NCBI Eukaryotic Genome Annotation Pipeline; A translation initiation site (TIS) with an optimal Kozak consensus sequence was identified in exon 1, but in tr3 this would extend an ORF of 147 nucleotides over the exons 1b and 2a, and reach a stop codon in exon 2 (Figure 7). This short transcript would likely be degraded by nonsense-mediated decay (NMD) [107]. If an alternative TIS was used in exon 2, tr3 would be in-frame with the other transcripts and produce a protein product of 455 amino acid residues featuring the complete TPR motif, which is involved in protein-protein interaction [108]. It is yet to be defined if this transcript is translated into a protein product, and if its expression is tissue specific.

The expression levels for all three *TTC8* transcripts found in this study were markedly reduced in the affected female dog. This was seen in the quantification of the cDNA sequencing data (Figure 8a–c), but also by the lack of read coverage of transcripts mapping to the *TTC8* locus in the dog reference genome sequence when manually inspecting the data in IGV. The highest read depth in the locus was 13× (TPM = 16.8), while the read coverage for the two unaffected dogs (250–500×, TPM = 60.6 and 99.8, respectively) was clearly higher than in the affected female. The reads detected in the affected dog appeared to be only partly spliced and none of the reads reached full-length over all exons. The low levels of *TTC8* transcripts in the affected dog was further supported by RT-qPCR (Figure 8d). The data suggested that the deletion in exon 7 (*TTC8*^{delA}) and the subsequent premature stop codon in exon 8 lead to degradation of the *TTC8* transcripts in the affected individual. To estimate the cell type constitution of the samples, we also studied the expression levels of retinal marker genes in the affected female compared to the two unaffected female dogs. As suggested by the histological sectioning of the affected male retina (Figure S1) and the fluorescence histochemistry of the affected female (Figure 9), the sequencing results showed a drastically lower expression of rod photoreceptor cell-specific genes, and cone photoreceptor cell marker expression was only one third compared to the levels detected in the two other dogs (Figure 8a–c, Table S4). The same pattern was observed in the RT-qPCR, where we quantified the relative expression of *RHO* and *OPN1LW* genes (Figure 8d). The retinal degeneration of both of these dogs (GR01 and GR02) was therefore likely advanced. BBSome deficiency has been shown to cause defects in the transport of phototransduction proteins between the inner and outer segments of the photoreceptors and, ultimately, these defects lead to photoreceptor cell death [96,109]. In addition to aberrant photoreceptor marker gene expression, our data also suggested that the expression of macroglial genes (Müller glia and astrocytes) was higher in the affected dog (Figure 8), most notably clusterin (*CLU*) and glial fibrillary acidic protein (*GFAP*) expression (Table S4), both of which are known to be upregulated under retinal stress and retinal degeneration [110–113].

5. Conclusions

The *TTC8* gene encodes for one of the proteins forming the BBSome, and has in humans been implicated in Bardet–Biedl syndrome (BBS). Long-read cDNA sequencing of non-affected dogs suggested the expression of three retinal *TTC8* transcripts and that the 1 bp deletion is a loss-of-function mutation. Golden retriever dogs homozygous for the deletion develop an autosomal recessive form of RP-like retinal degeneration (PRA), but it has hitherto been unclear if the affected dogs develop a non-syndromic PRA or a syndromic ciliopathy similar to human BBS. In addition to PRA, we have shown that the loss-of-function mutation indeed causes additional clinical features, such as obesity, renal and genital anomalies, anosmia, short stature, and dental anomalies. We therefore conclude that the deletion can result in a canine form of BBS. As in humans, BBS in dogs appear to be a heterogeneous disorder with variable severity of clinical and morphological signs. A canine model for BBS may be of importance for novel therapeutic management of human patients. Canine models have successfully been used to establish protocols for gene therapy of other inherited retinal diseases, and a *TTC8*-dog model could potentially be developed to restore vision and improve the quality of life for BBS patients.

Author Contributions: Conceptualization, S.M. and T.F.B.; methodology, S.M., M.H., A.D.v.d.H., E.A., E.T., B.S.H., J.H., I.L., C.M., F.H., G.A., B.E. and T.F.B.; software, S.M.; validation, S.M. and A.D.v.d.H.; formal analysis, S.M., M.H., A.D.v.d.H., E.A., E.T., B.S.H., B.E. and T.F.B.; investigation, S.M., M.H., A.D.v.d.H., E.A., E.T., B.S.H., J.H., I.L., C.M., F.H., G.A., B.E. and T.F.B.; resources, S.M., M.H., E.A., E.T., B.S.H., J.H., I.L., F.H., G.A., B.E. and T.F.B.; data curation, S.M., M.H., E.A., E.T., B.S.H., J.H., I.L., F.H., G.A., B.E. and T.F.B.; writing—original draft preparation, S.M. and T.F.B.; writing—review and editing, S.M., M.H., A.D., V.D.v.d.H., E.A., E.T., B.S.H., J.H., I.L., C.M., F.H., G.A., B.E. and T.F.B.; visualization, S.M., M.H., A.D.v.d.H., E.A., E.T., B.S.H., F.H., B.E. and T.F.B.; supervision, C.M., F.H., G.A., B.E. and T.B.; project administration, G.A. and T.F.B.; funding acquisition, G.A. and T.F.B. All authors have read and agreed to the published version of the manuscript.

Acknowledgments: The authors would like to acknowledge the support of the National Genomics Infrastructure (NGI)/Uppsala Genome Center and UPPMAX for providing computational infrastructure and the Swedish Bioinformatics Infrastructure Sweden at SciLifeLab for bioinformatics advice. We would also like to acknowledge Sofia Ryberg at the Department of Clinical Sciences, SLU for assisting in the ophthalmic examinations and support of the dedicated dog owners who allowed their dogs to take part in this study.

References

1. Downs, L.M.; Wallin-Håkansson, B.; Bergström, T.; Mellersh, C.S. A novel mutation in TTC8 is associated with progressive retinal atrophy in the golden retriever. *Canine Genet. Epidemiol.* **2014**, *1*, 4. [CrossRef] [PubMed]
2. Ansley, S.J.; Badano, J.L.; Blacque, O.E.; Hill, J.; Hoskins, B.E.; Leitch, C.C.; Kim, J.C.; Ross, A.J.; Eichers, E.R.; Teslovich, T.M.; et al. Basal body dysfunction is a likely cause of pleiotropic Bardet-Biedl syndrome. *Nature* **2003**, *425*, 628–633. [CrossRef] [PubMed]
3. Stone, E.M.; Andorf, J.L.; Whitmore, S.S.; DeLuca, A.P.; Giacalone, J.C.; Streb, L.M.; Braun, T.A.; Mullins, R.F.; Scheetz, T.E.; Sheffield, V.C.; et al. Clinically Focused Molecular Investigation of 1000 Consecutive Families with Inherited Retinal Disease. *Ophthalmology* **2017**, *124*, 1314–1331. [CrossRef] [PubMed]
4. Bardet, G. *Sur un Syndrome D'obesite Infantile avec Polydactylie et Retinite Pigmentaire (Contribution a L'etude des Formes Cliniques de L'obesite Hypophysaire)*; University of Paris: Paris, France, 1920.
5. Biedl, A. Ein Geschwisterpaar mit adiposo-genitaler Dystrophie. *Dtsch. Med. Wochenschr.* **1922**, *48*, 1630.
6. Forsythe, E.; Beales, P.L. Bardet-Biedl syndrome. *Eur. J. Hum. Genet.* **2013**, *21*, 8–13. [CrossRef]
7. Beales, P.L.; Elcioglu, N.; Woolf, A.S.; Parker, D.; Flinter, F.A. New criteria for improved diagnosis of Bardet-Biedl syndrome: Results of a population survey. *J. Med. Genet.* **1999**, *36*, 437–446.
8. Forsythe, E.; Beales, P.L. Bardet-Biedl Syndrome. In *GeneReviews((R))*; Adam, M.P., Ardinger, H.H., Pagon, R.A., Wallace, S.E., Bean, L.J.H., Stephens, K., Amemiya, A., Eds.; University of Washington: Seattle, WA, USA, 1993.
9. Niederlova, V.; Modrak, M.; Tsyklauri, O.; Huranova, M.; Stepanek, O. Meta-analysis of genotype-phenotype associations in Bardet-Biedl syndrome uncovers differences among causative genes. *Hum. Mutat* **2019**, *40*, 2068–2087. [CrossRef]
10. Wormser, O.; Gradstein, L.; Yogev, Y.; Perez, Y.; Kadir, R.; Goliand, I.; Sadka, Y.; El Riati, S.; Flusser, H.; Nachmias, D.; et al. SCAPER localizes to primary cilia and its mutation affects cilia length, causing Bardet-Biedl syndrome. *Eur. J. Hum. Genet.* **2019**, *27*, 928–940. [CrossRef]
11. Forsythe, E.; Kenny, J.; Bacchelli, C.; Beales, P.L. Managing Bardet-Biedl Syndrome-Now and in the Future. *Front. Pediatr.* **2018**, *6*, 23. [CrossRef]
12. Lindstrand, A.; Davis, E.E.; Carvalho, C.M.; Pehlivan, D.; Willer, J.R.; Tsai, I.C.; Ramanathan, S.; Zuppan, C.; Sabo, A.; Muzny, D.; et al. Recurrent CNVs and SNVs at the NPHP1 Locus Contribute Pathogenic Alleles to Bardet-Biedl Syndrome. *Am. J. Hum. Genet.* **2014**, *94*, 745–754. [CrossRef]
13. Lindstrand, A.; Frangakis, S.; Carvalho, C.M.; Richardson, E.B.; McFadden, K.A.; Willer, J.R.; Pehlivan, D.; Liu, P.; Pediaditakis, I.L.; Sabo, A.; et al. Copy-Number Variation Contributes to the Mutational Load of Bardet-Biedl Syndrome. *Am. J. Hum. Genet.* **2016**, *99*, 318–336. [CrossRef] [PubMed]
14. Stoetzel, C.; Laurier, V.; Davis, E.E.; Muller, J.; Rix, S.; Badano, J.L.; Leitch, C.C.; Salem, N.; Chouery, E.; Corbani, S.; et al. BBS10 encodes a vertebrate-specific chaperonin-like protein and is a major BBS locus. *Nat. Genet.* **2006**, *38*, 521–524. [CrossRef] [PubMed]

15. Katsanis, N. The oligogenic properties of Bardet–Biedl syndrome. *Hum. Mol. Genet.* **2004**, *13*, R65–R71. [CrossRef] [PubMed]

16. Mykytyn, K.; Nishimura, D.Y.; Searby, C.C.; Shastri, M.; Yen, H.J.; Beck, J.S.; Braun, T.; Streb, L.M.; Cornier, A.S.; Cox, G.F.; et al. Identification of the gene (BBS1) most commonly involved in Bardet-Biedl syndrome, a complex human obesity syndrome. *Nat. Genet.* **2002**, *31*, 435–438. [CrossRef] [PubMed]

17. Stoetzel, C.; Laurier, V.; Faivre, L.; Megarbane, A.; Perrin-Schmitt, F.; Verloes, A.; Bonneau, D.; Mandel, J.L.; Cossee, M.; Dollfus, H. BBS8 is rarely mutated in a cohort of 128 Bardet-Biedl syndrome families. *J. Hum. Genet.* **2006**, *51*, 81–84. [CrossRef] [PubMed]

18. Loktev, A.V.; Zhang, Q.; Beck, J.S.; Searby, C.C.; Scheetz, T.E.; Bazan, J.F.; Slusarski, D.C.; Sheffield, V.C.; Jackson, P.K.; Nachury, M.V. A BBSome subunit links ciliogenesis, microtubule stability, and acetylation. *Dev. Cell* **2008**, *15*, 854–865. [CrossRef]

19. Nachury, M.V.; Loktev, A.V.; Zhang, Q.; Westlake, C.J.; Peranen, J.; Merdes, A.; Slusarski, D.C.; Scheller, R.H.; Bazan, J.F.; Sheffield, V.C.; et al. A core complex of BBS proteins cooperates with the GTPase Rab8 to promote ciliary membrane biogenesis. *Cell* **2007**, *129*, 1201–1213. [CrossRef]

20. Jin, H.; White, S.R.; Shida, T.; Schulz, S.; Aguiar, M.; Gygi, S.P.; Bazan, J.F.; Nachury, M.V. The conserved Bardet-Biedl syndrome proteins assemble a coat that traffics membrane proteins to cilia. *Cell* **2010**, *141*, 1208–1219. [CrossRef]

21. Pretorius, P.R.; Baye, L.M.; Nishimura, D.Y.; Searby, C.C.; Bugge, K.; Yang, B.; Mullins, R.F.; Stone, E.M.; Sheffield, V.C.; Slusarski, D.C. Identification and functional analysis of the vision-specific BBS3 (ARL6) long isoform. *PLoS Genet.* **2010**, *6*, e1000884. [CrossRef]

22. Estrada-Cuzcano, A.; Koenekoop, R.K.; Senechal, A.; De Baere, E.B.W.; de Ravel, T.; Banfi, S.; Kohl, S.; Ayuso, C.; Sharon, D.; Hoyng, C.B.; et al. BBS1 Mutations in a Wide Spectrum of Phenotypes Ranging From Nonsyndromic Retinitis Pigmentosa to Bardet-Biedl Syndrome. *Arch. Ophthalmol.* **2012**, *130*, 1425–1432. [CrossRef]

23. Shevach, E.; Ali, M.; Mizrahi-Meissonnier, L.; McKibbin, M.; El-Asrag, M.; Watson, C.M.; Inglehearn, C.F.; Ben-Yosef, T.; Blumenfeld, A.; Jalas, C.; et al. Association Between Missense Mutations in the BBS2 Gene and Nonsyndromic Retinitis Pigmentosa. *JAMA Ophthalmol.* **2015**, *133*, 312–318. [CrossRef]

24. Riazuddin, S.A.; Iqbal, M.; Wang, Y.; Masuda, T.; Chen, Y.; Bowne, S.; Sullivan, L.S.; Waseem, N.H.; Bhattacharya, S.; Daiger, S.P.; et al. A splice-site mutation in a retina-specific exon of BBS8 causes nonsyndromic retinitis pigmentosa. *Am. J. Hum. Genet.* **2010**, *86*, 805–812. [CrossRef]

25. Ofri, R.; Ekesten, B. Baseline retinal OCT measurements in normal female beagles: The effects of eccentricity, meridian, and age on retinal layer thickness. *Vet. Ophthalmol.* **2020**, *23*, 52–60. [CrossRef] [PubMed]

26. Karlstam, L.; Hertil, E.; Zeiss, C.; Ropstad, E.O.; Bjerkås, E.; Dubielzig, R.R.; Ekesten, B. A slowly progressive retinopathy in the Shetland Sheepdog. *Vet. Ophthalmol.* **2011**, *14*, 227–238. [CrossRef] [PubMed]

27. Ekesten, B.; Komáromy, A.M.; Ofri, R.; Petersen-Jones, S.M.; Narfström, K. Guidelines for clinical electroretinography in the dog: 2012 update. *Doc. Ophthalmol.* **2013**, *127*, 79–87. [CrossRef] [PubMed]

28. Bane, A. Acrosomal abnormality associated with sterility in a boar. In Proceedings of the 4th International Congress of Animal Reproductives, The Hague, The Netherlands, 5–9 June 1961; pp. 810–817.

29. Thomas, W.P.; Gaber, C.E.; Jacobs, G.J.; Kaplan, P.M.; Lombard, C.W.; Moise, N.S.; Moses, B.L. Recommendations for standards in transthoracic two-dimensional echocardiography in the dog and cat. Echocardiography Committee of the Specialty of Cardiology, American College of Veterinary Internal Medicine. *J. Vet. Intern. Med.* **1993**, *7*, 247–252. [CrossRef]

30. Cornell, C.C.; Kittleson, M.D.; Della Torre, P.; Haggstrom, J.; Lombard, C.W.; Pedersen, H.D.; Vollmar, A.; Wey, A. Allometric scaling of M-mode cardiac measurements in normal adult dogs. *J. Vet. Intern. Med.* **2004**, *18*, 311–321. [CrossRef]

31. Hansson, K.; Haggstrom, J.; Kvart, C.; Lord, P. Left atrial to aortic root indices using two-dimensional and M-mode echocardiography in cavalier King Charles spaniels with and without left atrial enlargement. *Vet. Radiol. Ultrasound Off. J. Am. Coll. Vet. Radiol. Int. Vet. Radiol. Assoc.* **2002**, *43*, 568–575. [CrossRef]

32. Li, H. Minimap2: Pairwise alignment for nucleotide sequences. *Bioinformatics* **2018**, *34*, 3094–3100. [CrossRef]

33. Kovaka, S.; Zimin, A.V.; Pertea, G.M.; Razaghi, R.; Salzberg, S.L.; Pertea, M. Transcriptome assembly from long-read RNA-seq alignments with StringTie2. *Genome Biol.* **2019**, *20*, 278. [CrossRef]

34. Robinson, J.T.; Thorvaldsdóttir, H.; Winckler, W.; Guttman, M.; Lander, E.S.; Getz, G.; Mesirov, J.P. Integrative genomics viewer. *Nat. Biotechnol* **2011**, *29*, 24–26. [CrossRef] [PubMed]

35. Thorvaldsdóttir, H.; Robinson, J.T.; Mesirov, J.P. Integrative Genomics Viewer (IGV): High-performance genomics data visualization and exploration. *Brief. Bioinform.* **2013**, *14*, 178–192. [CrossRef]

36. Patro, R.; Duggal, G.; Love, M.I.; Irizarry, R.A.; Kingsford, C. Salmon provides fast and bias-aware quantification of transcript expression. *Nat. Methods* **2017**, *14*, 417–419. [CrossRef] [PubMed]

37. Kim, S.; Lowe, A.; Dharmat, R.; Lee, S.; Owen, L.A.; Wang, J.; Shakoor, A.; Li, Y.; Morgan, D.J.; Hejazi, A.A.; et al. Generation, transcriptome profiling, and functional validation of cone-rich human retinal organoids. *Proc. Natl. Acad. Sci. USA* **2019**, *116*, 10824–10833. [CrossRef] [PubMed]

38. Kohl, S.; Coppieters, F.; Meire, F.; Schaich, S.; Roosing, S.; Brennenstuhl, C.; Bolz, S.; van Genderen, M.M.; Riemslag, F.C.; European Retinal Disease, C.; et al. A nonsense mutation in PDE6H causes autosomal-recessive incomplete achromatopsia. *Am. J. Hum. Genet.* **2012**, *91*, 527–532. [CrossRef] [PubMed]

39. Nordstrom, K.; Larsson, T.A.; Larhammar, D. Extensive duplications of phototransduction genes in early vertebrate evolution correlate with block (chromosome) duplications. *Genomics* **2004**, *83*, 852–872. [CrossRef]

40. Renninger, S.L.; Gesemann, M.; Neuhauss, S.C. Cone arrestin confers cone vision of high temporal resolution in zebrafish larvae. *Eur. J. Neurosci.* **2011**, *33*, 658–667. [CrossRef]

41. Terakita, A. The opsins. *Genome Biol.* **2005**, *6*, 213. [CrossRef]

42. Mowat, F.M.; Petersen-Jones, S.M.; Williamson, H.; Williams, D.L.; Luthert, P.J.; Ali, R.R.; Bainbridge, J.W. Topographical characterization of cone photoreceptors and the area centralis of the canine retina. *Mol. Vis.* **2008**, *14*, 2518–2527.

43. Kaewkhaw, R.; Kaya, K.D.; Brooks, M.; Homma, K.; Zou, J.; Chaitankar, V.; Rao, M.; Swaroop, A. Transcriptome Dynamics of Developing Photoreceptors in Three-Dimensional Retina Cultures Recapitulates Temporal Sequence of Human Cone and Rod Differentiation Revealing Cell Surface Markers and Gene Networks. *Stem Cells* **2015**, *33*, 3504–3518. [CrossRef]

44. Chen, H.; Weber, A.J. Expression of glial fibrillary acidic protein and glutamine synthetase by Muller cells after optic nerve damage and intravitreal application of brain-derived neurotrophic factor. *Glia* **2002**, *38*, 115–125. [CrossRef] [PubMed]

45. Rauen, T.; Taylor, W.R.; Kuhlbrodt, K.; Wiessner, M. High-affinity glutamate transporters in the rat retina: A major role of the glial glutamate transporter GLAST-1 in transmitter clearance. *Cell Tissue Res.* **1998**, *291*, 19–31. [CrossRef] [PubMed]

46. Roesch, K.; Jadhav, A.P.; Trimarchi, J.M.; Stadler, M.B.; Roska, B.; Sun, B.B.; Cepko, C.L. The transcriptome of retinal Muller glial cells. *J. Comp. Neurol.* **2008**, *509*, 225–238. [CrossRef] [PubMed]

47. Macosko, E.Z.; Basu, A.; Satija, R.; Nemesh, J.; Shekhar, K.; Goldman, M.; Tirosh, I.; Bialas, A.R.; Kamitaki, N.; Martersteck, E.M.; et al. Highly Parallel Genome-wide Expression Profiling of Individual Cells Using Nanoliter Droplets. *Cell* **2015**, *161*, 1202–1214. [CrossRef]

48. Siegert, S.; Cabuy, E.; Scherf, B.G.; Kohler, H.; Panda, S.; Le, Y.Z.; Fehling, H.J.; Gaidatzis, D.; Stadler, M.B.; Roska, B. Transcriptional code and disease map for adult retinal cell types. *Nat. Neurosci.* **2012**, *15*, 487–495. [CrossRef]

49. Barnstable, C.J.; Drager, U.C. Thy-1 antigen: A ganglion cell specific marker in rodent retina. *Neuroscience* **1984**, *11*, 847–855. [CrossRef]

50. Erkman, L.; McEvilly, R.J.; Luo, L.; Ryan, A.K.; Hooshmand, F.; O'Connell, S.M.; Keithley, E.M.; Rapaport, D.H.; Ryan, A.F.; Rosenfeld, M.G. Role of transcription factors Brn-3.1 and Brn-3.2 in auditory and visual system development. *Nature* **1996**, *381*, 603–606. [CrossRef]

51. Fremeau, R.T., Jr.; Voglmaier, S.; Seal, R.P.; Edwards, R.H. VGLUTs define subsets of excitatory neurons and suggest novel roles for glutamate. *Trends Neurosci.* **2004**, *27*, 98–103. [CrossRef]

52. Huang, W.; Fileta, J.; Guo, Y.; Grosskreutz, C.L. Downregulation of Thy1 in retinal ganglion cells in experimental glaucoma. *Curr. Eye Res.* **2006**, *31*, 265–271. [CrossRef]

53. Rodriguez, A.R.; de Sevilla Muller, L.P.; Brecha, N.C. The RNA binding protein RBPMS is a selective marker of ganglion cells in the mammalian retina. *J. Comp. Neurol.* **2014**, *522*, 1411–1443. [CrossRef]

54. Ruiz-Ederra, J.; Garcia, M.; Hicks, D.; Vecino, E. Comparative study of the three neurofilament subunits within pig and human retinal ganglion cells. *Mol. Vis.* **2004**, *10*, 83–92. [PubMed]

55. Carr, A.J.; Vugler, A.A.; Yu, L.; Semo, M.; Coffey, P.; Moss, S.E.; Greenwood, J. The expression of retinal cell markers in human retinal pigment epithelial cells and their augmentation by the synthetic retinoid fenretinide. *Mol. Vis.* **2011** *17*, 1701–1715. [PubMed]

56. Cherry, T.J.; Trimarchi, J.M.; Stadler, M.B.; Cepko, C.L. Development and diversification of retinal amacrine interneurons at single cell resolution. *Proc. Natl. Acad. Sci. USA* **2009**, *106*, 9495–9500. [CrossRef] [PubMed]

57. Shekhar, K.; Lapan, S.W.; Whitney, I.E.; Tran, N.M.; Macosko, E.Z.; Kowalczyk, M.; Adiconis, X.; Levin, J.Z.; Nemesh, J.; Goldman, M.; et al. Comprehensive Classification of Retinal Bipolar Neurons by Single-Cell Transcriptomics. *Cell* **2016**, *166*, 1308–1323 e1330. [CrossRef]

58. Untergasser, A.; Cutcutache, I.; Koressaar, T.; Ye, J.; Faircloth, B.C.; Remm, M.; Rozen, S.G. Primer3—New capabilities and interfaces. *Nucleic Acids Res.* **2012**, *40*, e115. [CrossRef]

59. Koressaar, T.; Remm, M. Enhancements and modifications of primer design program Primer3. *Bioinformatics* **2007**, *23*, 1289–1291. [CrossRef]

60. Blom, E. A new sterilizing and hereditary defect (the "Dag defect") located in the bull sperm tail. *Nature* **1966**, *209*, 739–740. [CrossRef]

61. Laflamme, D. Development and validation of a body condition score system for dogs. *Canine Pract.* **1997**, *22*, 10–15.

62. Kozak, M. An analysis of vertebrate mRNA sequences: Intimations of translational control. *J. Cell Biol.* **1991**, *115*, 887–903. [CrossRef]

63. Hernández, G.; Osnaya, V.G.; Pérez-Martínez, X. Conservation and Variability of the AUG Initiation Codon Context in Eukaryotes. *Trends Biochem. Sci.* **2019**, *44*, 1009–1021. [CrossRef]

64. Chakraborty, D.; Conley, S.M.; Pittler, S.J.; Naash, M.I. Role of RDS and Rhodopsin in Cngb1-Related Retinal Degeneration. *Investig. Ophthalmol. Vis. Sci.* **2016**, *57*, 787–797. [CrossRef] [PubMed]

65. Downes, G.B.; Gautam, N. The G protein subunit gene families. *Genomics* **1999**, *62*, 544–552. [CrossRef] [PubMed]

66. Winkler, P.A.; Ekenstedt, K.J.; Occelli, L.M.; Frattaroli, A.V.; Bartoe, J.T.; Venta, P.J.; Petersen-Jones, S.M. A large animal model for CNGB1 autosomal recessive retinitis pigmentosa. *PLoS ONE* **2013**, *8*, e72229. [CrossRef] [PubMed]

67. Jain, V.; Ravindran, E.; Dhingra, N.K. Differential expression of Brn3 transcription factors in intrinsically photosensitive retinal ganglion cells in mouse. *J. Comp. Neurol.* **2012**, *520*, 742–755. [CrossRef]

68. Damiani, D.; Alexander, J.J.; O'Rourke, J.R.; McManus, M.; Jadhav, A.P.; Cepko, C.L.; Hauswirth, W.W.; Harfe, B.D.; Strettoi, E. Dicer inactivation leads to progressive functional and structural degeneration of the mouse retina. *J. Neurosci.* **2008**, *28*, 4878–4887. [CrossRef]

69. Moore, S.J.; Green, J.S.; Fan, Y.; Bhogal, A.K.; Dicks, E.; Fernandez, B.A.; Stefanelli, M.; Murphy, C.; Cramer, B.C.; Dean, J.C.; et al. Clinical and genetic epidemiology of Bardet-Biedl syndrome in Newfoundland: A 22-year prospective, population-based, cohort study. *Am. J. Med. Genet. A* **2005**, *132A*, 352–360. [CrossRef]

70. Ullah, A.; Umair, M.; Yousaf, M.; Khan, S.A.; Nazim-Ud-Din, M.; Shah, K.; Ahmad, F.; Azeem, Z.; Ali, G.; Alhaddad, B.; et al. Sequence variants in four genes underlying Bardet-Biedl syndrome in consanguineous families. *Mol. Vis.* **2017**, *23*, 482–494.

71. Smaoui, N.; Chaabouni, M.; Sergeev, Y.V.; Kallel, H.; Li, S.; Mahfoudh, N.; Maazoul, F.; Kammoun, H.; Gandoura, N.; Bouaziz, A.; et al. Screening of the eight BBS genes in Tunisian families: No evidence of triallelism. *Investig. Ophthalmol. Vis. Sci.* **2006**, *47*, 3487–3495. [CrossRef]

72. Sato, S.; Morimoto, T.; Hotta, K.; Fujikado, T.; Nishida, K. A novel compound heterozygous mutation in TTC8 identified in a Japanese patient. *Hum. Genome Var.* **2019**, *6*, 14. [CrossRef]

73. Janssen, S.; Ramaswami, G.; Davis, E.E.; Hurd, T.; Airik, R.; Kasanuki, J.M.; Van Der Kraak, L.; Allen, S.J.; Beales, P.L.; Katsanis, N.; et al. Mutation analysis in Bardet-Biedl syndrome by DNA pooling and massively parallel resequencing in 105 individuals. *Hum. Genet.* **2011**, *129*, 79–90. [CrossRef]

74. Redin, C.; Le Gras, S.; Mhamdi, O.; Geoffroy, V.; Stoetzel, C.; Vincent, M.C.; Chiurazzi, P.; Lacombe, D.; Ouertani, I.; Petit, F.; et al. Targeted high-throughput sequencing for diagnosis of genetically heterogeneous diseases: Efficient mutation detection in Bardet-Biedl and Alström syndromes. *J. Med. Genet.* **2012**, *49*, 502–512. [CrossRef] [PubMed]

75. Harville, H.M.; Held, S.; Diaz-Font, A.; Davis, E.E.; Diplas, B.H.; Lewis, R.A.; Borochowitz, Z.U.; Zhou, W.; Chaki, M.; MacDonald, J.; et al. Identification of 11 novel mutations in eight BBS genes by high-resolution homozygosity mapping. *J. Med. Genet.* **2010**, *47*, 262–267. [CrossRef] [PubMed]

76. M'Hamdi, O.; Redin, C.; Stoetzel, C.; Ouertani, I.; Chaabouni, M.; Maazoul, F.; M'Rad, R.; Mandel, J.L.; Dollfus, H.; Muller, J.; et al. Clinical and genetic characterization of Bardet-Biedl syndrome in Tunisia: Defining a strategy for molecular diagnosis. *Clin. Genet.* **2014**, *85*, 172–177. [CrossRef] [PubMed]

77. Goyal, S.; Jager, M.; Robinson, P.N.; Vanita, V. Confirmation of TTC8 as a disease gene for nonsyndromic autosomal recessive retinitis pigmentosa (RP51). *Clin. Genet.* **2016**, *89*, 454–460. [CrossRef] [PubMed]

78. Rizzo, J.F., III; Berson, E.L.; Lessell, S. Retinal and neurologic findings in the Laurence-Moon-Bardet-Biedl phenotype. *Ophthalmology* **1986**, *93*, 1452–1456. [CrossRef]

79. Dilan, T.L.; Singh, R.K.; Saravanan, T.; Moye, A.; Goldberg, A.F.X.; Stoilov, P.; Ramamurthy, V. Bardet-Biedl syndrome-8 (BBS8) protein is crucial for the development of outer segments in photoreceptor neurons. *Hum. Mol. Genet.* **2018**, *27*, 283–294. [CrossRef]

80. Bek, T.; Rosenberg, T. Clinical pathology and retinal vascular structure in the Bardet-Biedl syndrome. *Br. J. Ophthalmol.* **1995**, *79*, 76–80. [CrossRef]

81. Daniels, A.B.; Sandberg, M.A.; Chen, J.; Weigel-DiFranco, C.; Fielding Hejtmancic, J.; Berson, E.L. Genotype-phenotype correlations in Bardet-Biedl syndrome. *Arch. Ophthalmol.* **2012**, *130*, 901–907. [CrossRef]

82. Adkins, E.A.; Hendrix, D.V. Outcomes of dogs presented for cataract evaluation: A retrospective study. *J. Am. Anim. Hosp. Assoc.* **2005**, *41*, 235–240. [CrossRef]

83. Zigler, J.S., Jr.; Hess, H.H. Cataracts in the Royal College of Surgeons rat: Evidence for initiation by lipid peroxidation products. *Exp. Eye Res.* **1985**, *41*, 67–76. [CrossRef]

84. Deehr, A.J.; Dubielzig, R.R. A histopathological study of iridociliary cysts and glaucoma in Golden Retrievers. *Vet. Ophthalmol.* **1998**, *1*, 153–158. [CrossRef] [PubMed]

85. Nachury, M.V. The molecular machines that traffic signaling receptors into and out of cilia. *Curr. Opin. Cell Biol.* **2018**, *51*, 124–131. [CrossRef] [PubMed]

86. Ye, F.; Nager, A.R.; Nachury, M.V. BBSome trains remove activated GPCRs from cilia by enabling passage through the transition zone. *J. Cell Biol.* **2018**, *217*, 1847–1868. [CrossRef] [PubMed]

87. Satir, P.; Pedersen, L.B.; Christensen, S.T. The primary cilium at a glance. *J. Cell Sci.* **2010**, *123*, 499. [CrossRef]

88. Nonaka, S.; Shiratori, H.; Saijoh, Y.; Hamada, H. Determination of left-right patterning of the mouse embryo by artificial nodal flow. *Nature* **2002**, *418*, 96–99. [CrossRef]

89. Nonaka, S.; Tanaka, Y.; Okada, Y.; Takeda, S.; Harada, A.; Kanai, Y.; Kido, M.; Hirokawa, N. Randomization of left-right asymmetry due to loss of nodal cilia generating leftward flow of extraembryonic fluid in mice lacking KIF3B motor protein. *Cell* **1998**, *95*, 829–837. [CrossRef]

90. Olson, A.J.; Krentz, A.D.; Finta, K.M.; Okorie, U.C.; Haws, R.M. Thoraco-Abdominal Abnormalities in Bardet-Biedl Syndrome: Situs Inversus and Heterotaxy. *J. Pediatr.* **2019**, *204*, 31–37. [CrossRef]

91. Elbedour, K.; Zucker, N.; Zalzstein, E.; Barki, Y.; Carmi, R. Cardiac abnormalities in the Bardet-Biedl syndrome: Echocardiographic studies of 22 patients. *Am. J. Med. Genet.* **1994**, *52*, 164–169. [CrossRef]

92. Fox, P.R. Pathology of myxomatous mitral valve disease in the dog. *J. Vet. Cardiol.* **2012**, *14*, 103–126. [CrossRef]

93. Toomer, K.A.; Yu, M.; Fulmer, D.; Guo, L.; Moore, K.S.; Moore, R.; Drayton, K.D.; Glover, J.; Peterson, N.; Ramos-Ortiz, S.; et al. Primary cilia defects causing mitral valve prolapse. *Sci. Transl. Med.* **2019**, 11. [CrossRef]

94. Chew, T.; Haase, B.; Bathgate, R.; Willet, C.E.; Kaukonen, M.K.; Mascord, L.J.; Lohi, H.T.; Wade, C.M. A Coding Variant in the Gene Bardet-Biedl Syndrome 4 (BBS4) Is Associated with a Novel Form of Canine Progressive Retinal Atrophy. *G3* **2017**, *7*, 2327–2335. [CrossRef] [PubMed]

95. Davis, R.E.; Swiderski, R.E.; Rahmouni, K.; Nishimura, D.Y.; Mullins, R.F.; Agassandian, K.; Philp, A.R.; Searby, C.C.; Andrews, M.P.; Thompson, S.; et al. A knockin mouse model of the Bardet-Biedl syndrome 1 M390R mutation has cilia defects, ventriculomegaly, retinopathy, and obesity. *Proc. Natl. Acad. Sci. USA* **2007**, *104*, 19422–19427. [CrossRef] [PubMed]

96. Nishimura, D.Y.; Fath, M.; Mullins, R.F.; Searby, C.; Andrews, M.; Davis, R.; Andorf, J.L.; Mykytyn, K.; Swiderski, R.E.; Yang, B.; et al. Bbs2-null mice have neurosensory deficits, a defect in social dominance, and retinopathy associated with mislocalization of rhodopsin. *Proc. Natl. Acad. Sci. USA* **2004**, *101*, 16588–16593. [CrossRef]

97. Zhang, Q.; Nishimura, D.; Seo, S.; Vogel, T.; Morgan, D.A.; Searby, C.; Bugge, K.; Stone, E.M.; Rahmouni, K.; Sheffield, V.C. Bardet-Biedl syndrome 3 (Bbs3) knockout mouse model reveals common BBS-associated phenotypes and Bbs3 unique phenotypes. *Proc. Natl. Acad. Sci. USA* **2011**, *108*, 20678–20683. [CrossRef] [PubMed]

98. Mykytyn, K.; Mullins, R.F.; Andrews, M.; Chiang, A.P.; Swiderski, R.E.; Yang, B.; Braun, T.; Casavant, T.; Stone, E.M.; Sheffield, V.C. Bardet-Biedl syndrome type 4 (BBS4)-null mice implicate Bbs4 in flagella formation but not global cilia assembly. *Proc. Natl. Acad. Sci. USA* **2004**, *101*, 8664–8669. [CrossRef]

99.   Fath, M.A.; Mullins, R.F.; Searby, C.; Nishimura, D.Y.; Wei, J.; Rahmouni, K.; Davis, R.E.; Tayeh, M.K.; Andrews, M.; Yang, B.; et al. Mkks-null mice have a phenotype resembling Bardet-Biedl syndrome. *Hum. Mol. Genet.* **2005**, *14*, 1109–1118. [CrossRef]

100. Zhang, Q.; Nishimura, D.; Vogel, T.; Shao, J.; Swiderski, R.; Yin, T.; Searby, C.; Carter, C.S.; Kim, G.; Bugge, K.; et al. BBS7 is required for BBSome formation and its absence in mice results in Bardet-Biedl syndrome phenotypes and selective abnormalities in membrane protein trafficking. *J. Cell Sci.* **2013**, *126*, 2372–2380. [CrossRef]

101. Tadenev, A.L.D.; Kulaga, H.M.; May-Simera, H.L.; Kelley, M.W.; Katsanis, N.; Reed, R.R. Loss of Bardet–Biedl syndrome protein-8 (BBS8) perturbs olfactory function, protein localization, and axon targeting. *Proc. Natl. Acad. Sci. USA* **2011**, *108*, 10320. [CrossRef]

102. Kulaga, H.M.; Leitch, C.C.; Eichers, E.R.; Badano, J.L.; Lesemann, A.; Hoskins, B.E.; Lupski, J.R.; Beales, P.L.; Reed, R.R.; Katsanis, N. Loss of BBS proteins causes anosmia in humans and defects in olfactory cilia structure and function in the mouse. *Nat. Genet.* **2004**, *36*, 994–998. [CrossRef]

103. Bonnett, B.N.; Egenvall, A. Age patterns of disease and death in insured Swedish dogs, cats and horses. *J. Comp. Pathol.* **2010**, *142* (Suppl. 1), S33–S38. [CrossRef]

104. O'Dea, D.; Parfrey, P.S.; Harnett, J.D.; Hefferton, D.; Cramer, B.C.; Green, J. The importance of renal impairment in the natural history of Bardet-Biedl syndrome. *Am. J. Kidney Dis. Off. J. Natl. Kidney Found.* **1996**, *27*, 776–783. [CrossRef]

105. Murphy, D.; Singh, R.; Kolandaivelu, S.; Ramamurthy, V.; Stoilov, P. Alternative Splicing Shapes the Phenotype of a Mutation in BBS8 To Cause Nonsyndromic Retinitis Pigmentosa. *Mol. Cell Biol.* **2015**, *35*, 1860–1870. [CrossRef]

106. Klein, D.C. The 2004 Aschoff/Pittendrigh Lecture: Theory of the Origin of the Pineal Gland—A Tale of Conflict and Resolution. *J. Biol. Rhythm.* **2004**, *19*, 264–279. [CrossRef]

107. Lykke-Andersen, S.; Jensen, T.H. Nonsense-mediated mRNA decay: An intricate machinery that shapes transcriptomes. *Nat. Rev. Mol. Cell Biol.* **2015**, *16*, 665–677. [CrossRef]

108. Blatch, G.L.; Lassle, M. The tetratricopeptide repeat: A structural motif mediating protein-protein interactions. *Bioessays* **1999**, *21*, 932–939. [CrossRef]

109. Abd-El-Barr, M.M.; Sykoudis, K.; Andrabi, S.; Eichers, E.R.; Pennesi, M.E.; Tan, P.L.; Wilson, J.H.; Katsanis, N.; Lupski, J.R.; Wu, S.M. Impaired photoreceptor protein transport and synaptic transmission in a mouse model of Bardet-Biedl syndrome. *Vis. Res.* **2007**, *47*, 3394–3407. [CrossRef]

110. Lewis, G.P.; Fisher, S.K. Up-Regulation of Glial Fibrillary Acidic Protein in Response to Retinal Injury: Its Potential Role in Glial Remodeling and a Comparison to Vimentin Expression. In *International Review of Cytology*; Academic Press: Cambridge, MA, USA, 2003; Volume 230, pp. 263–290.

111. Jomary, C.; Ahir, A.; Agarwal, N.; Neal, M.J.; Jones, S.E. Spatio-temporal pattern of ocular clusterin mRNA expression in the rd mouse. *Brain Res. Mol. Brain Res.* **1995**, *29*, 172–176. [CrossRef]

112. Wong, P.; Borst, D.E.; Farber, D.; Danciger, J.S.; Tenniswood, M.; Chader, G.J.; van Veen, T. Increased TRPM-2/clusterin mRNA levels during the time of retinal degeneration in mouse models of retinitis pigmentosa. *Biochem. Cell Biol. Biochim. Biol. Cell.* **1994**, *72*, 439–446. [CrossRef] [PubMed]

113. Sarthy, P.V.; Fu, M.; Huang, J. Developmental expression of the glial fibrillary acidic protein (GFAP) gene in the mouse retina. *Cell. Mol. Neurobiol.* **1991**, *11*, 623–637. [CrossRef]

Mapping of Diabetes Susceptibility Loci in a Domestic Cat Breed with an Unusually High Incidence of Diabetes Mellitus

Lois Balmer [1,2,†], Caroline Ann O'Leary [3,†], Marilyn Menotti-Raymond [4], Victor David [5], Stephen O'Brien [6,7], Belinda Penglis [8], Sher Hendrickson [9], Mia Reeves-Johnson [3], Susan Gottlieb [3], Linda Fleeman [10], Dianne Vankan [3], Jacquie Rand [3,11,‡] and Grant Morahan [1,*,‡]

[1] Centre for Diabetes Research, Harry Perkins Institute for Medical Research, University of Western Australia, Nedlands 6009, Australia; l.balmer@ecu.edu.au

[2] School of Medical and Health Sciences, Edith Cowan University, Joondalup, Perth 6027, Australia

[3] School of Veterinary Science, the University of Queensland, Gottan 4343, Australia; c.oleary@uq.edu.au (C.A.O.); m.reevejohnson@uq.edu.au (M.R.-J.); susanalisongottlieb@gmail.com (S.G.); d.vankan@uq.edu.au (D.V.); j.rand@uq.edu.au (J.R.)

[4] Laboratory of Genomic Diversity, Center for Cancer Research (FNLCR), Frederick, MD 21702, USA; Marilyn.Menotti@gmail.com

[5] Laboratory of Basic Research, Center for Cancer Research (FNLCR), National Cancer Institute, Frederick, MD 21702, USA; davidvic@mail.nih.gov

[6] Laboratory of Genomics Diversity, Center for Computer Technologies, ITMO University, 197101 St. Petersburg, Russia; lgdchief@gmail.com

[7] Guy Harvey Oceanographic Center, Halmos College of Arts and Sciences, Nova Southeastern University, Ft Lauderdale, FL 33004, USA

[8] *IDEXX* Laboratories, East Brisbane 4169, Australia; belinda.penglis@bigpond.com

[9] Department of Biology, Shepherd University, Shepherdstown, WV 25443, USA; shendric@shepherd.edu

[10] Animal Diabetes Australia, Melbourne 3155, Australia; l.fleeman@AnimalDiabetesAustralia.com.au

[11] American College of Veterinary Internal Medicine, University of Zurich, 8006 Zurich, Switzerland

* Correspondence: grant.morahan@perkins.org.au

† These authors contributed equally to this work.

‡ Joint senior authors.

Abstract: Genetic variants that are associated with susceptibility to type 2 diabetes (T2D) are important for identification of individuals at risk and can provide insights into the molecular basis of disease. Analysis of T2D in domestic animals provides both the opportunity to improve veterinary management and breeding programs as well as to identify novel T2D risk genes. Australian-bred Burmese (ABB) cats have a 4-fold increased incidence of type 2 diabetes (T2D) compared to Burmese cats bred in the United States. This is likely attributable to a genetic founder effect. We investigated this by performing a genome-wide association scan on ABB cats. Four SNPs were associated with the ABB T2D phenotype with p values <0.005. All exons and splice junctions of candidate genes near significant single-nucleotide polymorphisms (SNPs) were sequenced, including the genes *DGKG, IFG2BP2, SLC8A1, E2F6, ETV5, TRA2B* and *LIPH*. Six candidate polymorphisms were followed up in a larger cohort of ABB cats with or without T2D and also in Burmese cats bred in America, which exhibit low T2D incidence. The original SNPs were confirmed in this cohort as associated with the T2D phenotype, although no novel coding SNPs in any of the seven candidate genes showed association with T2D. The identification of genetic markers associated with T2D susceptibility in ABB cats will enable preventative health strategies and guide breeding programs to reduce the prevalence of T2D in these cats.

Keywords: diabetes mellitus; Burmese cats; susceptibility; single-nucleotide polymorphism; genetic markers; LIPH

1. Introduction

Type 2 diabetes mellitus (T2D) is a polygenic disease with complex inheritance [1,2]. Studies of T2D in humans have identified over 80 genetic variants associated with disease susceptibility, but most of these contribute a small proportion of overall risk of disease, and the detailed molecular basis of how these contribute to disease is not well understood [3]. Animal models can provide additional evidence of the role of genes in T2D. For example, a polymorphism in the melanocortin 4 receptor gene (MC4R) was associated with T2D in overweight domestic cats, similar to humans [4]. Animal models can also provide a valuable opportunity to identify novel T2D genes. We demonstrated previously that Australian-bred Burmese (ABB) cats are at increased risk of developing T2D, and exhibit features typical of human T2D [5,6], including inadequate insulin secretion (dysfunctional β cells); impaired insulin action (insulin resistance) [7]; late age of onset; risk factors such as obesity and physical inactivity; islet vacuolation and amyloid deposition. Clinical features of diabetes in ABB cats are similar to atypical T2D in humans, which is most common in African-Americans, and includes presentation with very high blood glucose concentrations [8,9]. Diabetic ABB cats respond to insulin in a very similar way to human patients. Affected humans present with a history of polyuria, polydipsia and weight loss, but otherwise have a T2D phenotype and profile, and frequently have a family history of T2D. These patients respond to initial insulin treatment within days to weeks with long-lasting, insulin-free, near-normoglycaemic remission [9]. Similarly, cats with diabetes have high remission rates (67 to >80%) resulting in normoglycaemia without the need for insulin, if tight glycaemic control is instituted soon after diagnosis [10,11].

In a study of a cohort of 12,576 cats, the prevalence of diabetes was significantly higher in ABB cats than in domestic short or longhaired cats ($p < 0.001$), with the incidence rising to 10% in Burmese cats over eight years old [5]. Other Australian domestic cat breeds exhibit a diabetes incidence of ~0.25% to 1% [12]. American, European-and ABB cats have had distinct breeding histories since the 1970s [13]. Burmese cats bred in New Zealand and the UK, from where the ABB cats are believed to have originated, also demonstrate increased risk of diabetes [14,15]. However, Burmese cats in other countries such as the US do not show such increased T2D incidence [16,17]. US-bred Burmese cats did have different incidence rates for other genetic diseases [18].

Type 2 diabetes in ABB cats likely arises from a genetic founder effect. Several population bottlenecks have been experienced in cat evolution, including domestication and subsequently in the creation of breeds (mostly within the last 50–150 years) [19]. Of most relevance is the recent bottleneck associated with the establishment of the breed in Australia in 1957 from a very small number of individuals, possibly as few as five [13,20]. Founder effects can result in otherwise rare variants being established in a population and have had great utility in discovery of disease genes in domestic animal species. Thus, the genetic architecture of the ABB cat population provides an opportunity to identify novel genetic variants mediating T2D susceptibility. Identification of such genes could increase our understanding of molecular events leading to T2D and would be immediately applicable in the veterinary setting by identifying cats at risk of diabetes and improving breeding programs. Preventative management could also be implemented for at-risk individuals via dietary changes, weight loss and therapies to control glycaemia.

We hypothesize that genetic variant(s) predisposing to T2D demonstrate a higher frequency in ABB cats compared to American Burmese cats, thus providing a unique opportunity for discovery of diabetes-associated genes. We performed an exploratory case-control genome-wide association scan (GWAS), followed by validation of candidate SNPs in an expanded cohort. A similar approach identified candidate genes in other diseases [21,22].

2. Materials and Methods

This study was conducted in accordance with the Declaration of Helsinki and the protocol was approved by the Ethics Committee of The University of Queensland (AEC Approval Number: SVS/040/10/NCI/ABBOTT, date: 150910 to 150912; AEC Approval Number: SVS/200/12/NESTLE PURINA/ABBOT ANIMAL HEALTH, date: 180712 to 180715; AEC Approval Number: SVS/256/13/MEDINCELL/NCI, date: 311013 to 311016).

2.1. Characterisation of Australian-Bred Burmese Cats

Two ABB cat cohorts were studied. The first ("exploratory") cohort contained 10 cats diagnosed with T2D and 10 control non-diabetics with normal glucose tolerance. Of the diabetic cats, four were male. Samples were obtained for five of these from cat-specific practices in Brisbane, Australia, one individual from a general practice, and 4 individuals from a veterinary commercial diagnostic laboratory (*IDEXX*, Brisbane, Australia) that had received blood samples from veterinarians as part of the diagnostic work-up for cats that had clinical signs suggestive of diabetes.

Cats were classed as T2D if they were first diagnosed at 8 years of age or older based on hyperglycaemia (blood glucose concentrations over 15 mmol/L) and clinical signs of polydipsia and polyuria. At the time of sampling, 4 cats were in remission and maintained euglycaemia without insulin. Selecting cats above 8 years of age reduced the risk of including cats with type 1 diabetes, which develops at an earlier age [23] and is relatively rare [24]. Inclusion of cats with other types of diabetes causing insulin resistance, most commonly acromegaly, was unlikely as cats were treated with typical doses of insulin and were not reported to have consistent clinical and/or pathology findings of acromegaly [25]. Further, 5/7 cats had feline pancreatic lipase immunoreactivity (fPLI) below 8 µg/L [26] and two had values below 12 µg/L and therefore not consistent with a diagnosis of active pancreatitis [27]; 7/8 tested had normal total thyroxine (TT4) and one had hyperthyroidism (TT4 107), one had liver disease, 3 had mildly increased liver enzymes, and 4 had renal dysfunction.

The 10 control ABB cats (five males) were all older than 8 years and exhibited fasting and 2 h blood glucose concentrations in a glucose tolerance test within reference ranges for age-matched cats. They were clinically healthy based on history, physical examination, routine haematological, routine biochemical, feline pancreatic lipase, and TT4 testing. For the glucose tolerance test, cats were fasted overnight and 0.5 g/kg 50% glucose injection BP was injected via a cephalic catheter placed 3 h before and samples collected from the pinna or paw at 0, 2, 3 and 4 h. All cats had a 2 h glucose concentration <10 mmol/L (upper 95% for normal reference range for glucose concentration 2 h following 0.5 g/kg glucose) and all blood glucose concentrations had returned to <6.5 mmol/L (upper limit 95% reference range for fasting concentration) by 2 to 2.5 h. All control cats had fPLI measurements <7.6 µg/L, 8 of 8 tested had normal TT4, and all had normal haematology and biochemistry.

The second cohort consisted of 84 ABB; 37 with T2D and 47 controls. Of the T2D cases, 24 were male and 13 female. Eight were from a diabetes-specific practice in Melbourne and 4 from a cat-specific practice in Brisbane. Of these latter 12 cases, 5 were in remission and the remaining 7 were stable on insulin doses <1.5 U/kg. Evidence of renal dysfunction was present in 5/7, hyperthyroidism in 1/5, and liver disease in 1/7. Five of these 12 cats had fPLI values available, with 4 being below 8 µg/L. The remaining 25 samples were obtained Australia-wide by the veterinary diagnostic laboratory *IDEXX*. All cases were either diagnosed with blood glucose over 15 mmol/L; 8 were newly diagnosed, 2 were euthanased at diagnosis, 11 were on insulin <1.5 U/kg and 4 had unknown insulin treatment histories. Veterinarians caring for cats were contacted and the history, clinical details and therapeutic history of the cases were obtained to ensure these cats did not have other forms of diabetes, such as acromegaly. Further, 14/20 cats had fPLI <12 µg/L, 24/24 had normal total TT4. On haematology and biochemistry (and urinalysis where available), biochemical evidence of renal dysfunction was present in 6 of 26, liver disease in 7, renal and liver disease in 5, and there were no data for 1 animal.

ABB control cats in cohort two (*n* = 47) were eight years or older, with a screening blood glucose concentration (measured after entry to the clinic and any time in relation to eating) of <8.1

mmol/L measured from fluoride-oxalate samples on an automated serum chemistry analyser ($n = 42$ from *IDDEX*), or immediately after sample collection using a handheld glucose meter calibrated for cats (Abbott AlphaTRAK) ($n = 5$ from research projects) [28]. Of these, 14 were male, 33 female. Screening blood glucose concentration <8.1 mmol/L is lower than the upper limit of the screening blood glucose reference range (9.7 mmol/L) and in 45/47 cats, screening blood glucose was <6.5 mmol/L, a stringent cut-off point for aged, client-owned cats that have not been fasted and are potentially subject to stress (which may cause hyperglycaemia) [29]. Burmese cats without signs of diabetes have been shown to have fasting blood glucose concentrations on average 1.9 mmol/L higher ($p < 0.05$) than age-matched domestic cats [5]. Of these 47 cats, one had no haematology, biochemistry or urinalysis data available, evidence of renal dysfunction was present in 15, liver disease in 2, liver and renal disease in 6, and 23 had normal haematology and biochemistry (and urinalysis when available) findings.

2.2. US-Bred Burmese Cats

A third cohort comprised 84 DNA samples from American-bred Burmese cats; 37 female, 21 male and 26 of unknown sex. These cats were not tested for diabetes, but are representative of a population with a normal low risk of type 2 diabetes (~0.25% to 1%) [17].

2.3. Genome-Wide Association Mapping and Analyses for Association with Diabetes: Genomic

Genomic DNA was extracted using a QIAamp DNA Blood Mini Kit (QIAGEN, Hilde, Germany). Genotyping in the first cohort of cats was performed using the Illumina iSelect custom feline genome chip containing 58,444 SNPs. All SNPs were analysed with Illumina Genome Studio software and subjected to stringent quality control procedures. SNPs with GenTrain Scores <0.60, call rate <0.95, or failed genotype concordance in replicates were removed from analysis. SNPs were excluded if they exhibited a minor allele frequency (MAF) in cases <0.01 due to sample size, or case/control bias in missingness. In total, 38,487 SNPs remained after these cut offs. Association testing was performed in PLINK [30] using Fisher's Exact test, with *p* values corrected for multiple tests by Bonferroni correction. Correction for genetic admixture (caused by potential misrecorded matings) was assessed and corrected using Eigensoft [30]. The initial screening GWAS, with 10 cases and 10 controls, was regarded primarily as an exploratory study, with any suggestive findings to be followed in a subsequent cohort.

2.4. PCR, Gel, Digest and High-Resolution Melt Analysis

Targeted genotyping assays were developed to analyse the novel variants that we identified. Depending on the SNP, assays used were allele-specific PCR, single-strand conformation polymorphism PCR, restriction digestion or high-resolution melt analyses. Primer sequences are in Supplementary Table S1.

In general, 20 ng of genomic DNA from each sample was amplified by PCR in a 20 µL total PCR reaction mixture including 0.2 U Platinum Taq DNA polymerase (Life Technologies, Perth, Australia), 50 mM MgCl$_2$ (Life Technologies, Victoria, Australia), 10 mM nucleoside triphosphates (dNTPs) (SIGMA-Aldrich, Castle Hill, Australia) and 50 ng primers (SIGMA-Aldrich, Castle Hill, Australia). The cycling parameters were: one cycle at 96 °C for 5 min, then 34 cycles of 96 °C for 20 s, 58–66 °C for 20 s, 72 °C for 30 s and a final extension at 72 °C for 3 min. The PCR products were separated on a 3% agarose gel (BIO-RAD Laboratories, Hercules, CA, USA).

Genotyping was performed where possible by differential restriction enzyme digestion. After digesting 15 µL of PCR product for 3 h with the appropriate enzyme (Table 2), and manufacturers' instructions, the products were electrophoresed on a 3% agarose gel.

If PCR products (such as SNP6, chrC2:84361252+84361412), could not be distinguished by gel separation, they were tested by High Resolution Melt analysis. Briefly, they were amplified from 20 ng of genomic DNA in a 20 µL total PCR reaction mixture containing ResoLight Dye (Roche, Indianapolis, IN, USA), 0.2 U Platinum Taq DNA polymerase (Life Technologies, Victoria, Australia), 50 mM MgCl$_2$ (Life Technologies, Victoria, Australia), 10 mM dNTPs (SIGMA-Aldrich, Castle Hill, Australia) and

50 ng primer (SIGMA-Aldrich, Castle Hill, Australia). Following PCR, the samples were heated to 95 °C, rapidly cooled to 45 °C, reheated to 70–95 °C with a ramp rate of 0.2 °C/s, and analysis of melt curves was conducted using the Light Cycler 480 Software Release 1.5.0 SP3 (Roche, Sydney, Australia) [31].

Allele-specific PCRs were used to detect the G/A polymorphism in the *E2F6* gene. The allele-specific reaction mixture contained 20 µg of genomic DNA in a 20 µL PCR reaction mixture including 0.2 U Platinum Taq DNA polymerase (Life Technologies, Victoria, Australia), 40 mM MgCl$_2$ (Life Technologies, Victoria, Australia), 10 mM dNTPs (SIGMA-Aldrich, Castle Hill, Australia) and 50 ng allele specific primers (SIGMA-Aldrich, Castle Hill, Australia). Primer sequences are indicated in Supplementary Table S1. Forward primers were designed with a T-A nucleotide mismatch to create primer 3′ instability and increased allele specificity. The G and A 3′-terminal nucleotides of the allele-specific forward primers annealed to the G and A nucleotides of the *E2F6* gene. The reverse primer was designed to anneal to a highly conserved region of the *E2F6* gene in Australian-bred Burmese. The thermal profile consisted of one cycle at 96 °C for 5 min, then 34 cycles of 96 °C for 20 s, 58–66 °C for 20 s, 72 °C for 30 s, and a final extension at 72 °C for 3 min. Reactions were performed to determine AA/AG/GG status of all ABB DNA samples. The PCR products were separated on a 3% agarose gel (BIO-RAD Laboratories, Hercules, CA, USA).

2.5. Sequencing of Candidate Genes

Genes near the SNPs identified in the GWAS as loci of interest (Table 1) were inspected using the November 2017 ICGSC Felis_catus 9.0/felCat9 and candidate genes were chosen for sequencing On chromosome A3, SLC8A1 located within 20 Kb of SNP1 and E2F6 was within 20 Kb of SNP2. On chromosome C2, SNP4 was located adjacent to 3 candidate genes; ETV5 within 20 Kb, DGKG within 200 Kb, and TRA2B within 150 Kb. On chromosome C2, SNPs 5–6 were located near IGF2BP2 within 200 Kb, and LIPH within 100 Kb.

Table 1. Candidate SNPs identified from the exploratory GWAS. A1 indicates the minor allele (i.e., least frequently observed based on the whole sample); F_A and F_U indicate the frequency of the minor allele in the affected and unaffected cats, respectively. The *p* value is shown calculated by Fisher's Exact test and Bonferroni corrected by PLINK. No odds ratio could be calculated for SNP2 because the associated allele was not found in unaffected cats. SNPs were named in the Illumina array only as custom numbers; for convenience, they are named here as SNPs 1 to 6.

SNP	Illumina No.	A1	F_A	F_U	*p*	Odds Ratio
SNP1	10566	G	0.75	0.15	0.00014	17
SNP2	10762	G	0.5	0	0.00026	NA
SNP3	30747	G	0.1	0.65	0.00033	0.059
SNP4	36147	G	0.8	0.2	0.00015	16
SNP5	36165	A	0.1	0.65	0.00033	0.059
SNP6	36166	A	0.1	0.65	0.00033	0.059

Exons and the 5′ and 3′ untranslated regions (UTR) of all candidate genes were sequenced (primer sequences shown in Supplementary Table S2). To amplify the DGKG gene, M13 tails were added to all primers, and a touchdown PCR protocol was followed [32]. Sequencing for the DGKG gene was performed with Version 1.1 big dye terminator sequencing using M13 forward and reverse primers [33]; the remaining genes sequenced with the PCR primers. PCR products were cleaned using the PCR Clean up Kit (Qiagen), 20 ng/µL of this product was then mixed with 20 ng/µL of the forward or reverse primer (Sigma-Aldrich, Castle Hill, Australia), Big Dye Terminator (V1.3) and Buffer (×5) (Ambion). The cycling parameters were: one cycle at 96 °C for 3 min, then 25 cycles of 96 °C for 10 s, 50 °C for 2 s, 60 °C for 4 min. The sequencing reactions were cleaned and analysed on the ABI3730. Sequences were analysed using Sequence Scanner 2 software (Applied Biosystems, Victoria, Australia). Sequences were aligned using Clustal Omega 2019 (EMBL-EBI, Cambridge, UK) to identify SNPs. Variant protein sequences were submitted to Protein Variation Effect Analyser (PROVEAN V1.0) (Rockville, MD, USA) protein prediction software [34]. No further analysis was conducted on SNPs that did not result in protein coding changes.

3. Results

3.1. Search for Genetic Markers Associated with Type 2 Diabetes

Our strategy was to conduct an exploratory GWAS with 10 diabetic and 10 control ABB cats to characterise sequence polymorphisms between diabetic and non-diabetic Burmese which might be examined in a larger population sample, and to validate any candidate polymorphisms in a larger cohort. Genotyping was performed using custom Illumina arrays [35]. As expected for a sample this small, no SNP provided a p value below the threshold for significance after Bonferroni correction (i.e., $p\, 8 \times 10^{-7}$). However, six SNPs were identified with promising p values <0.0005 (Table 1). These SNPs tagged regions on cat chromosomes A3, C1 and C2. The SNPs on the custom Illumina chip had custom numerical annotations. For convenience, these six candidate SNPs are designated here as SNPs 1 through 6.

3.2. Validation of the Candidate Type 2 Diabetes Associated SNPs

The six candidate SNPs were genotyped in a second cohort of ABB cats supplemented with samples from Burmese cats from the low-prevalence US population. Only one (SNP6) was not significant in the validation cohort. SNPs 1–4 demonstrated significant association after Bonferroni correction while a further SNP (SNP5) had a p value of 0.01 (Table 2).

Table 2. Testing candidate SNPs in a validation cohort. DNA samples from a further 37 diabetic ABB cats, 47 normoglycaemic Australian-bred Burmese cats, and 84 Burmese cats from the low-prevalence US population were genotyped at the SNPs implicated by the GWAS. Results were analysed using Plink. A1 indicates the minor allele (i.e., least frequently observed based on the whole sample); F_A and F_U indicate the frequency of the minor allele in the affected and unaffected cats, respectively. The p value is shown calculated using Fisher's Exact test and Bonferroni correction. No odds ratio could be calculated for SNP2 because the associated allele was not found in the non-diabetic cats.

SNP	A1	F_A	F_U	p Value	OR	Chromosome Position
SNP1	T	0.59	0.38	0.00089	2.4	chrA3: 10995614
SNP2	G	0.29	0.52	0.00043	0.4	chrA3: 134626291
SNP3	C	0.17	0.46	5.35×10^{-6}	0.2	chrC1: 23237623
SNP4	C	0.63	0.41	0.0013	2.5	chrC2: 83660325
SNP5	T	0.32	0.49	0.012	0.5	chrC2: 84129862
SNP6	A	0.30	0.34	0.53	0.8	chrC2: 84135537

Haplotype analyses demonstrated that SNPs on chromosome C2 tagged intervals that were strongly associated with type 2 diabetes (Table 3). Even the SNP that was not significant as a singleton (SNP6), demonstrated a significant association when combined with SNP5, tagging a chromosome interval that showed association. As these SNPs span a genomic interval of well over 500 kb, these results suggest that they may tag a founder haplotype that increases the risk of type 2 diabetes, or that the individual variants near these SNPs interact to increase susceptibility.

Table 3. Haplotype analyses. Data from the validation cohort were analysed using the haplotype association test implemented in PLINK. Results for the most associated haplotype are shown.

Chr	SNPs	Haplotype	F (Diabetic)	F (Unaffected)	p Value	Chromosome Position
C2	4 and 5	CC	0.51	0.29	0.0006	93563976 and 94157910
C2	5 and 6	CC	0.55	0.34	0.001	94157910 and 94165023

3.3. Selection of Candidate Type 2 Diabetes Genes

Genes near the associated SNPs were inspected using the November 2017 ICGSC Felis_catus 9.0/felCat9. The two associated SNPs on chromosome A3, SNP1 and SNP2, were located within introns of *SLC8A1* and *E2F6*, respectively. There are no other known genes within 50 Kb 5' or 3' of these SNPs. Neither of these genes has previously been implicated in type 2 diabetes susceptibility. The most highly associated SNP, SNP3, resided in an area with no known coding genes within at least 300 Kb.

SNP4 is located in an intron of *ETV5*. The human orthologue of *ETV5* was reported to be associated with type 2 diabetes and obesity in several human populations [36,37]. SNPs 5 and 6 are within the same intron of the *LIPH* gene, which encodes a membrane-bound triglyceride lipase. The genomic region on chromosome C2 located between SNPs 4 and 6, contains only four other known genes based on sequence homology or conserved synteny with other species. These are: *TRA2B*, *CHCHD4*, *IGF2BP2* and *SENP2*. Of these, *TRA2B* (also known as SFRS10) has been linked in humans and mice to obesity and so to related metabolic syndromes including type 2 diabetes [38]. Studies have indicated the involvement of *IGF2BP2* in type 2 diabetes in humans [39].

3.4. Search for Polymorphisms within Candidate Genes

To identify genetic variants in the genes identified above, all coding regions of these genes were sequenced, including the 3' and 5' UTRs of each. Information about the genomic regions sequenced, any discovered SNPs, the nucleotide position of each SNP, any predicted amino acid change and the effect of the mutation as estimated by the PROVEAN algorithm is shown in Supplementary Table S3. Association results of selected SNPs with the diabetes trait are shown in Supplementary Table S4. Eleven SNPs were discovered in *SLC8A1*, of which two were found to contain a potentially deleterious amino acid substitution. Twelve SNPs were identified in *E2F6*, with one predicted to be deleterious. However, none of these SNPs were significantly associated with the disease phenotype, suggesting that they were commonly occurring in the Burmese cat breed but not the cat(s) used to establish the genome sequence of this species. No likely causal mutations, including non-synonymous substitutions, polymorphisms in splice junctions, introduction of premature stop codons or insertions/deletions resulting in frame-shifts were found in either *IGF2BP2* or *DGKG*. Fourteen SNPs were identified in *ETV5* with two predicted to be deleterious, but these also were not significantly associated with the disease phenotype. Two SNPs and one deletion were identified in the *TRAF2B* gene; all were found to reside within introns.

Finally, eight novel SNPs were identified in *LIPH*, none of which were in exons. One of these SNPs was significantly ($p = 1.6 \times 10^{-5}$) associated with diabetes, conferring a relative risk of 2.6. No feline transcripts of this gene have been sequenced, but by alignment of the cat genomic and human cDNA sequences, the significant SNP is located in the presumed 3'UTR region. This is reminiscent of the 3'UTR SNP in the *IL12B* gene which affects gene expression and is associated with susceptibility to type 1 diabetes and other diseases in humans [40,41]. This novel SNP was confirmed and was significantly associated with type 2 diabetes in the total cohort of ABB cats.

4. Discussion

Our exploratory GWAS found an association of six SNPs with type 2 diabetes. Seven candidate genes were investigated for the presence of variants that could contribute to type 2 diabetes. Of these candidates examined, only *LIPH* exhibited a novel disease-associated variant. Two genes near SNP 4, *ETV5* and *DGKD*, did not have disease-associated sequence variants. The region on Chr C2 near SNPs 5 and 6, contained four known genes (*TRA2B*, *CHCHD4*, *IGF2BP2* and *SENP2*) but none of these genes contained disease-associated protein-coding changes, despite *TRA2B* and *IGF2BP2* having association with type 2 diabetes in other species [39]. Thus, these gene variants compared to the reference cat genome sequence are found in the Burmese cat lineage but are not associated with T2D susceptibility.

SNP3, the most highly associated SNP, is in a genomic region of low gene density which has no known coding genes within at least 300 Kb. Many SNPs associated with disease risk occur in such "gene deserts". They may reside in enhancer elements [42] and regulate expression of distant genes, as shown for type 1 diabetes risk genes [43].

This study demonstrates the potential of ABB cats to identify novel genes involved in type 2 diabetes susceptibility. The ABB cat population originated from a small number of founders, with subsequent inbreeding leading to extensive linkage disequilibrium (LD) [44]. In US-bred Burmese cats, a more outbred population, average haplotype blocks have been reported to be 0.5 Mb [44], along with an average inbreeding coefficient of 0.22 and observed heterozygosity of 0.4 [45]. Extended LD observed in many domesticated animal breeds can be created by population bottlenecks, small effective population sizes and use of popular sires, and has proved highly beneficial in genetic mapping [45]. Thus, in this study, the ABB cat, with its genetic architecture and high prevalence of type 2 diabetes, allowed identification of genetic elements of large effect size using smaller sample sizes than required for outbred populations.

Up to 7% of Australian cats seen by veterinarians are Burmese [12], and up to 10% of ABB cats over 8 years old develop diabetes [5], so ABB cats comprise a significant proportion of the population of domesticated cats requiring veterinary care. Diabetes has major quality of life implications for cats and also major cost implications for owners [46]. Our results have clinical relevance for Burmese cats at increased risk of diabetes in Australia, and in other countries like the UK [14] and New Zealand [15], and possibly for other domestic cat populations.

Our results could reduce the burden of care on ABB cat owners by identifying cats carrying risk alleles. Identifying at-risk cats allows early intervention to identify pre-diabetic cats and prevent development of overt diabetes. Early identification of pre-diabetic cats is important, once cats are pre-diabetes (fasting blood glucose >7.5 mmol/L and 3 h glucose >14 mmol/L), they have an 88% probability of being diabetic within 9 months [47]. Potential interventions include weight control, a low carbohydrate diet to reduce postprandial increases in glycaemia, and insulin-sensitising drugs. Currently such drugs are not commonly used because of the difficulty in identifying at-risk pre-diabetic cats. Further, general dietary and body weight recommendations for cats are not always adopted by owners but may have increased uptake if owners knew their cat was genetically at risk. Identification of pre-diabetic and subclinical diabetic cats could result in these cats being managed without the need for insulin. Further, improved monitoring would expedite early diagnosis of diabetes and quick implementation of tight glycaemic control. This has benefits for diabetic cats and their owners because remission rates in excess of 80% can be achieved compared to 30–40% remission rates if tight glycaemic control is delayed [48].

This study, by identifying risk loci in the ABB cat population, particularly allows cat breeders to make informed choices to avoid type 2 diabetes risk in their breeding pedigrees. Cats are bred between 1 and 6 years, well before clinical signs of diabetes are evident, so identification of carriers of risk loci would help reduce type 2 diabetes prevalence. Further investigations may also show whether these loci may also contribute to diabetes in other cat breeds.

Type 2 diabetes in ABB cats is clearly not monogenic; while we have mapped a few loci, their susceptibility alleles are not present in all diabetic cats genotyped, and doubtless others with smaller effects are also involved. Despite this, our identification of risk alleles is a step toward a greater understanding of the metabolic basis of diabetes in cats. Identification of risk alleles in cats may also have relevance for the human disease [49], and this cat population could provide an animal model for studying the role of these genes in the disease process.

Author Contributions: L.B. and G.M. sequenced the genes, conducted the analysis and GWAS analysis and helped write the manuscript. L.B., G.M., C.A.O. and J.R. wrote the manuscript and devised the project, M.M.-R., V.D., S.O., B.P., S.H., M.R.-J., S.G., L.F. and D.V. helped with the design of the project, collection of data, DNA extraction and results coordination. All authors have read and agreed to the published version of the manuscript.

Acknowledgments: The authors thank C Bloom and T Evans, both of whom provided a sample of feline blood.

References

1. Pal, A.; McCarthy, M.I. The genetics of type 2 diabetes and its clinical relevance. *Clin. Genet.* **2013**, *83*, 297–306. [CrossRef] [PubMed]
2. Teslovich, T.M.; Fuchsberger, C.; Ramensky, V.; Yajnik, P.; Koboldt, D.C.; Larson, D.E.; Zhang, Q.; Lin, L.; Welch, R.; Ding, L.; et al. Re-sequencing expands our understanding of the phenotypic impact of variants at GWAS loci. *PLoS Genet.* **2014**, *10*, e1004147. [CrossRef]
3. Dorajoo, R.; Liu, J.; Boehm, B.O. Genetics of Type 2 Diabetes and Clinical Utility. *Genes* **2015**, *6*, 372–384. [CrossRef]
4. Forcada, Y.; Holder, A.; Church, D.B.; Catchpole, B. A polymorphism in the melanocortin 4 receptor gene (MC4R:c.92C>T) is associated with diabetes mellitus in overweight domestic shorthaired cats. *J. Vet. Intern. Med.* **2014**, *28*, 458–464. [CrossRef] [PubMed]
5. Lederer, R.; Rand, J.S.; Jonsson, N.N.; Hughes, I.P.; Morton, J.M. Frequency of feline diabetes mellitus and breed predisposition in domestic cats in Australia. *Vet. J.* **2009**, *179*, 254–258. [CrossRef] [PubMed]
6. Marshall, R.D.; Rand, J.S.; Morton, J.M. Treatment of newly diagnosed diabetic cats with glargine insulin improves glycaemic control and results in higher probability of remission than protamine zinc and lente insulins. *J. Feline Med. Surg.* **2009**, *11*, 683–691. [CrossRef] [PubMed]
7. Feldhahn, J.R.; Rand, J.S.; Martin, G. Insulin sensitivity in normal and diabetic cats. *J. Feline Med. Surg.* **1999**, *1*, 107–115. [CrossRef]
8. Mbanya, J.C.; Kengne, A.P.; Assah, F. Diabetes care in Africa. *Lancet* **2006**, *368*, 1628–1629. [CrossRef]
9. Mbanya, J.C.N.; Motala, A.A.; Sobngwi, E.; Assah, F.K.; Enoru, S.T. Diabetes in sub-Saharan Africa. *Lancet* **2010**, *375*, 2254–2266. [CrossRef]
10. Sieber-Ruckstuhl, N.S.; Kley, S.; Tschuor, F.; Zini, E.; Ohlerth, S.; Boretti, F.S.; Reusch, C.E. Remission of diabetes mellitus in cats with diabetic ketoacidosis. *J. Vet. Intern. Med.* **2008**, *22*, 1326–1332. [CrossRef]
11. Zini, E.; Hafner, M.; Osto, M.; Franchini, M.; Ackermann, M.; Lutz, T.A.; Reusch, C.E. Predictors of clinical remission in cats with diabetes mellitus. *J. Vet. Intern. Med.* **2010**, *24*, 1314–1321. [CrossRef] [PubMed]
12. Rand, J.S.; Bobbermien, L.M.; Hendrikz, J.K.; Copland, M. Over representation of Burmese cats with diabetes mellitus. *Aust. Vet. J.* **1997**, *75*, 402–405. [CrossRef] [PubMed]
13. Fogle, B. *The New Encyclopedia of the Cat*, 1st ed.; DK Publishing, Inc.: New York, NY, USA, 2001.
14. McCann, T.M.; Simpson, K.E.; Shaw, D.J.; Butt, J.A.; Gunn-Moore, D.A. Feline diabetes mellitus in the UK: The prevalence within an insured cat population and a questionnaire-based putative risk factor analysis. *J. Feline Med. Surg.* **2007**, *9*, 289–299. [CrossRef] [PubMed]
15. O'Leary, C.A.; Duffy, D.L.; Gething, M.A.; McGuckin, C.; Rand, J.S. Investigation of diabetes mellitus in Burmese cats as an inherited trait: A preliminary study. *N. Z. Vet. J.* **2013**, *61*, 354–358. [CrossRef] [PubMed]
16. Panciera, D.L.; Thomas, C.B.; Eicker, S.W.; Atkins, C.E. Epizootiologic patterns of diabetes mellitus in cats: 333 cases (1980–1986). *J. Am. Vet. Med. Assoc* **1990**, *197*, 1504–1508. [PubMed]
17. Prahl, A.; Guptill, L.; Glickman, N.W.; Tetrick, M.; Glickman, L.T. Time trends and risk factors for diabetes mellitus in cats presented to veterinary teaching hospitals. *J. Feline Med. Surg.* **2007**, *9*, 351–358. [CrossRef]
18. Gandolfi, B.; Alhaddad, H. Investigation of inherited diseases in cats: Genetic and genomic strategies over three decades. *J. Feline Med. Surg.* **2015**, *17*, 405–415. [CrossRef]
19. Menotti-Raymond, M.; David, V.A.; Pflueger, S.M.; Lindblad-Toh, K.; Wade, C.M.; O'Brien, S.J.; Johnson, W.E. Patterns of molecular genetic variation among cat breeds. *Genomics* **2008**, *91*, 1–11. [CrossRef]
20. Lease, K. A Trip Down Burmese Memory Lane. *R.A.S. Cat Control J.* **1997**, *28*, 17.
21. Alhaddad, H.; Gandolfi, B.; Grahn, R.A.; Rah, H.C.; Peterson, C.B.; Maggs, D.J.; Good, K.L.; Pedersen, N.C.; Lyons, L.A. Genome-wide association and linkage analyses localize a progressive retinal atrophy locus in Persian cats. *Mamm. Genome* **2014**, *25*, 354–362. [CrossRef]
22. Karyadi, D.M.; Karlins, E.; Decker, B.; Carpintero-Ramirez, G.; Parker, H.G.; Wayne, R.K.; Ostrander, E.A. A copy number variant at the KITLG locus likely confers risk for canine squamous cell carcinoma of the digit. *PLoS Genet.* **2013**, *9*, e1003409. [CrossRef] [PubMed]
23. Thoresen, S.I.; Bjerkås, E.; Aleksandersen, M.; Peiffer, R.L. Diabetes mellitus and bilateral cataracts in a kitten. *J. Feline Med. Surg.* **2002**, *4*, 115–122. [CrossRef] [PubMed]
24. Hackendahl, M.; Schaer, N. Insulin resistance in diabetic patients: Causes and management. *Compend. Contin. Educ. Pract. Vet.* **2006**, *28*, 271–284.

25. Niessen, S.J.M.; Church, D.B.; Forcada, Y. Hypersomatotropism, acromegaly, and hyperadrenocorticism and feline diabetes mellitus. *Vet. Clin. N. Am. Small Anim. Pract.* **2013**, *43*, 319–350. [CrossRef] [PubMed]

26. Xenoulis, P.G.; Steiner, J.M. Canine and feline pancreatic lipase immunoreactivity. *Vet. Clin. Pathol.* **2012**, *41*, 312–324. [CrossRef] [PubMed]

27. Steiner, J.M. Is it pancreatitis? *Vet. Med. Bonn. Springs Edw.* **2006**, *101*, 158.

28. Gottlieb, S.; Rand, J.S.; Marshall, R.; Morton, J. Glycemic status and predictors of relapse for diabetic cats in remission. *J. Vet. Intern. Med.* **2015**, *29*, 184–192. [CrossRef]

29. Animal–Cardiology, S.M.; Echocardiography, D.; Echocardiography, T.; Angiography, C.T.; Hearts, I.N. 2012 ACVIM Forum Research Abstracts Program. *J. Vet. Intern. Med.* **2012**, *26*, 690–822. [CrossRef]

30. Purcell, S.; Neale, B.; Todd-Brown, K.; Thomas, L.; Ferreira, M.A.; Bender, D.; Maller, J.; Sklar, P.; De Bakker, P.I.; Daly, M.J.; et al. PLINK: A tool set for whole-genome association and population-based linkage analyses. *Am. J. Hum. Genet.* **2007**, *81*, 559–575. [CrossRef]

31. Liew, M.; Pryor, R.; Palais, R.; Meadows, C.; Erali, M.; Lyon, E.; Wittwer, C. Genotyping of single-nucleotide polymorphisms by high-resolution melting of small amplicons. *Clin. Chem.* **2004**, *50*, 1156–1164. [CrossRef]

32. Menotti-Raymond, M.A.; David, V.A.; Wachter, L.L.; Butler, J.M.; O'Brien, S.J. An STR forensic typing system for genetic individualization of domestic cat (*Felis catus*) samples. *J. Forensic Sci.* **2005**, *50*, 1061–1070. [CrossRef] [PubMed]

33. Kehler, J.S.; David, V.A.; Schäffer, A.A.; Bajema, K.; Eizirik, E.; Ryugo, D.K.; Hannah, S.S.; O'Brien, S.J.; Menotti-Raymond, M. Four independent mutations in the feline fibroblast growth factor 5 gene determine the long-haired phenotype in domestic cats. *J. Hered.* **2007**, *98*, 555–566. [CrossRef] [PubMed]

34. Choi, Y.; Sims, G.E.; Murphy, S.; Miller, J.R.; Chan, A.P. Predicting the functional effect of amino acid substitutions and indels. *PLoS ONE* **2012**, *7*, e46688. [CrossRef] [PubMed]

35. Willet, C.E.; Haase, B. An updated felCat5 SNP manifest for the Illumina Feline 63k SNP genotyping array. *Anim. Genet.* **2014**, *45*, 614–615. [CrossRef]

36. Dorajoo, R.; Blakemore, A.I.; Sim, X.; Ong, R.T.; Ng, D.P.; Seielstad, M.; Wong, T.Y.; Saw, S.M.; Froguel, P.; Liu, J.; et al. Replication of 13 obesity loci among Singaporean Chinese, Malay and Asian-Indian populations. *Int. J. Obes.* **2012**, *36*, 159–163. [CrossRef]

37. Thorleifsson, G.; Walters, G.B.; Gudbjartsson, D.F.; Steinthorsdottir, V.; Sulem, P.; Helgadottir, A.; Styrkarsdottir, U.; Gretarsdottir, S.; Thorlacius, S.; Jonsdottir, I.; et al. Genome-wide association yields new sequence variants at seven loci that associate with measures of obesity. *Nat. Genet.* **2009**, *41*, 18–24. [CrossRef]

38. Pihlajamäki, J.; Lerin, C.; Itkonen, P.; Boes, T.; Floss, T.; Schroeder, J.; Dearie, F.; Crunkhorn, S.; Burak, F.; Jimenez-Chillaron, J.C.; et al. Expression of the splicing factor gene SFRS10 is reduced in human obesity and contributes to enhanced lipogenesis. *Cell Metab.* **2011**, *14*, 208–218. [CrossRef]

39. Benrahma, H.; Charoute, H.; Lasram, K.; Boulouiz, R.; Atig, R.K.; Fakiri, M.; Rouba, H.; Abdelhak, S.; Barakat, A. Association analysis of IGF2BP2, KCNJ11, and CDKAL1 polymorphisms with type 2 diabetes mellitus in a Moroccan population: A case-control study and meta-analysis. *Biochem. Genet.* **2014**, *52*, 430–442. [CrossRef]

40. Morahan, G.; Huang, D.; Ymer, S.I.; Cancilla, M.R.; Stephen, K.; Dabadghao, P.; Werther, G.; Tait, B.D.; Harrison, L.C.; Colman, P.G. Linkage disequilibrium of a type 1 diabetes susceptibility locus with a regulatory *IL12B* allele. *Nat. Genet.* **2001**, *27*, 218–221. [CrossRef]

41. Morahan, G.; Kaur, G.; Singh, M.; Rapthap, C.C.; Kumar, N.; Katoch, K.; Mehra, N.K.; Huang, D. Association of variants in the *IL12B* gene with leprosy and tuberculosis. *Tissue Antigens* **2007**, *69* (Suppl. 1), 234–236. [CrossRef]

42. Sur, I.; Tuupanen, S.; Whitington, T.; Aaltonen, L.A.; Taipale, J. Lessons from functional analysis of genome-wide association studies. *Cancer Res.* **2013**, *73*, 4180–4184. [CrossRef] [PubMed]

43. Ram, R.; Mehta, M.; Nguyen, Q.T.; Larma, I.; Boehm, B.O.; Pociot, F.; Concannon, P.; Morahan, G. Systematic Evaluation of Genes and Genetic Variants Associated with Type 1 Diabetes Susceptibility. *J. Immunol.* **2016**, *96*, 3043–3053. [CrossRef] [PubMed]

44. Pontius, J.U.; Mullikin, J.C.; Smith, D.R.; Team, A.S.; Lindblad-Toh, K.; Gnerre, S.; Clamp, M.; Chang, J.; Stephens, R.; Neelam, B.; et al. Initial sequence and comparative analysis of the cat genome. *Genome Res.* **2007**, *17*, 1675–1689. [CrossRef] [PubMed]

45. Lipinski, M.J.; Froenicke, L.; Baysac, K.C.; Billings, N.C.; Leutenegger, C.M.; Levy, A.M.; Longeri, M.; Niini, T.; Ozpinar, H.; Slater, M.R.; et al. The ascent of cat breeds: Genetic evaluations of breeds and worldwide random-bred populations. *Genomics* **2008**, *91*, 12–21. [CrossRef] [PubMed]

46. Gottlieb, S.; Rand, J. Managing feline diabetes: Current perspectives. *Vet. Med.* **2018**, *9*, 33–42. [CrossRef] [PubMed]

47. Gottlieb, S.; Rand, J.S. Remission in cats: Including predictors and risk factors. *Vet. Clin. N. Am. Small Anim. Pract.* **2013**, *43*, 245–249. [CrossRef]

48. Roomp, K.; Rand, J. Intensive blood glucose control is safe and effective in diabetic cats using home monitoring and treatment with glargine. *J. Feline Med. Surg.* **2009**, *11*, 668–682. [CrossRef]

49. Zini, E.; Linscheid, P.; Franchini, M.; Kaufmann, K.; Monnais, E.; Kutter, A.P.; Ackermann, M.; Lutz, T.A.; Reusch, C.E. Partial sequencing and expression of genes involved in glucose metabolism in adipose tissues and skeletal muscle of healthy cats. *Vet. J.* **2009**, *180*, 66–70. [CrossRef]

Whole Genome Sequencing Indicates Heterogeneity of Hyperostotic Disorders in Dogs

Anna Letko [1], **Fabienne Leuthard** [1], **Vidhya Jagannathan** [1], **Daniele Corlazzoli** [2], **Kaspar Matiasek** [3], **Daniela Schweizer** [4], **Marjo K. Hytönen** [5,6], **Hannes Lohi** [5,6], **Tosso Leeb** [1] and **Cord Drögemüller** [1,*]

[1]   Institute of Genetics, Vetsuisse Faculty, University of Bern, 3012 Bern, Switzerland; anna.letko@vetsuisse.unibe.ch (A.L.); fabileuthard@gmail.com (F.L.); vidhya.jagannathan@vetsuisse.unibe.ch (V.J.); tosso.leeb@vetsuisse.unibe.ch (T.L.)

[2]   Clinica Veterinaria Roma Sud, 00173 Roma, Italy; daniele.corlazzoli@me.com

[3]   Section of Clinical & Comparative Neuropathology, Centre for Clinical Veterinary Medicine, Ludwig Maximilians Universität Munich, 80539 Munich, Germany; matiasek@patho.vetmed.uni-muenchen.de

[4]   Division of Clinical Radiology, Vetsuisse Faculty, University of Bern, 3012 Bern, Switzerland; daniela.schweizer@vetsuisse.unibe.ch

[5]   Department of Medical and Clinical Genetics, and Department of Veterinary Biosciences, University of Helsinki, 00014 Helsinki, Finland; marjo.hytonen@helsinki.fi (M.K.H.); hannes.lohi@helsinki.fi (H.L.)

[6]   Folkhälsan Research Center, 00290 Helsinki, Finland

[*]   Correspondence: cord.droegemueller@vetsuisse.unibe.ch;

Abstract: Craniomandibular osteopathy (CMO) and calvarial hyperostotic syndrome (CHS) are proliferative, non-neoplastic disorders affecting the skull bones in young dogs. Different forms of these hyperostotic disorders have been described in many dog breeds. However, an incompletely dominant causative variant for CMO affecting splicing of *SLC37A2* has been reported so far only in three Terrier breeds. The purpose of this study was to identify further possible causative genetic variants associated with CHS in an American Staffordshire Terrier, as well as CMO in seven affected dogs of different breeds. We investigated their whole-genome sequences (WGS) and filtered variants using 584 unrelated genomes, which revealed no variants shared across all affected dogs. However, filtering for private variants of each case separately yielded plausible dominantly inherited candidate variants in three of the eight cases. In an Australian Terrier, a heterozygous missense variant in the *COL1A1* gene (c.1786G>A; p.(Val596Ile)) was discovered. A pathogenic missense variant in *COL1A1* was previously reported in humans with infantile cortical hyperostosis, or Caffey disease, resembling canine CMO. Furthermore, in a Basset Hound, a heterozygous most likely pathogenic splice site variant was found in *SLC37A2* (c.1446+1G>A), predicted to lead to exon skipping as shown before in *SLC37A2*-associated canine CMO of Terriers. Lastly, in a Weimaraner, a heterozygous frameshift variant in *SLC35D1* (c.1021_1024delTCAG; p.(Ser341ArgfsTer22)) might cause CMO due to the critical role of *SLC35D1* in chondrogenesis and skeletal development. Our study indicates allelic and locus heterogeneity for canine CMO and illustrates the current possibilities and limitations of WGS-based precision medicine in dogs.

Keywords: whole-genome sequencing; craniomandibular osteopathy; calvarial hyperostotic syndrome; Caffey disease; infantile cortical hyperostosis; rare disease; *SLC37A2*; *COL1A1*; *SLC35D1*

1. Introduction

Craniomandibular osteopathy (CMO) in dogs is a common type of a hyperostotic disorder, which mainly affects the mandible (OMIA 000236-9615). CMO is a developmental orthopedic disorder described in several dog breeds, and it is clinically equivalent to human infantile cortical hyperostosis, also known as Caffey disease [1] (OMIM 114000). The clinical signs in human patients appear under 6 months of age and are usually self-regressive. This includes swelling and inflammation of soft tissues, as well as hyperostosis of the facial bones, especially the mandible [2]. The disease typically follows an autosomal dominant mode of inheritance with reduced penetrance and has been associated with a common missense variant (NP_000079.2: p.Arg1014Cys) in the *COL1A1* gene [3]. However, genetic heterogeneity exists because this variant was not observed in some of the human Caffey-affected patients [3–5]. Furthermore, an autosomal recessive type of Caffey disease was recently described, reporting a nonsense variant in the *AHSG* gene that encodes alpha 2-HS glycoprotein involved in the formation of bone tissue [6].

CMO in dogs was first described in 1958 [7], and since then it has been observed in several dog breeds including Labrador Retriever, Doberman Pinscher, Great Dane, Boxer, English Bulldog, West Highland White Terrier, Shetland Sheepdog, Pyrenean Mountain Dog, Bullmastiff, Akita, Pit Bull Terrier, Airedale Terrier, Scottish Terrier, Cairn Terrier, and German Wirehaired Pointer (OMIA 000236-9615). This proliferative bone disorder is usually seen in young, growing dogs up to 12 months of age and affects both sexes equally. Clinically it is characterized by a painful swelling of the jaw and the consequent discomfort signs (e.g., difficulty in opening mouth, salivation, and dysphagia that might result in malnutrition) [8]. In addition, the inflammation of soft tissues often results in fever during the bone proliferation phase. The hyperostotic disorder is considered self-limiting, and all clinical signs usually resolve with time, when the regular bone growth and ossification are complete [7]. Calvarial hyperostotic syndrome (CHS) also belonging to the group of canine hyperostotic disorders clinically resembles canine craniomandibular osteopathy and is not histopathologically distinguishable from CMO. Both CHS and CMO may be associated with changes of the long bones, consistent with hypertrophic osteodystrophy. On the basis of histology, it has been proposed that CMO, calvarial hyperostosis, and hypertrophic osteodystrophy belong all to the same osteoproliferative or hyperostotic disorder complex depending on the bones affected [9].

Different modes of inheritance have been reported for canine CMO, suggesting heterogeneity and distinct breed-specific variants. Padgett and Mostosky [10] showed evidence for a recessive mode of inheritance in the West Highland White Terriers by retrospective pedigree analysis. In a genome-wide association study, a splicing variant in the *SLC37A2* gene (XM_005619600.3:c.1332C>T) was identified as causative in West Highland White Terriers, Cairn Terriers, and Scottish Terriers. CMO in these Terrier breeds is inherited with a dominant mode of inheritance with incomplete penetrance [11]. Recently, a more complex polygenic inheritance for CMO in German Wirehaired Pointers was suggested using statistical segregation analysis [12]. Therefore, the understanding of the underlying genetics of canine hyperostotic disorders might benefit from a precision medicine approach.

Germline genetic variation is a quite frequent causal factor in rare diseases in humans. Whole-genome sequencing (WGS) is a relatively inexpensive method to determine individual variation [13]. Precision medicine by using WGS has been proven suitable in recent years to help diagnose rare diseases in single patients and situations with limited access to patients [14]. The methodology has also been successfully adapted to veterinary medicine. For example, single dogs showing suspicious inherited disorders were sequenced and compared to hundreds of normal controls [15], which allowed a precise molecular diagnosis reporting the most likely disease-causing variants [16–18]. A similar approach has also been successfully applied to cats [19–21]. By applying short-read WGS as the current gold standard in precision medicine, we aimed to identify further plausible variants associated with canine hyperostotic disorders such as CMO and CHS to improve the understanding of the etiology of these rare genetic disorders.

2. Materials and Methods

2.1. Ethics Statement

All animal experiments were performed according to the local regulations. All animals in this study were examined with the consent of their owners. Sample collection was approved by the Cantonal Committee for Animal Experiments (Canton of Bern; permit 75/16).

2.2. Animals

Blood samples from a CHS-affected American Staffordshire Terrier and seven dogs affected by CMO of seven different breeds (Supplementary Table S1) were collected. Genomic DNA was isolated from EDTA blood samples using the Maxwell RSC Whole Blood DNA kit (Promega, Dübendorf, Switzerland). All dogs were diagnosed by respective veterinarians on the basis of clinical signs and imaging. Skull radiographs of four and CT scan images of two of the CMO-affected dogs were obtained.

2.3. Whole-Genome Resequencing

WGS data of the eight affected dogs were obtained after preparation of a PCR (polymerase chain reaction)-free fragment library at an average 26× coverage. Fastq-files were mapped to the dog reference genome assembly CanFam3.1. Single nucleotide and small indel variants were called and NCBI (National Center for Biotechnology Information) annotation release 105 was used to predict their functional effects, as described previously [15]. Private variants were identified by comparison with the variant catalog of 576 publically available dogs of 120 various breeds, as well as 8 wolves (Supplementary Table S1), provided by the Dog Biomedical Variant Database Consortium (DBVDC) [15]. The description of the sequence variants is in accordance with the recommendations of the Human Genome Variation Society [22]. Integrative genomics viewer (IGV) [23] was used for visual inspection and validation of the candidate variants found in the affected dogs' WGS data.

2.4. Protein and Splice Site Predictions

The Genome Aggregation Database (gnomAD) [24] was searched for corresponding variants in the human COL1A1, SLC37A2, and SLC35D1 genes. PredictSNP [25] and PROVEAN [26] were used to predict the biological consequences of the discovered COL1A1 variant on the protein. SpliceRack tools [27] were used to evaluate the SLC37A2 splice site variant. All references to the canine COL1A1, SLC37A2, and SLC35D1 genes correspond to the accessions NC_006591.3 (chromosome 9) and NC_006587.3 (chromosome 5) (NCBI accession); NM_001003090.1, XM_005619600.3, and XM_003434643.2 (mRNA); and NP_001003090.1, XP_005619657.1, and XP_003434691.1 (protein), respectively. The canine COL1A1 protein has 1460 amino acids compared to the human protein (NP_000079.2) with 1464 amino acids, from which 98% are identical between dog and human. The canine SLC37A2 protein has 508 amino acids compared to the human protein (NP_001138762.1) with 501 amino acids, from which 86% are identical between dog and human. The canine SLC35D1 protein has the same length of 355 amino acids compared to the human protein (NP_055954.1), from which 98% are identical between dog and human. For the multi-species COL1A1 protein alignment, the following NCBI accession numbers for each species were used: NP_001003090.1 (Canis familiaris), NP_000079.2 (Homo sapiens), NP_001029211.1 (Bos taurus), NP_031768.2 (Mus musculus), NP_445756.1 (Rattus norvegicus), NP_001011005.1 (Xenopus tropicalis), and NP_954684.1 (Danio rerio).

2.5. Availability of Data and Material

The WGS data of all affected as well as comparison cohort dogs/wolves have been made freely available at the European Nucleotide Archive (ENA). All ENA accession numbers are given in the Supplementary Table S1.

3. Results

3.1. Phenotype

We investigated a CHS-affected American Staffordshire Terrier and seven CMO-affected dogs of different breeds (Australian Terrier, Basset Hound, Cairn Terrier, Curly Coated Retriever, German Wirehaired Pointer, Old English Sheepdog, and Weimaraner). The diagnosis was made by veterinarians observing the typical clinical signs including persistent and sharp pain when opening mouth, painful swelling of the jaw, fever, and in some cases also severe pain of ulna and radius bones. Age of onset of the clinical signs ranged from 3 to 7 months of age, and skull radiographs/computed tomographic (CT) images were available for six of the affected dogs (Supplementary Table S1). The imaging findings of one dog was consistent with CHS and in four dogs with CMO (Figure 1), in the remaining dog, no changes were identified on radiographs, but clinical signs were consistent with the diagnosis of CMO. Due to the self-regressive course of the disorder, the remission of clinical signs appeared in all cases soon after the diagnosis and symptomatic treatment. On the basis of the previously published gene test, all eight collected dogs were genotyped negative for the reported CMO-causing variant in *SLC37A2* (XM_005619600.3:c.1332C>T) [11]. In addition, for all eight dogs, the region of the *SLC37A2* gene was also manually inspected in IGV to confirm no candidate variants were missed in the functional annotation and to rule out obvious, large structural variants including copy number variation affecting this gene.

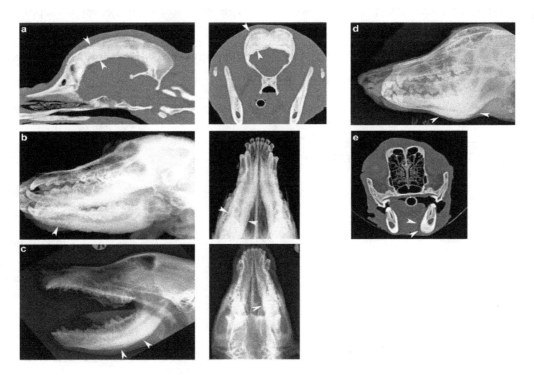

Figure 1. Radiographs/computed tomographic (CT) images of the craniomandibular osteopathy (CMO)/calvarial hyperostotic syndrome (CHS)-affected dogs. (**a**) Sagittal and transverse CT images of an American Staffordshire Terrier showing severe thickening of the calvarial diploic bone (arrowheads). (**b**) Ventrolateral-dorsolateral oblique and ventrodorsal skull radiographs illustrating a palisading periosteal new bone formation along the mandible of a Basset Hound (arrowheads). (**c**) Open mouth laterolateral and ventrodorsal view of the skull of a German Wirehaired Pointer showing periosteal new bone formation along the mandible (arrowheads). (**d**) Slightly oblique laterolateral view of the mandible of an Old English Sheepdog showing similar periosteal new bone formation along the mandible (arrowheads). (**e**) Transverse CT image of a Weimeraner with the arrowheads pointing towards the periosteal new bone formation at the ventral and medial aspect of the left mandibular corpus.

3.2. Identification of Private Candidate Variants

We considered both the autosomal dominant and autosomal recessive modes of inheritance when analyzing the WGS data. Filtering for private variants present in a homozygous or heterozygous state in all eight affected dogs and absent in 584 publicly available dog and wolf genomes revealed no variants shared across all cases. However, filtering for private variants of each of the cases separately yielded possible dominantly inherited candidate protein-changing variants in three cases (Figures 2–4). In the remaining five affected dogs, no variants in obvious functional candidate genes were found. Therefore, we report a catalog of each dog's private variants (Supplementary Tables S2–S9). The total number of variants per genome, when compared to the CanFam3.1 reference, ranged from 4.9 million in the American Staffordshire Terrier to 5.6 million in the Basset Hound (Table 1). After filtering against the public genomes, on average ≈9200 variants were left with the least count observed in American Staffordshire Terrier (4582 variants) and the highest in the Basset Hound (13,370 variants), as shown in Table 1. In total, most of the called variants were located in non-coding intergenic (50.7%) or intronic (48.3%) regions, whereas on average 64.5 (34–96) protein-changing (0.7%) variants were found in each genome.

Table 1. Private variants detected in the individual genomes of the 8 affected dogs and absent in the 584 comparison cohort genomes. The table gives total counts of private variants divided into classes on the basis of their predicted effect. The counts of homozygous/heterozygous genotypes separately are shown in parentheses.

Affected Dog	Total Variants in the Whole Genome	Private Variants after Filtering against 584 Publically Available Genomes				
		Total	Protein-Changing	Synonymous	Intronic	Intergenic
American Staffordshire Terrier (CHS)	4,861,208	4582	76 (67/9)	71 (69/2)	2217 (1832/385)	2218 (1831/387)
Australian Terrier (CMO)	5,495,830	13,147	79 (73/6)	30 (24/6)	6527 (6012/515)	6511 (5875/636)
Basset Hound (CMO)	5,573,559	13,370	96 (87/9)	30 (28/2)	6535 (5917/618)	6709 (6073/636)
Cairn Terrier (CMO)	5,425,950	7373	55 (45/10)	17 (16/1)	3486 (3066/420)	3815 (3344/471)
Curly Coated Retriever (CMO)	5,326,349	4960	34 (34/0)	15 (15/0)	2405 (2248/157)	2506 (2260/246)
German Wirehaired Pointer (CMO)	5,519,945	11,713	63 (52/11)	28 (25/3)	5706 (5137/569)	5916 (5291/625)
Old English Sheepdog (CMO)	5,283,629	10,711	59 (52/7)	22 (17/5)	4966 (4175/791)	5664 (4558/1106)
Weimaraner (CMO)	5,201,857	8056	54 (48/6)	26 (21/5)	3859 (3183/676)	4117 (3307/810)

In the CMO-affected Australian Terrier, a missense variant in exon 26 of the alpha 1 chain of type I collagen (COL1A1) gene was discovered. The detected variant (NM_001003090.1:c.1786G>A) alters the encoded amino acid residue 596 of COL1A1 (NP_001003090.1:p.(Val596Ile)) with a predicted moderate impact on the resulting protein (Figure 2). The missense variant affects the triple helix domain of COL1A1 protein, which typically consists of the invariant Gly-X-Y repeat motif. The amino acid is conserved across species but the valine to isoleucine substitution was predicted neutral and tolerated by in silico prediction tools [25,26]. In humans, a similar missense variant has been described in exon 41, also changing the X residue in the triple repeat motif (Figure 2). There is no non-synonymous variant in the human COL1A1 coding region reported at the corresponding position in the gnomAD [24].

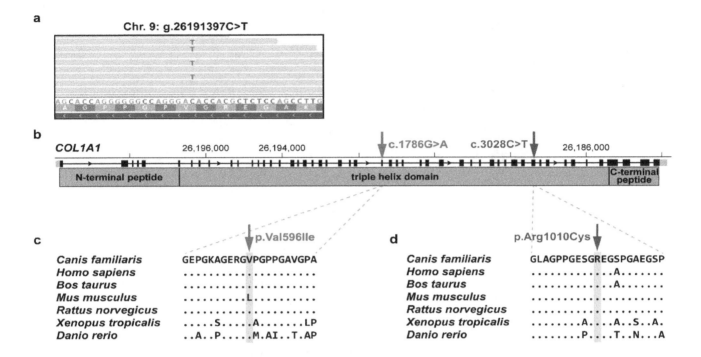

Figure 2. Characterization of the identified functional candidate variant in *COL1A1* in the CMO-affected Australian Terrier. (**a**) Integrative genomics viewer (IGV) snapshot showing the heterozygous missense candidate variant (NC_006591.3:g.26191397C>T). (**b**) Schematic representation of *COL1A1* indicating the c.1786G>A variant location in exon 26 (red) and the previously described human variant (position with respect to the canine *COL1A1*) in exon 41 (blue) encoding the triple helix domain. Note that the canine *COL1A1* gene is annotated on the reverse complementary strand. (**c**) Multispecies protein alignment of the canine CMO-associated missense variant identified herein (red). (**d**) Multispecies protein alignment of the human disease-causing missense variant (blue) [3] with respect to the canine COL1A1 position.

In the CMO-affected Basset Hound, a splice site variant was found in the solute carrier family 37 member 2 (*SLC37A2*) gene. This single nucleotide variant (XM_005619600.3:c.1446+1G>A) affects an evolutionary strongly conserved donor splice site at the beginning of intron 16 and was predicted to disrupt splicing (Figure 3). The human consensus sequence for the U2-type GT-AG donor splice site corresponds to a perfect base pairing to the 5' end of U1 small nuclear RNA [27]. The variant changes this canonical dinucleotide sequence (Figure 3c) and therefore most likely eliminates the splice site and leads to skipping of exon 16 and a shortened transcript. One human variant (rs1278346722) alters the same position of the human *SLC37A2* donor splice site as the dog variant; however, the guanine is exchanged by cytosine (c.1425+1G>C), not by adenine as found here. This human variant is present in only 2 out of 125,127 patients in a heterozygous state (allele frequency of 7.99×10^{-6}) [24].

Lastly, a frameshift variant in the solute carrier family 35 member D1 (*SLC35D1*) gene (XM_003434643.2:c.1021_1024delTCAG) was found in a CMO-affected Weimaraner. The schematic representation indicates that the 4 bp deletion is located in exon 12 and leads to a frameshift affecting the last 15 amino acids of the SLC35D1 protein, and was predicted to produce a novel 22 amino acid long C-terminus of SLC35D1 (XP_003434691.1:p.(Ser341ArgfsTer22); Figure 4). There is no non-synonymous variant in the human *SLC35D1* coding region at the corresponding position described in the gnomAD [24].

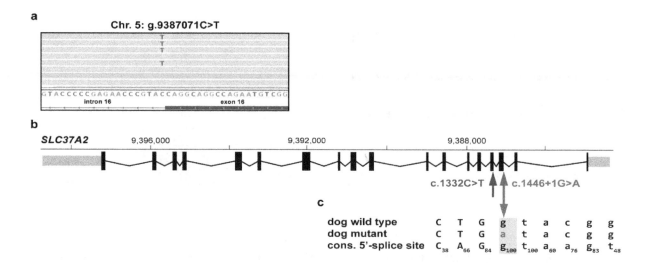

Figure 3. Characterization of the most likely pathogenic variant in *SLC37A2* in the CMO-affected Basset Hound. (**a**) IGV snapshot showing the heterozygous splice site candidate variant (NC_006587.3:g.9387071C>T). (**b**) Schematic representation of the *SLC37A2* transcript (XM_005619600.3) including the location of previously identified canine splicing variant at the end of exon 15 [11] (blue), as well as the newly reported variant at the beginning of intron 16 (red). Note that the *SLC37A2* gene is annotated on the reverse complementary strand. (**c**) Wild type and mutant allele compared to the human consensus sequence for the U2-type GT-AG donor splice sites [27]. The uppercase letters indicate exon 16 and lowercase letters intron 16 sequence, whereas the subscript numbers show the percentage of the respective conserved nucleotide in 186,630 investigated U2-type GT-AG human 5'-splice site motifs. The base at position +1 is a highly conserved G (100%) [27].

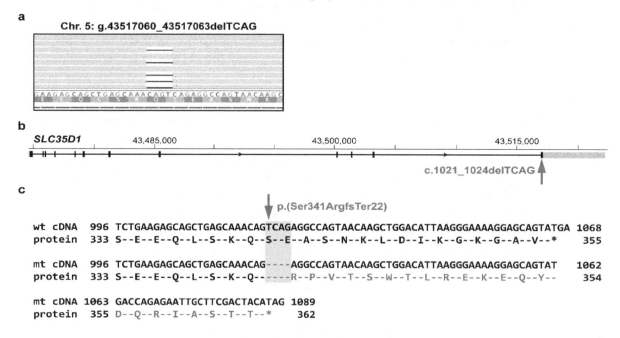

Figure 4. Characterization of the identified functional candidate variant in *SLC35D1* in the CMO-affected Weimaraner. (**a**) IGV snapshot showing the heterozygous frameshift candidate variant (NC_006587.3:g.43517060_435178063delTCAG), note that the variant description is adapted to the 3' rule [22]. (**b**) Schematic representation of the *SLC35D1* gene with the variant affecting the last exon. (**c**) Comparison of wild type and the predicted mutant C-terminus protein sequence based on cDNA entry XM_003434643.2. The variant (XP_003434691.1:p.(Ser341ArgfsTer22)) affects the last 15 amino acids of SLC35D1.

4. Discussion

On the basis of clinical signs and/or radiography analyses, eight dogs of eight different breeds were diagnosed with different forms of hyperostotic disorders such as CHS or CMO. Because all eight affected dogs were homozygous wild type for the previously described variant causing CMO in three different Terrier breeds [11], whole-genome sequencing of the individual cases was performed to investigate the underlying genetics.

No variants shared across all 8 affected dogs and absent from 584 publically available genomes were discovered, which was in accordance with the expectation of several breed-specific types. The total number of private variants varied greatly between the individual genomes. This might be partially the consequence of different levels of inbreeding in different breeds, as well as the variable numbers of breed controls present in the studied dataset [15]. By prioritization of functional candidate genes, three possible causative variants in *COL1A1*, *SCL37A2*, and SLC35D1 were identified when searching for private variants in the Australian Terrier, the Basset Hound, and the Weimaraner, respectively.

The identified *COL1A1*:c.1786G>A variant in a CMO-affected Australian Terrier was predicted to result in a substitution of valine by isoleucine in the triple helix domain of alpha 1 chain of type I collagen (*COL1A1*). The structure of connective tissues includes collagens, proteoglycans, and non-collagenous proteins, as well as enzymes that are necessary for precise extracellular matrix assembly and degradation. Mutations in genes encoding these distinct components of the matrix result in similar phenotypes [28]. The triple-helical domain in collagen proteins consists of a Gly-X-Y repeating motif that is essential for the helix folding [29]. Mutations of the Gly residues lead to more severe defects such as osteogenesis imperfecta (OMIM 120150, OMIA 002126-9615, OMIA 002127-9913). On the other hand, substitutions of the X or Y residues result in milder phenotypes and are associated with Ehlers–Danlos syndrome and Caffey disease (OMIM 120150) [28]. The autosomal dominant form of infantile cortical hyperostosis in humans (OMIM 114000) is described as a collagenopathy caused by a single heterozygous missense variant in *COL1A1* with incomplete penetrance. This variant affects the X residue in a triple-helical domain of COL1A1 (Figure 2), but the exact pathogenesis of how it leads to self-limiting hyperostotic bone lesions is still unclear [3]. Therefore, we speculate that the identified missense variant in canine *COL1A1* might represent a candidate variant of uncertain significance for CMO in the affected Australian Terrier. However, as the predicted amino acid substitution involves two chemically similar, hydrophobic amino acids, this result should be considered preliminary and requires further confirmation.

The detected splice site variant in *SLC37A2* is the most likely pathogenic variant for CMO in the affected Basset Hound. *SLC37A2* has been shown to be associated with CMO in Terriers [11]. Belonging to the glucose-phosphate transporter family, it is expressed in bone-related tissues including bone marrow or osteoclasts. In mice, *Slc37a2* was shown to have an important role in osteoclast differentiation and function [30]. The previously identified synonymous variant causes altered splicing, resulting in a frameshift and premature stop codon [11]. This likely affects the function of SLC37A2 and leads to disturbed glucose homeostasis in osteoclasts in the developing bones, potentially explaining the hyperostosis phenotype of CMO-affected Terriers [11]. The process of splicing consists of the recognition of exon-intron boundaries by spliceosome complex and the subsequent excision of an intron and is highly conserved across eukaryotes [31]. Splice sites are classified in four major subtypes on the basis of components of the spliceosome and the introns' terminal dinucleotides. The majority of all human splice sites are the U2-type GT-AG subtype. The highly conserved bases at the first and second positions of the 5' motif of U2-type splice sites are G and T (100%) [27]. The herein reported splice site variant (c.1446+1G>A) detected in a CMO-affected Basset Hound changes this canonical dinucleotide sequence. Therefore, it most likely disrupts the correct splicing of intron 16.

The *SLC35D1* protein-changing variant (c.1021_1024delTCAG) found in a CMO-affected Weimaraner leads to a frameshift affecting the last 15 amino acids of the SLC35D1 protein. The solute carrier family 35 member D1 (*SLC35D1*) gene encodes another nucleotide-sugar transporter, which has a crucial role in chondroitin sulfate biosynthesis [32]. Chondroitin sulfate chains are an important part of cartilage proteoglycans, which are needed for chondrogenesis and skeletal development [33]. Impairment of the proteoglycan synthesis was confirmed in the *Slc35d1*-knockout mice, which showed severe chondrodysplasia, including hypoplastic craniofacial bones and extremely short long bones. The heterozygous *Slc35d1*$^{+/-}$ mice were phenotypically apparently normal [32]. In humans, autosomal recessive mutations in *SLC35D1* have been described in a rare lethal skeletal dysplasia (OMIM 269250). On the basis of these comparative data, it seems possible that the canine frameshift variant represents a likely causative variant for CMO phenotype in the affected Weimaraner. This might be either due to haploinsufficiency or a dominant negative function of the mutant protein on the residual wildtype SLC35D1.

The success rate of WGS-based identification of rare disease-causing genes is difficult to determine because about two-thirds of studied human diseases discover too many credible candidate variants and in the remaining one-third there are none [13]. Similarly, the comparisons described herein, using the recently presented DBVDC variant catalog, reduced the ≈5,000,000 variants per genome identified from WGS to <100 protein-changing variants per genome. Even though the DBVDC variant catalog is a great resource for identification of potential causal variants in dogs, the numbers of identified private protein-changing variants per genome are probably overestimated because of the still imperfect status and annotation of the current CanFam3.1 reference genome, and prioritization of causal variants remains challenging. For example, there is a gap in the reference assembly in the 5′-region of *SLC37A2*. Therefore, sequencing of additional genomes of well-phenotyped breed-matched obligate carriers and/or affected dogs may help unravel the complete molecular etiology of canine hyperostotic disorders such as CHS or CMO in the remaining cases by reducing the number of private candidate variants shared in cases of the same breed. De novo mutations causing autosomal dominant disorders are easier to identify when parents' data is available because each individual carries fewer variants that are not also found in the parents [16]. Unfortunately, for the examined cases in this study, we had no access to samples of the parents to evaluate the possibility of spontaneously occurring mutations causing the hyperostotic disorder. Furthermore, analyzing the transcriptome of biopsies or even better relevant cells from affected tissue by RNAseq methods would be an excellent option to get further insights into the development of this transient disease phenotype. Despite the availability of the molecular methods, studying possible temporal and/or cell-specific expression changes remains challenging due to the practical and ethical limitations of accessing the appropriate samples in privately-owned dogs.

Considering the relatively mild and self-limiting phenotype, some cases may remain undiagnosed, which together with lower penetrance possibly prevented the identification of further disease-causing variants. Comparison cohort dogs used for variant filtering were assumed to be non-affected. However, in light of the fact that the affected individuals with CHS or CMO spontaneously recover, we cannot rule out the possibility that pathogenic alleles were present in the publically available genomes, which would obviously limit the power of the WGS-based precision medicine approach.

5. Conclusions

We propose that the novel splicing variant *SLC37A2*:c.1446+1G>A is most likely pathogenic for CMO. We report two other candidate causative variants of uncertain significance with less evidence for pathogenicity in compelling functional candidate genes (*COL1A1* and *SLC35D1*). Further functional studies are needed to confirm the causality of the described variants, whereas additional genetic and/or environmental factors might also influence the manifestation of the disorder. In addition, the detection of structural variants such as larger-sized indels or segmental duplications is strongly limited. The sensitivity of our variant detection might have been compromised by the presence of gaps in the reference genome and the employed short-read sequencing technology. Consequently, long-read sequencing improved reference assembly and annotation quality, and better algorithms for indels and structural variant calling might overcome these issues in the future. Nevertheless, our study demonstrates allelic and locus heterogeneity of different forms of canine hyperostotic disorders and indicates the current possibilities and limitations of precision medicine in dogs.

Supplementary Materials:
Table S1: Detailed information of all whole-genome sequences. Table S2: List of private variants of the sequenced CMO-affected Australian Terrier. Table S3. List of private variants of the sequenced CHS-affected American Staffordshire Terrier. Table S4. List of private variants of the sequenced CMO-affected Basset Hound. Table S5. List of private variants of the sequenced CMO-affected Cairn Terrier. Table S6. List of private variants of the sequenced CMO-affected Curly Coated Retriever. Table S7. List of private variants of the sequenced CMO-affected German Wirehaired Pointer. Table S8. List of private variants of the sequenced CMO-affected Old English Sheepdog. Table S9. List of private variants of the sequenced CMO-affected Weimaraner.

Author Contributions: Conceptualization, C.D.; data curation, V.J.; formal analysis, A.L.; funding acquisition, C.D.; investigation, A.L., F.L., and D.S.; methodology, A.L.; project administration, C.D.; resources, D.C., K.M., M.K.H., and H.L.; software, V.J.; supervision, C.D.; visualization, A.L. and F.L.; writing—original draft, A.L.; writing—review and editing, A.L., F.L., T.L., and C.D. All authors have read and agreed to the published version of the manuscript.

Acknowledgments: The authors are grateful to the owners of the affected dogs, who provided samples and shared valuable information about their dogs. Furthermore, we would like to thank all the veterinarians, in particular, Jean-Baptiste Fabre, for their expertise in diagnosing the cases. We acknowledge the Next Generation Sequencing Platform of the University of Bern for performing the whole-genome resequencing experiments, and the Interfaculty Bioinformatics Unit of the University of Bern for providing computational infrastructure.

References

1. Thornburg, L.P. Infantile cortical hyperostosis (Caffey-Silverman syndrome). Animal model: Craniomandibular osteopathy in the canine. *Am. J. Pathol.* **1979**, *95*, 575–578. [PubMed]

2. Kamoun-Goldrat, A.; Le Merrer, M. Infantile Cortical Hyperostosis (Caffey Disease): A Review. *J. Oral Maxillofac. Surg.* **2008**, *66*, 2145–2150. [CrossRef] [PubMed]

3. Gensure, R.C.; Cole, W.G.; Jüppner, H.; Gensure, R.C.; Mäkitie, O.; Barclay, C.; Chan, C.; Depalma, S.R.; Bastepe, M.; Abuzahra, H.; et al. A novel COL1A1 mutation in infantile cortical hyperostosis (Caffey disease) expands the spectrum of collagen-related disorders. *J. Clin. Investig.* **2005**, *115*, 1250–1257. [CrossRef] [PubMed]

4. Kamoun-Goldrat, A.; Martinovic, J.; Saada, J.; Sonigo-Cohen, P.; Razavi, F.; Munnich, A.; Le Merrer, M. Prenatal Cortical Hyperostosis With COL1A1 Gene Mutation. *Am. J. Med. Genet.* **2008**, *146*, 1820–1824. [CrossRef] [PubMed]

5. Kitaoka, T.; Miyoshi, Y.; Namba, N.; Miura, K.; Jüppner, H.; Kubota, T.; Ohata, Y.; Fujiwara, M.; Takagi, M.; Hasegawa, T.; et al. Two Japanese familial cases of Caffey disease with and without the common COL1A1 mutation and normal bone density, and review of the literature. *Eur. J. Pediatr.* **2014**, *173*, 799–804. [CrossRef] [PubMed]

6. Merdler-rabinowicz, R.; Grinberg, A.; Jacobson, J.M.; Somekh, I.; Klein, C.; Lev, A.; Ihsan, S.; Habib, A.; Somech, R.; Simon, A.J. Fetuin-A deficiency is associated with infantile cortical hyperostosis (Caffey disease). *Pediatr. Res.* **2019**. [CrossRef]

7. Newton, C.D.; Nunamaker, D.M. *Textbook of Small Animal Orthopaedics*; Lippincott: Philadelphia, PA, USA, 1985; ISBN 9780397520985.

8. Alexander, J.W. Selected Skeletal Dysplasias: Craniomandibular Osteopathy, Multiple Cartilaginous Exostoses, and Hypertrophic Osteodystrophy. *Vet. Clin. North Am. Small Anim. Pract.* **1983**, *13*, 55–70. [CrossRef]

9. Pastor, K.F.; Boulay, J.P.; Schelling, S.H.; Carpenter, J.L. Idiopathic hyperostosis of the calvaria in five young bullmastiffs. *J. Am. Anim. Hosp. Assoc.* **2000**, *36*, 439–445. [CrossRef]

10. Padgett, G.A.; Mostosky, U.V. Animal Model: The Mode of Inheritance of Craniomandibular Osteopathy in West Highland White Terrier Dogs. *Am. J. Med. Genet.* **1986**, *13*, 9–13. [CrossRef]

11. Hytönen, M.K.; Arumilli, M.; Lappalainen, A.K.; Owczarek-Lipska, M.; Jagannathan, V.; Hundi, S.; Salmela, E.; Venta, P.; Sarkiala, E.; Jokinen, T.; et al. Molecular Characterization of Three Canine Models of Human Rare Bone Diseases: Caffey, van den Ende-Gupta, and Raine. *PLoS Genet.* **2016**, *12*, 1–20. [CrossRef]

12. Vagt, J.; Distl, O. Complex segregation analysis of craniomandibular osteopathy in Deutsch Drahthaar dogs. *Vet. J.* **2018**, *231*, 30–32. [CrossRef] [PubMed]

13. Boycott, K.M.; Vanstone, M.R.; Bulman, D.E.; MacKenzie, A.E. Rare-disease genetics in the era of next-generation sequencing: Discovery to translation. *Nat. Rev. Genet.* **2013**, *14*, 681. [CrossRef] [PubMed]

14. Ashley, E.A. Towards precision medicine. *Nat. Rev. Genet.* **2016**, *17*, 507–522. [CrossRef] [PubMed]

15. Jagannathan, V.; Drögemüller, C.; Leeb, T. Dog Biomedical Variant Database Consortium (DBVDC) A comprehensive biomedical variant catalogue based on whole genome sequences of 582 dogs and 8 wolves. *Anim. Genet.* **2019**. [CrossRef] [PubMed]

16. Bauer, A.; Waluk, D.P.; Galichet, A.; Timm, K.; Jagannathan, V.; Sayar, B.S.; Wiener, D.J.; Dietschi, E.; Muller, E.J.; Roosje, P.; et al. A de novo variant in the *ASPRV1* gene in a dog with ichthyosis. *PLoS Genet.* **2017**, *13*, e1006651. [CrossRef]

17. Hadji Rasouliha, S.; Bauer, A.; Dettwiler, M.; Welle, M.M.; Leeb, T. A frameshift variant in the *EDA* gene in Dachshunds with X-linked hypohidrotic ectodermal dysplasia. *Anim. Genet.* **2018**, *49*, 651–654. [CrossRef]

18. Caduff, M.; Bauer, A.; Jagannathan, V.; Leeb, T. A single base deletion in the *SLC45A2* gene in a Bullmastiff with oculocutaneous albinism. *Anim. Genet.* **2017**, *48*, 619–621. [CrossRef]

19. Spycher, M.; Bauer, A.; Jagannathan, V.; Frizzi, M.; De Lucia, M.; Leeb, T. A frameshift variant in the COL5A1 gene in a cat with Ehlers-Danlos syndrome. *Anim. Genet.* **2018**, *49*, 641–644. [CrossRef]

20. Bridavsky, M.; Kuhl, H.; Woodruff, A.; Kornak, U.; Timmermann, B.; Mages, N.; Lupianez, D.G.; Symmons, O.; Ibrahim, D.M.; 99 Lives Consortium. Crowdfunded whole-genome sequencing of the celebrity cat Lil BUB identifies causal mutations for her osteopetrosis and polydactyly. *bioRxiv* **2019**, 556761. [CrossRef]

21. Mauler, D.A.; Gandolfi, B.; Reinero, C.R.; Spooner, J.L.; Lyons, L.A.; 99 Lives Consortium. Precision Medicine in Cats: Novel Niemann-Pick Type C1 Diagnosed by Whole-Genome Sequencing. *J. Vet. Intern. Med.* **2017**, 539–544. [CrossRef]

22. den Dunnen, J.T.; Dalgleish, R.; Maglott, D.R.; Hart, R.K.; Greenblatt, M.S.; McGowan-Jordan, J.; Roux, A.-F.; Smith, T.; Antonarakis, S.E.; Taschner, P.E.M. HGVS Recommendations for the Description of Sequence Variants: 2016 Update. *Hum. Mutat.* **2016**, *37*, 564–569. [CrossRef] [PubMed]

23. Thorvaldsdóttir, H.; Robinson, J.T.; Mesirov, J.P. Integrative Genomics Viewer (IGV): High-performance genomics data visualization and exploration. *Brief. Bioinform.* **2013**, *14*, 178–192. [CrossRef] [PubMed]

24. Karczewski, K.J.; Francioli, L.C.; Tiao, G.; Cummings, B.B.; Alföldi, J.; Wang, Q.; Collins, R.L.; Laricchia, K.M.; Ganna, A.; Birnbaum, D.P.; et al. Variation across 141,456 human exomes and genomes reveals the spectrum of loss-of-function intolerance across human protein-coding genes. *bioRxiv* **2019**, 531210. [CrossRef]

25. Bendl, J.; Stourac, J.; Salanda, O.; Pavelka, A.; Wieben, E.D.; Zendulka, J.; Brezovsky, J.; Damborsky, J. PredictSNP: Robust and Accurate Consensus Classifier for Prediction of Disease-Related Mutations. *PLOS Comput. Biol.* **2014**, *10*, e1003440. [CrossRef] [PubMed]

26. Choi, Y.; Chan, A.P. PROVEAN web server: A tool to predict the functional effect of amino acid substitutions and indels. *Bioinformatics* **2015**, *31*, 2745–2747. [CrossRef]

27. Sheth, N.; Roca, X.; Hastings, M.L.; Roeder, T.; Krainer, A.R.; Sachidanandam, R. Comprehensive splice-site analysis using comparative genomics. *Nucleic Acids Res.* **2006**, *34*, 3955–3967. [CrossRef]

28. Nistala, H.; Mäkitie, O.; Jüppner, H. Caffey disease: New perspectives on old questions. *Bone* **2014**, *60*, 246–251. [CrossRef]

29. Campbell, B.G.; Wootton, J.A.M.; MacLeod, J.N.; Minor, R.R. Sequence of Normal Canine COL1A1 cDNA 1 and Identification of a Heterozygous alpha1 (I) Collagen Gly208Ala Mutation in a Severe Case of Canine Osteogenesis Imperfecta. *Arch. Biochem. Biophys.* **2000**, *384*, 37–46. [CrossRef]

30. Ha, B.G.; Hong, J.M.; Park, J.-Y.; Ha, M.-H.; Kim, T.-H.; Cho, J.-Y.; Ryoo, H.-M.; Choi, J.-Y.; Shin, H.-I.; Chun, S.Y.; et al. Proteomic profile of osteoclast membrane proteins: Identification of Na+/H+ exchanger domain containing 2 and its role in osteoclast fusion. *Proteomics* **2008**, *8*, 2625–2639. [CrossRef]

31. Reese, M.G.; Eeckman, F.H.; Kulp, D.; Haussler, D. Improved Splice Site Detection in Genie. *J. Comput. Biol.* **1997**, *4*, 311–323. [CrossRef]

32. Hiraoka, S.; Furuichi, T.; Nishimura, G.; Shibata, S.; Yanagishita, M.; Rimoin, D.L.; Superti-Furga, A.; Nikkels, P.G.; Ogawa, M.; Katsuyama, K.; et al. Nucleotide-sugar transporter SLC35D1 is critical to chondroitin sulfate synthesis in cartilage and skeletal development in mouse and human. *Nat. Med.* **2007**, *13*, 1363–1367. [CrossRef] [PubMed]

33. Sugahara, K.; Kitagawa, H. Recent advances in the study of the biosynthesis and functions of sulfated glycosaminoglycans. *Curr. Opin. Struct. Biol.* **2000**, *10*, 518–527. [CrossRef]

13

Mitochondrial PCK2 Missense Variant in Shetland Sheepdogs with Paroxysmal Exercise-Induced Dyskinesia (PED)

Jasmin Nessler [1,†], Petra Hug [2,†], Paul J. J. Mandigers [3], Peter A. J. Leegwater [3], Vidhya Jagannathan [2], Anibh M. Das [4], Marco Rosati [5], Kaspar Matiasek [5], Adrian C. Sewell [6], Marion Kornberg [7], Marina Hoffmann [8], Petra Wolf [9], Andrea Fischer [10], Andrea Tipold [1] and Tosso Leeb [2,*]

[1] Department of Small Animal Medicine and Surgery, University of Veterinary Medicine Hannover Foundation, 30559 Hannover, Germany; jasmin.nessler@tiho-hannover.de (J.N.); andrea.tipold@tiho-hannover.de (A.T.)

[2] Institute of Genetics, Vetsuisse Faculty, University of Bern, 3001 Bern, Switzerland; petrahug@bluewin.ch (P.H.); vidhya.jagannathan@vetsuisse.unibe.ch (V.J.)

[3] Department of Clinical Sciences, Faculty of Veterinary Medicine, Utrecht University, 3584 CM Utrecht, The Netherlands; p.j.j.mandigers@veterinair-neuroloog.nl (P.J.J.M.); P.A.J.Leegwater@uu.nl (P.A.J.L.)

[4] Department of Pediatrics, Hannover Medical School, 30625 Hannover, Germany; Das.Anibh@mh-hannover.de

[5] Section of Clinical and Comparative Neuropathology, Institute of Veterinary Pathology at the Centre for Clinical Veterinary Medicine, Ludwig-Maximilians-Universität, 80539 Munich, Germany; marco.rosati@neuropathologie.de (M.R.); kaspar.matiasek@neuropathologie.de (K.M.)

[6] Biocontrol, Labor für Veterinärmedizinische Diagnostik, 55218 Ingelheim, Germany; a.sewell@freenet.de

[7] AniCura Tierklinik Trier GbR, 54294 Trier, Germany; Kornberg@t-online.de

[8] Tierklinik Stommeln, 50259 Puhlheim, Germany; dr.marinahoffmann@googlemail.com

[9] Nutritional Physiology and Animal Nutrition, University of Rostock, 18059 Rostock, Germany; petra.wolf@uni-rostock.de

[10] Section of Neurology, Clinic of Small Animal Medicine, Ludwig-Maximilians-Universität, 80539 Munich, Germany; A.Fischer@medizinische-kleintierklinik.de

* Correspondence: tosso.leeb@vetsuisse.unibe.ch;
† These authors contributed equally to this work.

Abstract: Four female Shetland Sheepdogs with hypertonic paroxysmal dyskinesia, mainly triggered by exercise and stress, were investigated in a retrospective multi-center investigation aiming to characterize the clinical phenotype and its underlying molecular etiology. Three dogs were closely related and their pedigree suggested autosomal dominant inheritance. Laboratory diagnostic findings included mild lactic acidosis and lactaturia, mild intermittent serum creatine kinase (CK) elevation and hypoglycemia. Electrophysiological tests and magnetic resonance imaging of the brain were unremarkable. A muscle/nerve biopsy revealed a mild type II fiber predominant muscle atrophy. While treatment with phenobarbital, diazepam or levetiracetam did not alter the clinical course, treatment with a gluten-free, home-made fresh meat diet in three dogs or a tryptophan-rich, gluten-free, seafood-based diet, stress-reduction, and acetazolamide or zonisamide in the fourth dog correlated with a partial reduction in, or even a complete absence of, dystonic episodes. The genomes of two cases were sequenced and compared to 654 control genomes. The analysis revealed a case-specific missense variant, c.1658G>A or p.Arg553Gln, in the *PCK2* gene encoding the mitochondrial phosphoenolpyruvate carboxykinase 2. Sanger sequencing confirmed that all four cases carried the mutant allele in a heterozygous state. The mutant allele was not found in 117 Shetland Sheepdog controls and more than 500 additionally genotyped dogs from various other breeds. The p.Arg553Gln substitution affects a highly conserved residue in close proximity to the GTP-binding site of PCK2. Taken together, we describe a new form of paroxysmal exercise-induced dyskinesia (PED) in dogs. The genetic findings suggest that PCK2:p.Arg553Gln should be further investigated as putative candidate causal variant.

Keywords: *Canis lupus familiaris*; whole genome sequencing; dog; mitochondrion; phosphoenolpyruvate-carboxykinase; inborn error of metabolism; precision medicine

---

1. Introduction

Paroxysmal movement disorders are a group of diverse neurological conditions characterized by the episodic occurrence of involuntary movements. In most cases with such disorders, patients have a normal interictal examination [1]. In human medicine, paroxysmal movement disorders are classified into paroxysmal dyskinesias (PxDs) and episodic ataxias (EAs). The PxDs are further subdivided into four related forms, paroxysmal kinesigenic dyskinesia (PKD), paroxysmal non-kinesigenic dyskinesia (PNKD), paroxysmal hypnogenic dyskinesia (PHD), and paroxysmal exercise-induced dyskinesia (PED) [1].

PED in humans is most frequently due to genetic variants in the *SLC2A1* gene encoding the GLUT1 transporter mediating glucose transfer across the blood–brain barrier [1–4]. Dominant and recessive forms of *SLC2A1* related PED have been described. Depending on the specific variant, the PED may occur isolated [2,3] or in combination with other phenotypes, such as epilepsy, delayed development and mental retardation [4]. In other human patients with isolated or syndromic PED forms, genetic variants in *GCH1* or *PARKN* have been described [5,6].

In veterinary medicine, several breed-specific episodic movement disorders characterized by spasticity have been reported [7]. Their etiopathophysiology is heterogenous in different breeds and the causal genetic variants are only partially known. The so-called Scottie Cramp in Scottish Terriers was already recognized 50 years ago and is characterized by generalized or hind limb spasticity. The molecular cause has not yet been reported in the scientific literature [8–10]. Related phenotypes also with unclear causative genetic defects were reported in Bichon Frisé [11,12], Border Terriers [13–15], Boxers [16], Chinooks [17], German Shorthair Pointers [18], Jack Russell Terriers [19] and Maltese dogs [20].

In Soft-Coated Wheaten Terriers, an autosomal recessive paroxysmal dyskinesia is caused by a variant in the *PIGN* gene encoding the phosphatidylinositol glycan anchor biosynthesis class N (OMIA 002084-9615) [21]. Episodic falling syndrome in Cavalier King Charles Spaniels is an autosomal recessive disorder caused by variants in the *BCAN* gene encoding the brain-specific extracellular matrix proteoglycan brevican (OMIA 001592-9615) [22,23].

In this manuscript, we describe the clinical and diagnostic findings, treatment and outcome of four Shetland Sheepdogs with a paroxysmal movement disorder classified as PED together with our efforts to elucidate the underlying causative genetic defect. The study was conducted as a retrospective multi-center investigation.

2. Materials and Methods

2.1. Ethics Statement

All animal experiments were performed according to local regulations. All dogs in this study were privately owned and examined with the consent of their owners. The "Cantonal Committee for Animal Experiments" approved the collection of blood samples (Canton of Bern; permit 75/16).

2.2. Animal Selection

This study included four PED affected Shetland Sheepdogs, one from Germany and three related cases from the Netherlands (Figure 1). In the Dutch family, one of the cases is the mother of the other two cases, who are full siblings. A half sibling to the two cases with similar clinical signs died before blood samples could be drawn. For the genetic analyses, we used 117 additional blood samples of Shetland Sheepdogs without any reports of neurological disease and 515 dogs of various other breeds, which had been donated to the Vetsuisse Biobank. Additional details on the samples are given in Tables S1 and S2.

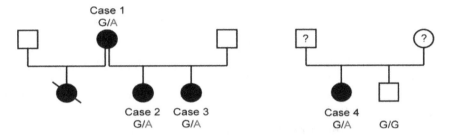

Figure 1. Pedigrees of the four affected Shetland Sheepdogs. Squares represent males and circles represent females. Filled symbols indicate affected dogs and open symbols indicate non-affected dogs. Symbols with question marks indicate dogs of an unknown phenotype. The strike-through symbol represents a dog that died before the beginning of the investigation. According to the owner, this dog had similar clinical signs as the other affected Shetland Sheepdogs. The genotypes at the PCK2:c.1658G>A variant are given for dogs, from which samples were available (see Section 3.5).

2.3. Clinical Examinations

Clinical examinations were performed at the University of Veterinary Medicine Hannover, Foundation, Utrecht University, Department of Clinical Sciences of Companion Animals, AniCura Veterinary Clinic Trier GbR, and Veterinary Clinic Neandertal GbR. All examinations were performed after written informed owner´s consent according to the ethical guidelines of the University of Veterinary Medicine Hannover, Foundation and Utrecht University. A resident or diplomate of the European College of Veterinary Neurology performed the examinations in every dog.

Stress tests were performed to aggravate clinical signs by playing with the dogs for up to 30 min or by applying different external stressful stimuli ($n = 3$). Heart rate, rectal body temperature, blood glucose, lactate, creatinine kinase (CK) and electrolytes were measured before and after playing.

2.4. Laboratory Examinations

Blood examinations were performed immediately after blood sampling and included blood cell count (ADVIA 120 Hematology System, Siemens Healthcare GmbH, Erlangen, Germany), biochemistry (Cobas c 311 analyzer, Roche Deutschland Holding GmbH, Mannheim, Germany) and electrolytes (RAPIDLab 1260, Siemens Healthcare GmbH). Plasma was examined for total thyroxine content via electro-chemiluminescence immunoassay (ECLI, $n = 3$). Serum for insulin measurements was frozen at $-4\,°C$ immediately after sampling and was examined within 24 h via chemiluminescent Immunoassay (CLIA, $n = 1$, Biocontrol, Ingelheim am Rhein, Germany). Urine samples were taken via cystocentesis and immediately frozen at $-20\,°C$ until examination. Analysis of urinary organic acids ($n = 3$) was performed by gas chromatography and mass spectroscopy (Biocontrol, and Biochemical Genetics Laboratory, San Diego, CA, USA). For detailed case information, see Table S3.

2.5. Cardiac Examinations

Cardiac sonography was performed in an awake state in all 4 cases [24]. Ambulatory electrocardiography (ECG) was performed for 24 hours in case 4 with a bipolar triaxial lead system via telemetric ECG on a holter (Televet 100 Version 4.2, Engel Engineering Service GmbH, Heusenstamm, Germany) [25].

2.6. Muscle Examinations and Histopathology

Electrodiagnostic examinations of the axial and abaxial muscles and peripheral nerves in all 4 cases were performed using a Vicking Quest electrodiagnostic device (Nicolet Viking Quest IV, Nicolet EBE GmbH, Kleinostheim Germany). Recordings of the compound muscle action potentials (CMAP) and measurement of the motor nerve conduction velocity (mNCV) and the amplitude of the CMAP as well as repetitive nerve stimulation were performed with 0.5, 2, 3, 10 and 30 Hz of the radial and peroneal nerves. Muscle and nerve biopsies were taken from the extensor carpi radialis and tibialis cranialis muscles of case 4 under general anesthesia according to Platt and Olby [26] and were sent to the Clinical and Comparative Neuropathology Laboratory of the Ludwig-Maximilians-Universität, Munich. Samples underwent routine cryohistological processing, including enzyme histochemistry for cytochrome oxidase and nicotinamide adenine dinucleotide tetrazolium reductase, myofiber typing and special stains for the detection of polysaccharides (periodic acid Schiff) and lipids (oil red O), mitochondria and protein aggregates (Engel´s modified Gomori stain). Further samples of both muscles were subjected to transmission electron microscopy following glutaraldehyde fixation, embedding in epoxy resin, ultrasectioning and contrasting with lead citrate and uranyl acetate.

2.7. Additional Diagnostic Examinations

Electroencephalography (EEG, NicoletOne nEEG, Nicolet) of case 4 was obtained in an awake state with a montage according to Brauer et al. [27].

Low field magnetic resonance imaging (MRI) of the brain of case 4 was performed by the referring veterinarian. T2weighted (T2w), T1weighted (T1w) and fluid attenuation inversion recovery (FLAIR) sequences were available for review.

Cerebrospinal fluid (CSF) was sampled from case 4 in general anesthesia from the cisterna magna and was immediately examined for protein (Cobas c 311 analyzer) and cell content [26].

2.8. Autoantibodies

Serum and CSF of case 4 were screened for known and novel nervous system autoantibodies with cell-based assays (GAD65, NMDAR, GABABR, AMPARI, AMPAR2, DPPX, LGl1, CASPR2, GlyR, mGlu5) and immunofluorescence test (IFT) on mice hippocampi (Epilepsiezentrum Bethel, Bielefeld, Germany).

2.9. Fibroblast Culture

Dermal fibroblasts from case 4 were cultured to further examine mitochondrial function according to [28]. A skin biopsy as a starting material was taken from case 4 under local anesthesia (Lidocain 2 mL subcutaneously with 2 cm of spatial distance to the biopsy site; Lidocard 2% Mini-Plasco; B. Braun Melsungen AG, Melsungen, Germany).

2.10. Tryptophan Content of Therapeutic Diet

Tryptophan contents of a conventional gluten-containing diet (Markus Mühle®, Langenhahn, Germany), a conventional gluten-free diet (Wildkind®, Das Futterhaus-Franchise GmbH & Co. KG, Elmshorn, Germany) and a gluten- and grain-free, seafood-based diet (Purizon Fisch®, Matina GmbH, München, Germany) fed to case 4 were measured (Routine Laboratory, University of Rostock).

2.11. Whole Genome Sequencing of Two Affected Shetland Sheepdogs

Genomic DNA was isolated from the EDTA blood of affected dogs and healthy controls with the Maxwell RSC Whole Blood Kit using a Maxwell RSC instrument (Promega, Dübendorf, Switzerland). Illumina TruSeq PCR-free DNA libraries with 350 bp insert size of one affected Shetland Sheepdog from each of the two families were prepared (cases 2 and 4). We collected 331 and 321 million 2×150 bp paired-end reads on a NovaSeq 6000 instrument (37.4× and 38.0× coverage). Mapping and alignment were performed as described [29]. The sequence data were deposited under the study accession

PRJEB16012 and the sample accessions SAMEA104091573 and SAMEA4867921 at the European Nucleotide Archive.

2.12. Variant Calling

Variant calling was performed as described [29]. To predict the functional effects of the called variants, the SnpEFF [30] software together with NCBI annotation release 105 for CanFam 3.1 was used. For variant filtering, we used 654 control genomes, which were publicly available. The control genomes were derived from 648 dogs of genetically diverse breeds and 8 wolves (Table S2).

2.13. Gene Analysis

We used the dog CanFam 3.1 reference genome assembly for all analyses. Numbering within the canine PCK2 gene corresponds to the NCBI RefSeq accessions XM_537379.6 (mRNA) and XP_537379.2 (protein).

2.14. Sanger Sequencing

To genotype the PCK2:c.1658G>A variant, a 468 bp PCR product was amplified from genomic DNA using the AmpliTaqGold360Mastermix (Thermo Fisher Scientific, Waltham, MA, USA) together with primers 5'-GCT ACA ACT TTG GGC GCT AC-3' (Primer F) and 5'- ATG AGG GGT AGG AAG GGA TG-3' (Primer R). After treatment with exonuclease I and alkaline phosphatase, amplicons were sequenced on an ABI 3730 DNA Analyzer (Thermo Fisher Scientific, Waltham, MA, USA). Sanger sequences were analyzed using the Sequencher 5.1 software (GeneCodes, Ann Arbor, MI, USA).

3. Results

3.1. Clinical Examinations and Family History

Four female Shetland Sheepdogs (age 2–6 years) were presented due to progressive dyskinetic episodes. Three of the four dogs were closely related, suggesting an inherited disorder. Although not conclusive, the pedigrees were compatible with an autosomal dominant mode of inheritance (Figure 1).

The episodes were characterized by generalized ataxia with hypermetria and muscular hypertonia of all limbs, dystonia, normal to mildly reduced mentation, and a mild tremor. In the more severe episodes, the dogs were no longer ambulatory. No signs of autonomic dysfunction were visible (normal size of pupils, no salivation, no defecation or urination, no signs of increased gastro-intestinal motility) (Video S1). The episodes varied from minutes to hours and could start while at rest, or during activity. In case 4, they were triggered by excitement or stress, like playing or after being startled by noise, according to the owner. Episodes in this dog were more intense and of longer duration after physical exercise. In cases 1–3, hot weather seemed to aggravate the clinical signs.

General and neurological examination was normal in all dogs, except for mild generalized muscle atrophy in case 4. Stress tests led to intermittent stiff gait in cases 1 and 2 but could not provoke a dystonic episode in case 4. The findings were consistent with a movement disorder or paroxysmal dyskinesia. Encephalopathy or neuromuscular disorders were also considered. All clinical examination results are summarized in Table S3.

3.2. Laboratory Examinations

Interictal blood cell count, biochemistry, and electrolytes were mostly within the reference range in all four affected dogs. Mildly increased creatine kinase activity (CK) was seen in cases 2 and 3 ($n = 2/4$, 221 U/l and 350 U/l, respectively, reference: <220 U/l). Total thyroxine (tT4) was normal in all tested dogs ($n = 3/3$, Table S3).

In case 4, fasted blood glucose was at the lower boundary of the reference range (72 mg/dL, reference: 70–110 mg/dL) and lactate at the upper reference limit (21.7 mg/dL, reference: 4.5–22.5 mg/dL). In venous blood, the base excess (BE) was −8.5 mmol/L (reference: −4 to 4 mmol/L) with a HCO_3^-

of 13 mmol/L (reference: 20–30 mmol/L), decreased pCO_2 (19.7 mm Hg, reference: 35–55 mm Hg) with normal pH (7.44, reference: 7.3–7.45). These findings are consistent with a metabolic acidosis with respiratory compensation. Blood examination after the stress test showed increased CK values in cases 1 and 2 ($n = 2/3$), and mildly decreased blood glucose (69 mg/dL) and the deterioration of BE (−10 mmol/L) in case 4 ($n = 1/3$). The parallel insulin measurement in case 4 was normal (6.8 µU/mL, reference: 5–25 µU/mL; glucose-insulin-ratio 10.14, reference: <30).

Urinary organic acid analysis an showed increased excretion of lactate ($n = 3/3$) and 2-hydroxybutyrate ($n = 1/3$) or 3-hydroxybutyrate ($n = 2/3$) compared to normal control (Figure 2). A full overview of all clinical and diagnostic findings in the four affected dogs is given in Table S3.

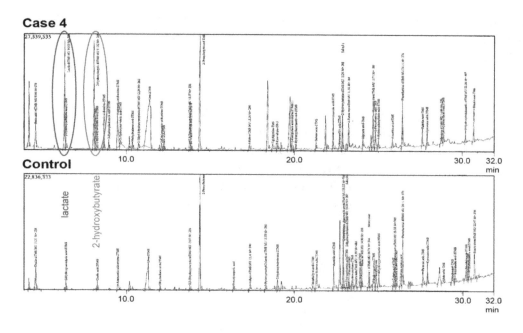

Figure 2. Metabolic screening of urinary organic acids in case 4. Gas chromatographic examination of a 3-year-old paroxysmal exercise-induced dyskinesia (PED)-affected dog's urine showed an increased excretion of lactate (red circle) and 2-hydroxybutyrate (blue circle) compared to a healthy control dog.

3.3. Additonal Examinations

Cardiac sonography and ECG were normal between episodes. ECG immediately before an episode revealed normal sinus rhythm with mild tachycardia (120–180 bpm). When a dyskinetic episode started, ECG was overlapped by muscle artefacts. ECG did not reveal cardiac pathology (Figure S1).

EEG in case 4 while the dog was awake showed mostly muscle artefacts and otherwise predominantly normal low voltage beta-rhythm.

Low-field MRI of the brain was performed in case 4 by the referring veterinarian and was available for review. No pathological abnormality was visible.

A CSF tap was performed in case 4 and was unremarkable: no cells were present, protein content was 11.8 mg/dL (reference <25 mg/dL), and glucose was 69 mg/dL (reference 42–77 mg/dL).

Electromyography (EMG) showed normal insertional discharge in all examined muscles without pathological spontaneous activity. Nerve-conduction studies showed normal nerve conduction velocities with normal CMAP amplitudes in all four dogs.

A search for autoantibodies in case 4 did not reveal any pathological findings.

3.4. Histopathology

Histopathological muscle changes in case 4 were sparse and featured a diffuse type II fiber predominant muscle atrophy. There was no evidence of mitochondrial changes and/or substrate accumulation on histology, enzyme histochemistry, or electron microscopy.

3.5. Clinical Management

Treatment with oral phenobarbital up to 3 mg/kg twice daily (cases 1–4) and levetiracetam 60 mg/kg three times daily (case 4) did not decrease the frequency of episodes according to the owners. Diazepam 2 mg/kg rectally did not seem to decrease the length of the episodes (case 4). Acetazolamid 50 mg/kg three times daily initially was reported to improve the clinical signs in case 4, but only for 6 months when the frequency started to increase again. Changing to zonisamide 10 mg/kg three times daily seemed to have an impact on episode frequency in the long term.

Supplementation with L-carnitine and multivitamins did not improve clinical signs in any of the four affected dogs.

A number of various commercial diets and gluten-free diets were tried but appeared to be unsuccessful in three dogs (case 1–3). However, in case 4, the feeding of a gluten-free, home-made fresh meat diet improved clinical signs. In case 4, the frequency of episodes improved with a commercially available gluten-free diet. Interruption of this diet led to the recurrence of an increased frequency of the episodes. A further change in diet to a seafood-based, gluten- and grain-free diet markedly improved the clinical signs again, even better than before. The last diet had the highest tryptophan content (Table 1).

Table 1. Tryptophan content in three different commercially available food samples and owners' subjective perception of clinical signs.

Diet	Dry Matter	Tryptophan	Clinical Response
normal	921 g/kg	1.52 g/kg	worsening of clinical signs
gluten-free	950 g/kg	1.65 g/kg	improved clinical signs
seafood gluten- and grain free	951 g/kg	2.97 g/kg	markedly improved clinical signs

Additional supplementation with tryptophan 50 mg/kg twice daily in case 4 combined with the prevention of stress and exhausting exercise further decreased clinical signs according to the owner. A summary of treatments in all four cases is given in Table S3.

3.6. Outcome

We were able to monitor all four affected dogs over a period of 5 to 12 years and the dogs remained stable (Table S3). Two dogs were event-free, one dog suffered from only one to two events per year. Exercise- and stress-management in combination with zonisamide, a seafood-based, gluten-free diet and tryptophan helped the fourth dog to stabilize on a low-level frequency of episodes. The dog continued to display one short episode every 2–3 days, during which she was still ambulatory (Figure 3). Six years after diagnosis, case 3 died of an acute renal failure, case 1 died of old age at 15 years of age. Cases 2 and 4 were still alive at the time of writing (Table S3).

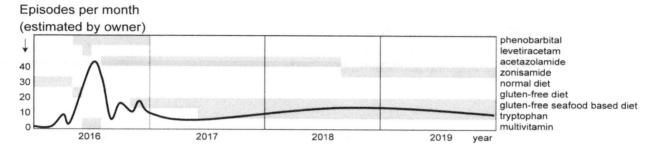

Figure 3. Frequency of dyskinetic episodes in case 4. The estimated frequency of episodes per month (black line), contemporaneous medications and diets are displayed with green and blue bars, respectively. A combination of seafood-based, gluten-free diet with supplementation of tryptophan and treatment with acetazolamide or zonisamide seemed to reduce frequency of episodes.

3.7. Genetic Analysis

We sequenced the genomes of cases 2 and 4 at 37.4× and 38.0× coverage and called SNVs and short indels with respect to the CanFam 3.1 reference genome assembly. We then searched for shared heterozygous and homozygous variants in the genome sequence of the two affected dogs that were not present in 654 control genomes. This analysis yielded 1066 variants that were exclusively shared by the two cases and not present in any of the control genomes (Table S4). None of the shared homozygous variants were predicted to have a protein-changing effect, but 10 heterozygous variants shared by the two cases were predicted to be protein changing (Table 2).

Table 2. Shared variants in the two sequenced cases.

Filtering Step	Heterozygous Variants	Homozygous Variants
Case-specific variants	1030	36
Case-specific protein-changing variants	10	0

We then prioritized the 10 private protein-changing variants according to the functional knowledge on the altered genes. We considered the *PCK2* gene encoding the mitochondrial phosphoenolpyruvate carboxykinase 2 the most likely candidate gene for the observed clinical phenotype (Table 3).

Table 3. Heterozygous protein-changing variants shared by the 2 PED cases and absent in 654 controls.

Gene	Protein	Variant
C7	complement C7	p.Glu799*
CDH24	cadherin 24	p.Asp669Asn
CNNM1	cyclin and CBS domain divalent metal cation transport mediator 1	p.Asp170Tyr
LOC485317		p.Lys270Asn
LOC106559343		p.Ala179Gly
LOC111097338		p.Arg182Trp
OR2A14	olfactory receptor family 2 subfamily A member 14	p.Ser56Arg
OR2A14	olfactory receptor family 2 subfamily A member 14	p.Leu54Gln
PCK2	phosphoenolpyruvate carboxykinase 2, mitochondrial	p.Arg553Gln
TM9SF1	transmembrane 9 superfamily member 1	p.His362Tyr

The top candidate variant on the genomic level was Chr8:4,107,413G>A. The corresponding variant designations on the cDNA and protein level are XM_537379.6:c.1658G>A or XP_537379.2:p.(Arg553Gln), respectively. We confirmed the variant by Sanger sequencing. (Figure 4A). The variant is predicted to alter a positively charged arginine close to the GTP-binding site of PCK2 into a neutral glutamine without major changes to the threedimensional structure of the enzyme. The wildtype arginine is strictly conserved across animals from *C. elegans* up to mammals (Figure 4B).

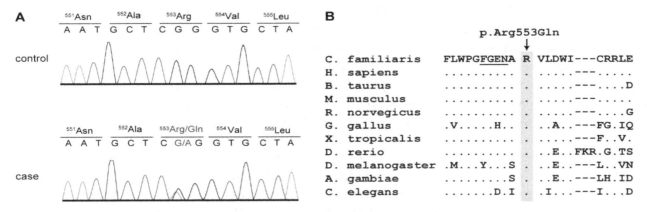

Figure 4. Details of the PCK2:c.1658G>A variant. (**A**) Representative Sanger sequencing electropherograms of two dogs with the different genotypes are shown. (**B**) Evolutionary conservation of the arginine residue at position 553 of the PCK2 protein. A multiple species alignment illustrates that this residue is strictly conserved across animals from worms to mammals. Amino acids 548-551 form part of the GTP-binding site of PCK2 and are underlined [31].

We then genotyped all four affected dogs, 117 Shetland Sheepdog controls without any movement disorder or seizures and 515 control dogs from 71 genetically diverse dog breeds for the PCK2:c.1658G>A variant and found a perfect genotype-phenotype association. All four cases carried one copy of the mutant allele, while all control dogs were homozygous for the reference allele (Table 4; Table S1). The segregation of the genotypes in the available family was compatible with an autosomal dominant inheritance (Figure 1). An attempt to establish a fibroblast culture from case 4 to perform analyses on mitochondrial function was unsuccessful. While fibroblasts from a healthy control dog grew as expected, fibroblasts from case 4 did not grow appropriately to allow biochemical studies.

Table 4. Association of the genotypes at *PCK2*:c.1658G>A with paroxysmal dyskinesia.

Dogs	G/G	G/A
Cases Shetland Sheepdogs (*n* = 4)	0	4
Controls Shetland Sheepdogs (*n* = 117)	117	0
Controls other breeds (*n* = 515) [1]	515	0

[1] Independent from the 654 controls of the variant discovery.

4. Discussion

The present article describes the clinical and diagnostic findings of an inherited PED in four Shetland Sheepdogs with a suspected deficiency in the mitochondrial phosphoenolpyruvate carboxykinase 2 (PCK2). There are two isoforms of phosphoenolpyruvate carboxykinase, a cytosolic isoform, encoded by the *PCK1* gene, and a mitochondrial isoform, encoded by the *PCK2* gene. The tissue specificity of these isoforms has been described [32]. PCK1 is hormonally regulated, with insulin switching the enzyme off, whereas PCK2 does not seem to be regulated by hormones, but rather by mitochondrial GTP levels [32–35].

Our genetic analysis revealed a *PCK2* missense variant in the affected dogs, which was predicted to change an evolutionarily conserved amino acid located close to the GTP-binding site of PCK2 [31]. The mutant allele was exclusively found in a heterozygous state in the four studied PED cases and absent in more than one thousand control dogs. As PCK2 is a monomeric enzyme, we consider it unlikely that the p.Arg553Gln substitution will have a dominant negative effect. We speculate that haploinsufficiency during periods of high energy demand may be causing the phenotype in the affected dogs. We have to caution that our genetic analysis was strictly based on the assumption of a shared causative genetic variant between the two sequenced cases. If the phenotypes in the studied dogs are due to different genetic and/or environmental causes, the detected PCK2 variant might be functionally neutral. We also have to caution that our bioinformatics analysis considered only small genetic variants and would not have detected any large structural variants involving more than ~25 consecutive nucleotides.

We did not succeed in proving the functional relevance of the genetic variant by enzyme activity assay as fibroblasts from a PED-affected dog did not proliferate appropriately, whereas a parallel culture of control fibroblasts from a healthy dog grew sufficiently. We have observed this phenomenon before in some human diseased fibroblasts (personal observation, A.M.D.).

Few human patients with primary phosphoenolpyruvate carboxykinase deficiency have been reported in the literature, mainly with isolated variants in PCK1 [36–38]. These patients suffer from liver dysfunction, sometimes leading to liver failure, hypoglycemia, lactic acidosis and sometimes complex symptoms [36–38]. To the best of our knowledge, no PCK2 variants have been described in human patients. Some reports in the older literature claim a deficiency of mitochondrial phosphoenolpyruvate carboxykinase in human patients [39,40]; however, later on, these diagnoses were withdrawn or revised. One publication reports a patient with a complex phenotype suffering from both cytosolic and mitochondrial phosphoenolpyruvate carboxykinase deficiency [41].

The current human genome and exome data of the gnomAD browser do not indicate any intolerance of heterozygous PCK2 loss of function variants [42,43]. Interestingly, the variant found in the affected Shetland Sheepdogs, p.Arg553Gln, also represents a rare variant in humans. The gnomAD data lists 27 heterozygotes for the ^{553}Gln-allele, which has a frequency of 9.55×10^{-5} in the dataset [43]. It is unknown whether these persons have any clinical phenotype.

In the four affected dogs, paroxysmal hypertonic dyskinetic episodes often being triggered by stress, excitement or hot weather were the prominent clinical signs. Transient hypoglycemia, lactaturia, ketonuria and subsequent metabolic acidosis were noted. A muscle biopsy showed mild type II fiber predominant muscle atrophy, which is common in metabolic disease [44]. No cardiac abnormalities, structural changes of brain parenchyma, or signs of hepatopathy were seen in our canine patients. Similar clinical signs were described in a Shetland Sheepdog in 1992, but at this time the etiopathology remained obscure [45].

We suggest that decreased PCK2 activity may have led to impaired gluconeogenesis and energy metabolism in the affected Shetland Sheepdogs. The most severely affected dog (case 4) showed borderline low glucose. We suggest that clinical signs are therefore most pronounced in times of stress or exercise, when the body has an increased demand for energy. The resulting shortage of energy might first affect those organs with a high energetic turnover, such as muscles and the brain. This might result in the paroxysmal dyskinetic events seen in the Shetland Sheepdogs similar to glucose transporter GLUT1 deficiency where gait abnormalities are observed [46]. Phosphoenolpyruvate carboxykinase is expressed in astrocytes [47] and impaired gluconeogenesis may have a similar effect. GTP levels in neuronal cells may be altered, which may affect the production of tetrahydrobiopterin [48] and thus synthesis of neurotransmitters and NO.

As not all dogs had measurable episodes of hypoglycemia, another albeit highly speculative pathomechanism should be considered: PCK2 acts as a sensor of the citric acid cycle ('Krebs cycle') flux by removing oxaloacetate [34]. A reduced PCK2 activity could result in the accumulation of oxaloacetate hampering the citric acid cycle flux. PCK2 is the only isoform providing phosphoenolpyruvate carboxykinase activity in pancreas and possibly other tissues, linking the production of mitochondrial GTP to anaplerotic phosphoenolpyruvate cycling [35]. PCK2 also has pyruvate kinase activity, which theoretically could enhance mitochondrial pyruvate formation and transformation into oxaloacetate when energy levels in the mitochondrion are low, thus contributing to the citric acid cycle, a situation suggested to be stress-related [49]. We have to caution that our two mechanistic hypotheses so far are not supported by any experimental data. As heterozygous PCK2 loss-of-function variants have not yet been identified as causative for a corresponding phenotype in human patients, functional validation will be of the utmost importance to further evaluate the hypothetical link of canine PCK2 deficiency and PED.

In human medicine, a ketogenic diet with a low glycemic index is recommended for diseases that affect energy metabolism to avoid high insulin peaks [50,51]. In humans, ketogenic diets classically include high amounts of fat and low amounts of carbohydrates, which forces the body to change to a ketogenic metabolism, to provide ketone bodies as an alternative energy source for the brain and muscles [52,53]. In contrast, dogs do not tend to change into a ketogenic metabolism as easily as humans [54]. Additionally, a diet with a high amount of fat may cause pancreatitis in dogs [55]. Therefore, it is common practice in veterinary medicine to use a gluten- and grain-free diet as a more compatible form of a diet with a low glycemic index. This was also successfully applied in the presented Shetland Sheepdogs, whose clinical signs improved after being fed a gluten-free, high-protein diet. In one dog, a seafood-based diet showed the best results. This diet was rich in tryptophan, which is an essential amino acid involved in the production of serotonin [56]. Increased serotonin levels in the brain reduce stress [57]—an important trigger of dyskinetic episodes observed in this dog. Tryptophan may enhance de novo synthesis of NAD [58], an important metabolic regulator for energy metabolism. However, these mechanisms are highly speculative as we did not measure tryptophan nor neurotransmitter levels. Additionally, in one dog, antiepileptic drugs of the class of carbonic anhydrase inhibitors (acetazolamide or zonisamide) were used and correlated with improved clinical signs. Successful treatment with acetazolamide has been described in Soft-coated Wheaten Terriers and Golden Retrievers with paroxysmal dyskinesia [59,60]. The exact mechanism of action is not clear yet, but it is thought that acetazolamide supports ion transport across the blood–brain barrier, modifying the intracellular pH and, therefore, the transmembrane potential, which lowers the excitability of neurons [51].

5. Conclusions

We describe a new PED with presumed autosomal dominant inheritance in Shetland Sheepdogs. Stress management, a specific diet and pharmacological therapy resulted in the partial or complete suppression of hypertonic dyskinetic episodes and enabled a good quality of life. The genetic analysis suggested that the *PCK2*:p.Arg553Gln missense variant should be considered and further evaluated as potential candidate causal variant for this phenotype. This study provides an interesting potential link between exercise-induced hypoglycemia, mitochondrial energy metabolism and paroxysmal dyskinesia that warrants further investigation.

Supplementary Materials:
Figure S1: Long-term electrocardiography (ECG) of case 4 before a dyskinetic episode and at the beginning of an episode, Table S1: PCK2:c.1658G>A genotypes of 636 dogs from 69 different dog breeds; Table S2: Accession numbers of 648 dog and 8 wolf genome sequences; Table S3: Summary of clinical and diagnostic findings in the 4 affected dogs. Table S4: List of heterozygous private variants that were shared in the two sequenced cases and absent from 654 control genomes. Video S1: 3 year old PED-affected female Shetland Sheepdog experiencing a hypertonic dyskinetic episode triggered by excitement while playing at the beach.

Author Contributions: Conceptualization, J.N. and T.L.; investigation, J.N., P.H., P.J.J.M., V.J., K.M., M.R., M.K., P.W., A.F., A.T.; resources, J.N., P.J.J.M., P.A.J.L.; data curation, V.J.; writing—original draft preparation, J.N., P.H., A.M.D., M.R., K.M., M.K., T.L.; writing—review and editing, J.N., P.H., P.J.J.M., P.A.J.L., V.J., A.M.D., M.R., K.M., A.C.S., M.K., M.H., P.W., A.F., A.T., T.L.; supervision, T.L. All authors have read and agreed to the published version of the manuscript.

Acknowledgments: We would like to acknowledge the owners of the dogs for donating samples and data including precise recording of clinical signs and video recording. We thank Nathalie Besuchet Schmutz, Catia Coito, Marion Ernst and Daniela Steiner for expert technical assistance, the Next Generation Sequencing Platform of the University of Bern for performing the high-throughput sequencing experiments, and the Interfaculty Bioinformatics Unit of the University of Bern for providing high performance computing infrastructure. We thank the Dog Biomedical Variant Database Consortium (Gus Aguirre, Catherine André, Danika Bannasch, Doreen Becker, Brian Davis, Cord Drögemüller, Kari Ekenstedt, Kiterie Faller, Oliver Forman, Steve Friedenberg, Eva Furrow, Urs Giger, Christophe Hitte, Marjo Hytönen, Vidhya Jagannathan, Tosso Leeb, Frode Lingaas, Hannes Lohi, Cathryn Mellersh, Jim Mickelson, Leonardo Murgiano, Anita Oberbauer, Sheila Schmutz, Jeffrey Schoenebeck, Kim Summers, Frank van Steenbeek, Claire Wade) for sharing whole genome sequencing data from control dogs. We also acknowledge all canine researchers who deposited dog whole genome sequencing data into public databases.

References

1.   Xu, Z.; Lim, C.K.; Tan, L.C.S.; Tan, E.-K. Paroxysmal Movement Disorders: Recent Advances. *Curr. Neurol. Neurosci. Rep.* **2019**, *19*, 48. [CrossRef]

2.   Weber, Y.G.; Storch, A.; Wuttke, T.V.; Brockmann, K.; Kempfle, J.; Maljevic, S.; Margari, L.; Kamm, C.; Schneider, S.A.; Huber, S.M.; et al. GLUT1 mutations are a cause of paroxysmal exertion-induced dyskinesias and induce hemolytic anemia by a cation leak. *J. Clin. Investig.* **2008**, *118*, 2157–2168. [CrossRef]

3.   Weber, Y.G.; Kamm, C.; Suls, A.; Kempfle, J.; Kotschet, K.; Schüle, R.; Wuttke, T.V.; Maljevic, S.; Liebrich, J.; Gasser, T.; et al. Paroxysmal choreoathetosis/spasticity (DYT9) is caused by a GLUT1 defect. *Neurology* **2011**, *77*, 959–964. [CrossRef]

4.   Seidner, G.; Alvarez, M.G.; Yeh, J.-I.; O'Driscoll, K.R.; Klepper, J.; Stump, T.S.; Wang, N.; Spinner, N.B.; Birnbaum, M.; De Vivo, D.C. GLUT-1 deficiency syndrome caused by haploinsufficiency of the blood-brain barrier hexose carrier. *Nat. Genet.* **1998**, *18*, 188–191. [CrossRef] [PubMed]

5.   Ichinose, H.; Ohye, T.; Takahashi, E.-I.; Seki, N.; Hori, T.-A.; Segawa, M.; Nomura, Y.; Endo, K.; Tanaka, H.; Tsuji, S.; et al. Hereditary progressive dystonia with marked diurnal fluctuation caused by mutations in the GTP cyclohydrolase I gene. *Nat. Genet.* **1994**, *8*, 236–242. [CrossRef]

6.   Méneret, A.; Roze, E. Paroxysmal movement disorders: An update. *Rev. Neurol.* **2016**, *172*, 433–445. [CrossRef] [PubMed]

7.   Urkasemsin, G.; Olby, N.J. Canine Paroxysmal Movement Disorders. *Vet. Clin. Small Anim. Pract.* **2014**, *44*, 1091–1102. [CrossRef] [PubMed]

8.   Meyers, K.M.; Padgett, G.A.; Dickson, W.M. The Genetic Basis of a Kinetic Disorder of Scottish Terrier Dogs. *J. Hered.* **1970**, *61*, 189–192. [CrossRef]

9.   Geiger, K.M.; Klopp, L.S. Use of a selective serotonin reuptake inhibitor for treatment of episodes of hypertonia and kyphosis in a young adult Scottish Terrier. *J. Am. Vet. Med. Assoc.* **2009**, *235*, 168–171. [CrossRef]

10. Urkasemsin, G.; Olby, N.J. Clinical characteristics of Scottie Cramp in 31 cases. *J. Small Anim. Pract.* **2015**, *56*, 276–280. [CrossRef]

11. Penderis, J.; Franklin, R. Dyskinesia in an adult bichon frise. *J. Small Anim. Pract.* **2001**, *42*, 24–25. [CrossRef] [PubMed]

12. Lowrie, M.; Varejão, A.S.P. Paroxysmal dyskinesia in the bichon frise. *Vet. Rec.* **2018**, *182*, 578. [CrossRef] [PubMed]

13. Black, V.L.; Garosi, L.; Lowrie, M.; Harvey, R.J.; Gale, J. Phenotypic characterisation of canine epileptoid cramping syndrome in the Border terrier. *J. Small Anim. Pract.* **2013**, *55*, 102–107. [CrossRef] [PubMed]

14. Stassen, Q.E.M.; Koskinen, L.; Van Steenbeek, F.; Seppälä, E.; Jokinen, T.; Prins, P.; Bok, H.; Zandvliet, M.M.; Vos-Loohuis, M.; Leegwater, P.; et al. Paroxysmal Dyskinesia in Border Terriers: Clinical, Epidemiological, and Genetic Investigations. *J. Vet. Intern. Med.* **2017**, *31*, 1123–1131. [CrossRef] [PubMed]

15. Lowrie, M.; Garden, O.; Hadjivassiliou, M.; Sanders, D.; Powell, R.; Garosi, L. Characterization of Paroxysmal Gluten-Sensitive Dyskinesia in Border Terriers Using Serological Markers. *J. Vet. Intern. Med.* **2018**, *32*, 775–781. [CrossRef] [PubMed]

16. Ramsey, I.; Chandler, K.E.; Franklin, R.J.M. A movement disorder in boxer pups. *Vet. Rec.* **1999**, *144*, 179–180. [CrossRef]

17. Packer, R.; Patterson, E.; Taylor, J.; Coates, J.; Schnabel, R.D.; O'Brien, D. Characterization and Mode of Inheritance of a Paroxysmal Dyskinesia in Chinook Dogs. *J. Vet. Intern. Med.* **2010**, *24*, 1305–1313. [CrossRef]

18. Harcourt-Brown, T. Anticonvulsant responsive, episodic movement disorder in a German shorthaired pointer. *J. Small Anim. Pract.* **2008**, *49*, 405–407. [CrossRef]

19. Shelton, G.D. Muscle pain, cramps and hypertonicity. *Vet. Clin. Small Anim. Pract.* **2004**, *34*, 1483–1496. [CrossRef]

20. Polidoro, D.; Van Ham, L.; Santens, P.; Cornelis, I.; Charalambous, M.; Broeckx, B.J.G.; Bhatti, S.F.M. Phenotypic characterization of paroxysmal dyskinesia in Maltese dogs. *J. Vet. Intern. Med.* **2020**. [CrossRef]

21. Kolicheski, A.L.; Johnson, G.S.; Mhlanga-Mutangadura, T.; Taylor, J.F.; Schnabel, R.D.; Kinoshita, T.; Murakami, Y.; O'Brien, D.P. A homozygous PIGN missense mutation in Soft-Coated Wheaten Terriers with a canine paroxysmal dyskinesia. *Neurogenetics* **2016**, *18*, 39–47. [CrossRef] [PubMed]

22. Garosi, L.S.; Platt, S.R.; Shelton, G.D. Hypertonicity in Cavalier King Charles spaniel. *J. Vet. Intern. Med.* **2002**, *16*, 330.

23. Forman, O.P.; Penderis, J.; Hartley, C.; Hayward, L.J.; Ricketts, S.L.; Mellersh, C.S. Parallel Mapping and Simultaneous Sequencing Reveals Deletions in BCAN and FAM83H Associated with Discrete Inherited Disorders in a Domestic Dog Breed. *PLoS Genet.* **2012**, *8*, e1002462. [CrossRef] [PubMed]

24. Crippa, L.; Ferro, E.; Melloni, E.; Brambilla, P.; Cavalletti, E. Echocardiographic parameters and indices in the normal Beagle dog. *Lab. Anim.* **1992**, *26*, 190–195. [CrossRef] [PubMed]

25. Miller, R.H.; Lehmkuhl, L.B.; Bonagura, J.D.; Beall, M.J. Retrospective analysis of the clinical utility of ambulatory electrocardiographic (Holter) recordings in syncopal dogs: 44 cases (1991–1995). *J. Vet. Intern. Med.* **1999**, *13*, 111–122.

26. Platt, S.R.; Olby, N.J. *BSAVA Manual of Canine and Feline Neurology*, 4th ed.; British Small Animal Veterinary Association: Quedgeley, UK, 2014; pp. 47–55.

27. Brauer, C.; Kästner, S.B.; Rohn, K.; Schenk, H.C.; Tünsmeyer, J.; Tipold, A. Electroencephalographic recordings in dogs suffering from idiopathic and symptomatic epilepsy: Diagnostic value of interictal short time EEG protocols supplemented by two activation techniques. *Vet. J.* **2012**, *193*, 185–192. [CrossRef] [PubMed]

28. Das, A.M.; Byrd, D.J.; Brodehl, J. Regulation of the mitochondrial ATP-synthase in human fibroblasts. *Clin. Chim. Acta* **1994**, *231*, 61–68. [CrossRef]

29. Jagannathan, V.; Drögemüller, C.; Leeb, T.; Aguirre, G.; André, C.; Bannasch, D.; Becker, D.; Davis, B.; Ekenstedt, K.; Faller, K.; et al. A comprehensive biomedical variant catalogue based on whole genome sequences of 582 dogs and eight wolves. *Anim. Genet.* **2019**, *50*, 695–704. [CrossRef]

30. Cingolani, P.; Platts, A.E.; Wang, L.L.; Coon, M.; Nguyen, T.; Wang, L.; Land, S.J.; Lu, X.; Ruden, D.M. A program for annotating and predicting the effects of single nucleotide polymorphisms, SnpEff. *Fly* **2012**, *6*, 80–92. [CrossRef]

31. Holyoak, T.; Sullivan, S.M.; Nowak, T. Structural Insights into the Mechanism of PEPCK Catalysis. *Biochemistry* **2006**, *45*, 8254–8263. [CrossRef]

32. Chakravarty, K.; Cassuto, H.; Reshef, L.; Hanson, R.W. Factors That Control the Tissue-Specific Transcription of the Gene for Phosphoenolpyruvate Carboxykinase-C. *Crit. Rev. Biochem. Mol. Biol.* **2005**, *40*, 129–154. [CrossRef]

33. Quinn, P.G.; Yeagley, D. Insulin regulation of PEPCK gene expression: A model for rapid and reversible modulation. *Curr. Drug Targets Immuneendocr. Metab. Disord.* **2005**, *5*, 423–437. [CrossRef] [PubMed]

34. Stark, R.; Kibbey, R.G. The mitochondrial isoform of phosphoenolpyruvate carboxykinase (PEPCK-M) and glucose homeostasis: Has it been overlooked? *Biochim. Biophys.* **2014**, *1840*, 1313–1330. [CrossRef] [PubMed]

35. Stark, R.; Pasquel, F.; Turcu, A.; Pongratz, R.L.; Roden, M.; Cline, G.W.; Shulman, G.I.; Kibbey, R.G. Phosphoenolpyruvate cycling via mitochondrial phosphoenolpyruvate carboxykinase links anaplerosis and mitochondrial GTP with insulin secretion. *J. Biol. Chem.* **2009**, *284*, 26578–26590. [CrossRef]

36. Santra, S.; Cameron, J.M.; Shyr, C.; Zhang, L.; Drogemoller, B.; Ross, C.; Wasserman, W.W.; Wevers, R.A.; Rodenburg, R.J.; Gupte, G.; et al. Cytosolic phosphoenolpyruvate carboxykinase deficiency presenting with acute liver failure following gastroenteritis. *Mol. Genet. Metab.* **2016**, *118*, 21–27. [CrossRef] [PubMed]

37. Vieira, P.; Cameron, J.; Rahikkala, E.; Keski-Filppula, R.; Zhang, L.-H.; Santra, S.; Matthews, A.; Myllynen, P.; Nuutinen, M.; Moilanen, J.; et al. Novel homozygous PCK1 mutation causing cytosolic phosphoenolpyruvate carboxykinase deficiency presenting as childhood hypoglycemia, an abnormal pattern of urine metabolites and liver dysfunction. *Mol. Genet. Metab.* **2017**, *120*, 337–341. [CrossRef]

38. Adams, D.R.; Yuan, H.; Holyoak, T.; Arajs, K.H.; Hakimi, P.; Markello, T.C.; Wolfe, L.A.; Vilboux, T.; Burton, B.K.; Fajardo, K.F.; et al. Three rare diseases in one Sib pair: RAI1, PCK1, GRIN2B mutations associated with Smith-Magenis Syndrome, cytosolic PEPCK deficiency and NMDA receptor glutamate insensitivity. *Mol. Genet. Metab.* **2014**, *113*, 161–170. [CrossRef] [PubMed]

39. Clayton, P.T.; Hyland, K.; Brand, M.; Leonard, J.V. Mitochondrial phosphoenolpyruvate carboxykinase deficiency. *Eur. J. Nucl. Med. Mol. Imaging* **1986**, *145*, 46–50. [CrossRef] [PubMed]

40. Leonard, J.V.; Hyland, K.; Furukawa, N.; Clayton, P.T. Mitochondrial phosphoenolpyruvate carboxykinase deficiency. *Eur. J. Nucl. Med. Mol. Imaging* **1991**, *150*, 198–199. [CrossRef] [PubMed]

41. Robinson, B.H.; Taylor, J.; Sherwood, W.G. The Genetic Heterogeneity of Lactic Acidosis: Occurrence of Recognizable Inborn Errors of Metabolism in a Pediatric Population with Lactic Acidosis. *Pediatr. Res.* **1980**, *14*, 956–962. [CrossRef] [PubMed]

42. Karczewski, K.J.; Francioli, L.C.; Tiao, G.; Cummings, B.B.; Alföldi, J.; Wang, Q.; Collins, R.L.; Laricchia, K.M.; Ganna, A.; Birnbaum, D.P.; et al. The mutational constraint spectrum quantified from variation in 141,456 humans. *Nature* **2020**, *581*, 434–443. [CrossRef] [PubMed]

43. GnomAD–Genome Aggregation Database. Available online: https://gnomad.broadinstitute.org/ (accessed on 2 June 2020).

44. Lorenz, M.D.; Coates, J.; Kent, M. *Handbook of Veterinary Neurology-E-Book*; Elsevier Health Sciences: Amsterdam, The Netherlands, 2010; pp. 209–211.

45. Nakahata, K.; Uzuka, Y.; Matsumoto, H.; Gotoh, N.; Sasaki, K. Hyperkinetic involuntary movements in a young Shetland sheepdog. *J. Am. Anim. Hosp. Assoc.* **1992**, *28*, 347–348.

46. Pons, R.; Collins, A.; Rotstein, M.; Engelstad, K.; De Vivo, D.C. The spectrum of movement disorders in Glut-1 deficiency. *Mov. Disord.* **2010**, *25*, 275–281. [CrossRef]

47. Yip, J.; Geng, X.; Shen, J.; Ding, Y. Cerebral Gluconeogenesis and Diseases. *Front. Pharmacol.* **2017**, *7*, 1547. [CrossRef]

48. Thöny, B.; Auerbach, G.; Blau, N. Tetrahydrobiopterin biosynthesis, regeneration and functions. *Biochem. J.* **2000**, *347 Pt 1*, 1–16. [CrossRef]

49. Escós, M.; Latorre, P.; Hidalgo, J.; Hurtado-Guerrero, R.; Carrodeguas, J.A.; López-Buesa, P. Kinetic and functional properties of human mitochondrial phosphoenolpyruvate carboxykinase. *Biochem. Biophys. Rep.* **2016**, *7*, 124–129. [CrossRef]

50. Maalouf, M.A.; Rho, J.M.; Mattson, M.P. The neuroprotective properties of calorie restriction, the ketogenic diet, and ketone bodies. *Brain Res. Rev.* **2009**, *59*, 293–315. [CrossRef] [PubMed]

51. Anheim, M.; Maillart, E.; Vuillaumier-Barrot, S.; Flamand-Rouvière, C.; Pineau, F.; Ewenczyk, C.; Riant, F.; Apartis, E.; Roze, E. Excellent response to acetazolamide in a case of paroxysmal dyskinesias due to GLUT1-deficiency. *J. Neurol.* **2010**, *258*, 316–317. [CrossRef] [PubMed]

52. Mayorandan, S.; Meyer, U.; Hartmann, H.; Das, A. Glycogen storage disease type III: Modified Atkins diet improves myopathy. *Orphanet J. Rare Dis.* **2014**, *9*, 196. [CrossRef] [PubMed]

53. Freeman, J.M.; Kossoff, E.H.; Hartman, A. The Ketogenic Diet: One Decade Later. *Pediatrics* **2007**, *119*, 535–543. [CrossRef]

54. Keller, U.; Cherrington, A.D.; Liljenquist, J.E. Ketone body turnover and net hepatic ketone production in fasted and diabetic dogs. *Am. J. Physiol. Metab.* **1978**, *235*, E238. [CrossRef] [PubMed]

55. Packer, R.M.; Shihab, N.K.; Torres, B.B.J.; Volk, H.A. Responses to successive anti-epileptic drugs in canine idiopathic epilepsy. *Vet. Rec.* **2015**, *176*, 203. [CrossRef] [PubMed]

56. Schaechter, J.D.; Wurtman, R.J. Serotonin release varies with brain tryptophan levels. *Brain Res.* **1990**, *532*, 203–210. [CrossRef]

57. Putman, P.; Roelofs, K. Effects of single cortisol administrations on human affect reviewed: Coping with stress through adaptive regulation of automatic cognitive processing. *Psychoneuroendocrinology* **2011**, *36*, 439–448. [CrossRef]

58. Okabe, K.; Yaku, K.; Tobe, K.; Nakagawa, T. Implications of altered NAD metabolism in metabolic disorders. *J. Biomed. Sci.* **2019**, *26*, 34. [CrossRef]

59. Royaux, E.; Bhatti, S.; Harvey, R.J.; Garosi, L.; Shelton, G.D.; Van Ham, L. Acetazolamide-responsive paroxysmal dyskinesia in a 12-week-old female golden retriever dog. *Vet. Q.* **2015**, *36*, 1–12. [CrossRef]

60. O'Brien, D.; Kolicheski, A.; Packer, R.; Thomovsky, S.; Taylor, J.; Schnabel, R.; Berg, J.; Vasquez, L.; Johnson, G. Paroxysmal non-kinesogenic dyskinesia in soft coated Wheaten terriers is associated with a missense mutation in PIGN and responds to acetazolamide therapy. *J. Vet. Intern. Med.* **2015**, *29*, 1267.

SLC19A3 Loss-of-Function Variant in Yorkshire Terriers with Leigh-Like Subacute Necrotizing Encephalopathy

Michaela Drögemüller [1,†], Anna Letko [1,†], Kaspar Matiasek [2,†], Vidhya Jagannathan [1], Daniele Corlazzoli [3], Marco Rosati [2], Konrad Jurina [4], Susanne Medl [5], Thomas Gödde [6], Stefan Rupp [7], Andrea Fischer [8], Alejandro Luján Feliu-Pascual [9] and Cord Drögemüller [1,*]

[1]   Institute of Genetics, Vetsuisse Faculty, University of Bern, 3012 Bern, Switzerland; michaela.droegemueller@vetsuisse.unibe.ch (M.D.); anna.letko@vetsuisse.unibe.ch (A.L.); vidhya.jagannathan@vetsuisse.unibe.ch (V.J.)

[2]   Section of Clinical & Comparative Neuropathology, Centre for Clinical Veterinary Medicine, Ludwig Maximilians Universität Munich, 80539 Munich, Germany; kaspar.matiasek@neuropathologie.de (K.M.); marco.rosati@neuropathologie.de (M.R.)

[3]   Neurology & Neurosurgery Unit, Policlinico Veterinario Roma Sud, 00173 Roma, Italy; daniele.corlazzoli@me.com

[4]   Small Animal Hospital, Tierklinik Haar, 85540 Haar, Germany; datenschutz.haar@anicura.de

[5]   Small Animal Hospital, Anicura Kleintierklinik Babenhausen, 87727 Babenhausen, Germany; smedl@tierklinik-medl.de

[6]   Small Animal Referral Practice, Veterinary Health Centre, 83451 Piding, Germany; t.goedde@tierarzt-piding.com

[7]   Small Animal Hospital, Tierklinik Hofheim, 65719 Hofheim, Germany; s.rupp@tierklinik-hofheim.de

[8]   Section of Neurology, Centre for Clinical Veterinary Medicine, Ludwig-Maximilians-Universität, 80539 Munich, Germany; a.fischer@medizinische-kleintierklinik.de

[9]   Aúna Especialidades Veterinarias, 46980 Valencia, Spain; alf@aunaespecialidadesveterinarias.es

*   Correspondence: cord.droegemueller@vetsuisse.unibe.ch

†   These authors contributed equally to the work.

Abstract: Sporadic occurrence of juvenile-onset necrotizing encephalopathy (SNE) has been previously reported in Yorkshire terriers. However, so far, no causative genetic variant has been found for this breed-specific form of suspected mitochondrial encephalomyopathy. Affected dogs showed gait abnormalities, central visual defects, and/or seizures. Histopathological analysis revealed the presence of major characteristics of human Leigh syndrome and SNE in Alaskan huskies. The aim of this study was to characterize the genetic etiology of SNE-affected purebred Yorkshire terriers. After SNP genotyping and subsequent homozygosity mapping, we identified a single loss-of-function variant by whole-genome sequencing in the canine *SLC19A3* gene situated in a 1.7 Mb region of homozygosity on chromosome 25. All ten cases were homozygous carriers of a mutant allele, an indel variant in exon 2, that is predicted to lead to a frameshift and to truncate about 86% of the wild type coding sequence. This study reports a most likely pathogenic variant in *SLC19A3* causing a form of SNE in Yorkshire terriers and enables selection against this fatal neurodegenerative recessive disorder. This is the second report of a pathogenic alteration of the *SLC19A3* gene in dogs with SNE.

Keywords: *Canis familiaris*; whole-genome sequencing; rare disease; precision medicine; neurometabolic disorder

1. Introduction

Subacute necrotizing encephalomyelopathy (SNE), also termed Leigh syndrome (LS; OMIM 256000) represents a devastating neurodegenerative disorder in people, characterized by a wide variety of clinical signs, ranging from severe neurologic problems to a near absence of abnormalities with the central nervous system most frequently affected [1]. Originally, Archibald Denis Leigh, a British neuropsychiatrist described the condition in 1951 [2]. SNE is characterized by focal and bilaterally symmetrical, necrotic lesions involving the thalamus, brainstem, and posterior columns of the spinal cord [3]. In SNE, various mutations in mitochondrial respiratory chain complexes lead to the disruption of ATP synthesis resulting in the characteristic pathology of SNE [4]. Mitochondrial encephalomyelopathies, such as SNE or LS, represent rare inherited neurometabolic disorders showing considerable genetic heterogeneity and associated pathogenic variants affecting over 85 different genes of the mitochondrial or nuclear genome [3]. Therefore, they represent mitochondrial disorders with the largest genetic heterogeneity [1].

As human SNE is rare and heterogeneous, studying domestic animal species showing resembling conditions might add to the understanding of such a complex group of disorders. Rare forms of SNE were described e.g., in cattle [5–7] and dogs (OMIA 001097-9615). The first report of this disorder was described in Alaskan huskies [8,9] and subsequently, a similar form of SNE was reported in Yorkshire terriers [10] and American Staffordshire bull terriers [11]. Neuropathologically, SNE in Yorkshire terriers is nearly identical to the Alaskan husky form and very similar to human Leigh syndrome [10]. An initial genetic investigation of SNE-affected Yorkshire terriers revealed no indication for disease-causing variants in the mitochondrial genome [10], whereas more recently in Alaskan huskies the pathogenesis of recessively inherited SNE was unraveled [12,13]. This breed-specific fatal brain disorder in Alaskan huskies is associated with a deleterious loss-of-function variant in *SLC19A3* encoding for a thiamine transporter 2 (THTR2) with a predominately central nervous system (CNS) distribution [12,13]. The *SLC19A3* gene product controls the uptake of thiamine in the CNS via expression of the thiamine transporter protein THTR2. Pathogenic variants are associated with thiamine metabolism dysfunction syndrome-2 in people (THMD2; OMIM 607483), also known as biotin-responsive basal ganglia disease (BBGD) or thiamine-responsive encephalopathy [14]. This *SLC19A3*–related condition is an autosomal recessive disorder with childhood-onset that presents as a subacute encephalopathy and progresses to severe cogwheel rigidity, dystonia, quadriparesis, and eventually death if left untreated (OMIM 606152). The *SLC19A3*–related SNE of Alaskan huskies was proposed as a possible large animal model that may allow prospective investigations into the mechanisms of *SLC19A3*-related syndromes and the potential role of thiamine and/or biotin as a therapeutic strategy [12,13].

To elucidate the disease mechanism underlying monogenic autosomal recessive inherited SNE in Yorkshire terriers, we applied homozygosity mapping and whole-genome sequencing revealing a most likely pathogenic variant in the canine *SLC19A3* gene.

2. Materials and Methods

2.1. Ethics Statement

All animal experiments were performed according to the local regulations. All animals in this study were examined with the consent of their owners. Sample collection was approved by the Cantonal Committee for Animal Experiments (Canton of Bern; permit 71/19).

2.2. Animals

In total, 172 blood samples of Yorkshire terriers were collected. Ten dogs were diagnosed with Leigh-like subacute necrotizing encephalopathy (SNE) according to Baiker et al. [10]. These affected dogs were unrelated, apart from two full siblings for which their sire and dam (obligate carriers) as well as a single normal littermate were also available. The remaining 159 dogs represented unrelated purebred controls. Genomic DNA was isolated from EDTA blood samples using the Maxwell RSC Whole Blood DNA kit (Promega, Dübendorf, Switzerland).

2.3. Single Nucleotide Polymorphism Array Genotyping

Four selected SNE-affected Yorkshire terriers were genotyped on Illumina CanineHD BeadChip array (Illumina, San Diego, CA, USA). PLINK v1.9 [15] was used to perform the quality control filtering steps of the obtained genotyping data and the subsequent homozygosity analysis. Single nucleotide polymorphisms (SNP) with a call rate <90% were removed leaving 167,185 markers. All individuals had call rates >90%. Homozygosity analysis was carried out with PLINK v1.9 [15] to determine intervals of extended homozygous regions with alleles shared by all four affected dogs.

2.4. Whole-Genome Sequencing

Whole-genome sequence (WGS) data of a single affected dog was obtained at 19.7× coverage in order to identify the causative variant for SNE. The sequence data analysis and calling of single nucleotide variants and small indels (SNVs) including the prediction of functional effects were described before [16]. The dog reference genome assembly CanFam3.1 and NCBI annotation release 105 was used. Additionally, a publicly available control genomes cohort of 720 dogs from 130 various breeds, and 9 wolves [16] was used to filter variants private in the sequenced SNE-affected dog; this also included 60 unrelated Yorkshire terriers (Supplementary Table S1). The Integrative genomics viewer (IGV) software [17] was used for visual inspection and screening for structural variants in the associated regions.

2.5. Sanger Sequencing and Targeted Genotyping

Polymerase chain reaction (PCR) and Sanger sequencing were used to validate and characterize the SLC19A3 indel variant (XM_022409850.1:c.205_210delins35) identified from whole-genome sequencing. PCR primers were designed using primer 3 [18]. PCR products from genomic DNA were amplified using AmpliTaqGold360 MasterMix (Thermo Fisher Scientific, Waltham, MA, USA) and the purified PCR amplicons were directly sequenced on an ABI3730 capillary sequencer (Thermo Fisher Scientific) using the following primers: GGCAGTCACCATCCCATAGA (forward) and GATATTGGGCAAGCCACCTA (reverse) generating 309 bp products. The sequence data were analyzed with Sequencher 5.1 software (GeneCodes, Ann Arbor, MI, USA). Diagnostic genotyping was performed by fragment length analysis using a different forward primer (ATCCCTTGCAGGATGATGAC) to produce amplicons of 218 bp or 247 bp representing the wild type or variant allele, respectively. The 29 bp size difference was visualized on a Fragment Analyzer capillary gel electrophoresis instrument (Advanced Analytical Technologies, Ames, IA, USA).

2.6. Availability of Data and Material

The whole-genome data of an SNE-affected Yorkshire terrier are freely available at the European Nucleotide Archive (ENA) under sample accession number SAMEA3928145. All accession numbers of the used control genomes are available in Supplementary Table S1.

All genome positions are reported with respect to dog reference genome assembly CanFam3.1 and NCBI annotation release 105. All references to the canine SLC19A3 gene correspond to the accessions NC_006607.3 (NCBI accession), XM_022409850.1 (mRNA), and XP_022265558.1 (protein).

3. Results

3.1. Homozygosity Analysis

Based on the clinicopathological diagnosis of Leigh-like subacute necrotizing encephalopathy (SNE) in all examined Yorkshire terriers and the similarities to the recessively inherited conditions in SNE-affected Alaskan husky dogs and THMD2-affected humans, as well as the available pedigree information of the two SNE-affected siblings, a recessive mode of inheritance was postulated. Therefore, homozygosity mapping assuming identity-by-descent (IBD) was used to determine critical genomic regions shared across four SNP array genotyped cases. This revealed five genome regions with a total of ~4.1 Mb located on five different dog chromosomes (Table 1), representing 0.17% of the canine reference sequence. Visual inspection of these regions in the WGS of the affected dog did not reveal any evidence for copy number variants or large structural rearrangements.

Table 1. Regions of shared homozygosity detected in four subacute necrotizing encephalomyelopathy (SNE)-affected Yorkshire terriers.

Chromosome	Position [1]		Length (kb)	Number of Annotated Protein-Coding Genes in the Region
	Start	End		
3	44,184,889	44,286,148	101.3	0
6	71,329,720	71,552,171	222.5	1
10	20,608,121	22,376,735	1768.6	22
25	39,477,619	41,191,570	1714.0	13
31	33,337,422	33,591,249	253.8	2

[1] in respect to dog reference genome assembly CanFam3.1.

3.2. Identification of the Causative Variant

Filtering the variants of a single affected Yorkshire terrier against 729 public control genomes [16], including 60 breed controls, for single-nucleotide variants (SNVs) and short indels present in the five identified IBD-regions resulted in only a single private protein-changing variant (Figure 1a). The indel affecting ~45 bp is located in exon 2 of the *thiamine transporter 2* (*LOC486151*) gene, also known as solute carrier family 19 members 3 (*SLC19A3*) gene (Figure 1b). PCR and subsequent Sanger sequencing confirmed the homozygous presence of this small structural variant in SNE-affected Yorkshire terriers and revealed the detailed features of the indel: a 35 bp insertion replacing 6 bp and thereby disturbing the correct reading frame (Figure 1c). There are 15 currently annotated transcript isoforms for the canine *SLC19A3*, which is in reverse complementary orientation with respect to the canine reference genome. While the canine SLC19A3 protein length is 495 amino acids, the human protein (NP_001358340.1) has 496 amino acids, from which 408 (82.3%) are identical between dog and human. The Yorkshire terrier variant leads to a frameshift and a premature stop codon (c.205_210delins35; p.Pro69Ilefs*45) truncating ~86% of the wild type coding sequence (Figure 1c).

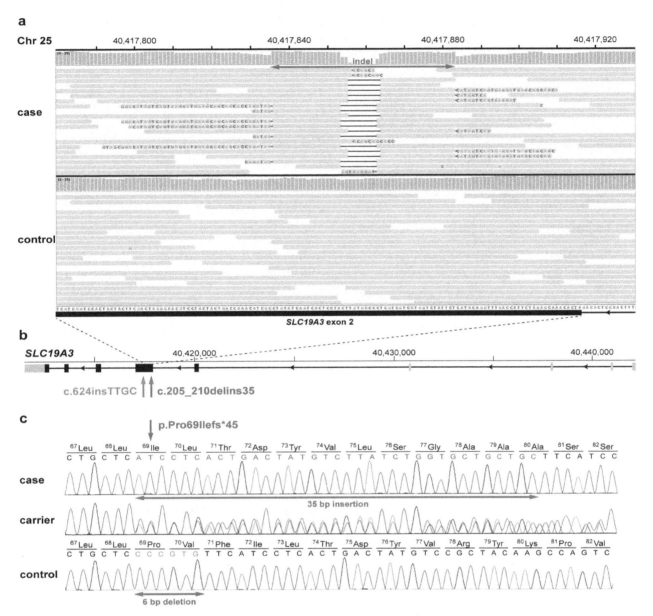

Figure 1. Subacute necrotizing encephalopathy (SNE)-associated *SLC19A3* loss-of-function variant in Yorkshire terriers. (**a**) IGV [17] screenshots of the genome region on canine chromosome 25 with the *SLC19A3*:c.205_210delins35 variant in an affected and a control Yorkshire terrier (NC_006607.3:40417780-40417930); The indel variant detected in the SNE-affected dog is indicated by a red arrow. (**b**) Schematic representation of the canine *SLC19A3* gene showing the location of both pathogenic variants in exon 2 (XM_022409850.1): the herein identified indel (red arrow) and the insertion previously described in encephalopathy-affected Alaskan huskies (blue arrow) [12]. Note that the number of 5′-untranslated exons (grey) varies between transcript isoforms, whereas the five protein-coding 3′-exons (black) are more conserved; (**c**) Sanger sequencing electropherograms illustrate sequences of a homozygous SNE-affected Yorkshire terrier, a heterozygous carrier, and a homozygous wild type dog. The red arrows indicate that the 35 bases shown in red are inserted, whereas the 6 bases in blue are deleted in the mutant allele. The predicted consequence of the shift in the reading frame altering the amino acid sequence of the SLC19A3 protein and leading to a premature stop is shown above.

3.3. Targeted Genotyping of the Variant

Genotyping by fragment size analysis of the 172 available Yorkshire terriers confirmed perfect segregation of the detected *SLC19A3* variant with the observed disease phenotype. Only the ten

SNE-affected dogs were homozygous for the variant allele (Table 2). Two obligate carriers and one tested normal littermate were heterozygous carriers of the variant, while 162 controls tested homozygous for the wild type allele (Table 2).

Table 2. Segregation of the *SLC19A3*: c.205_210delins35 genotypes with subacute necrotizing encephalopathy in Yorkshire terriers.

SNE Status	wt/wt	wt/var	var/var
Affected (*n* = 10)	0	0	10
Non-affected (*n* = 222) [1]	219	3 [2]	0

[1] including 60 dogs with WGS data [2] includes 2 obligate carriers and 1 normal littermate of the affected dogs.

4. Discussion

In this study, the obtained genetic results elucidate the underlying aetiology of the previous clinical and pathological characterization of a Leigh-like subacute necrotizing encephalopathy in the affected Yorkshire terriers, which resembles the human Leigh syndrome. The *SLC19A3* variant found by a combination of SNP genotyping-based homozygosity mapping and whole-genome sequencing, confirmed by Sanger sequencing, segregated perfectly in the investigated cohort of >200 unrelated Yorkshire terriers.

Numerous homozygous as well as compound heterozygous variants have been reported before in different regions of *SLC19A3* in human patients suffering from thiamine metabolism dysfunction syndrome-2 [19]. *SLC19A3* is a member of solute carrier family 19 and encodes thiamine transporter 2. Together with thiamine transporter 1, it is necessary for transport and homeostasis of thiamine that is important in brain development. [20]. *Slc19a3*-knockout mice showed progressive wasting and lethargy leading to a premature death as well as a significant decrease in thiamin uptake, even though there were no obvious histological changes in the brain [21].

The herein-described most likely pathogenic variant (XP_022265558.1:p.Pro69Ilefs*45) lies within the second of 12 transmembrane domains of the SLC19A3 protein and, therefore, affects ~86% of the wild type sequence. The *SLC19A3* gene probability of loss-of-function intolerance is pLI = 0.104 [22], which indicates variants in *SLC19A3* leading to a loss of gene function are most likely recessive, where loss of a single copy is often tolerated but the loss of both copies is not. The herein-described variant leads to an insertion of a premature termination in the second out of five coding exons, suggesting that any synthesized mRNA would likely be degraded through nonsense-mediated decay, unlikely to produce a fully functional protein. Heterozygous carriers did not show a visible clinical phenotype, as they can most likely compensate due to the presence of the normal protein, albeit at a decreased amount.

In conclusion, our results provide strong evidence for a breed-specific deleterious variant in *SLC19A3* as the most likely genetic cause of monogenic autosomal recessive Leigh-like subacute necrotizing encephalopathy in Yorkshire terriers, and they enable the development of a genetic test for veterinary diagnostic and breeding decisions. Finally, this presents the second, most likely breed-specific pathogenic variant in the canine *SLC19A3* gene in SNE-affected dogs.

Author Contributions: Conceptualization, K.M. and C.D.; methodology, M.D.; data curation, V.J.; formal analysis, M.D. and A.L.; investigation, M.D.; resources, K.M., D.C., M.R., K.J., S.M., T.G., S.R., A.F. and A.L.F.-P.; writing—original draft preparation, A.L., M.D., K.M. and C.D.; writing—review and editing, M.D., A.L., K.M. and C.D.; visualization, A.L. and C.D.; software, V.J.; supervision, C.D.; funding acquisition, C.D. All authors have read and agreed to the published version of the manuscript.

Acknowledgments: The authors are grateful to the owners of all dogs who provided samples and shared valuable information. The Next Generation Sequencing Platform and the Interfaculty Bioinformatics Unit of the University of Bern are acknowledged for performing the WGS and providing high-performance computational infrastructure.

References

1. Finsterer, J. Leigh and Leigh-Like Syndrome in Children and Adults. *Pediatr. Neurol.* **2008**, *39*, 223–235. [CrossRef] [PubMed]

2. Leigh, D. Subacute necrotizing encephalomyelopathy in an infant. *J. Neurol. Neurosurg. Psychiatry* **1951**, *14*, 216–221. [CrossRef] [PubMed]

3. Chang, X.; Wu, Y.; Zhou, J.; Meng, H.; Zhang, W.; Guo, J. A meta-analysis and systematic review of Leigh syndrome: Clinical manifestations, respiratory chain enzyme complex deficiency, and gene mutations. *Medicine* **2020**, *99*, e18634. [CrossRef] [PubMed]

4. Fecek, C.; Samanta, D. Subacute Necrotizing Encephalomyelopathy (Leigh Syndrome). Available online: http://www.ncbi.nlm.nih.gov/pubmed/32644590 (accessed on 14 September 2020).

5. Steffen, D.J.; Vestweber, J.G.; Cash, W.; El-Hamidi, M.; Leipold, H.W. Multifocal Subacute Necrotizing Encephalomyelopathy in Simmental Calves. *J. Vet. Diagn. Investig.* **1994**, *6*, 466–472. [CrossRef]

6. Desjardins, I.; Fecteau, G.; Hélie, P.; Desrochers, A. Multifocal subacute necrotizing encephalomyelopathy in a Simmental calf. *Can. Vet. J.* **2001**, *42*, 375–377.

7. Philbey, A.W.; Martel, K.S. A multifocal symmetrical necrotising encephalomyelopathy in Angus calves. *Aust. Vet. J.* **2003**, *81*, 226–229. [CrossRef] [PubMed]

8. Wakshlag, J.J.; de Lahunta, A.; Robinson, T.; Cooper, B.J.; Brenner, O.; O'Toole, T.D.; Olson, J.; Beckman, K.B.; Glass, E.; Reynolds, A.J. Subacute necrotising encephalopathy in an Alaskan husky. *J. Small Anim. Pract.* **1999**, *40*, 585–589. [CrossRef]

9. Brenner, O.; Wakshlag, J.J.; Summers, B.A.; de Lahunta, A. Alaskan Husky encephalopathy—A canine neurodegenerative disorder resembling subacute necrotizing encephalomyelopathy (Leigh syndrome). *Acta Neuropathol.* **2000**, *100*, 50–62. [CrossRef] [PubMed]

10. Baiker, K.; Hofmann, S.; Fischer, A.; Gödde, T.; Medl, S.; Schmahl, W.; Bauer, M.F.; Matiasek, K. Leigh-like subacute necrotising encephalopathy in Yorkshire Terriers: Neuropathological characterisation, respiratory chain activities and mitochondrial DNA. *Acta Neuropathol.* **2009**, *118*, 697–709. [CrossRef] [PubMed]

11. Collins, D.; Angles, J.M.; Christodoulou, J.; Spielman, D.; Lindsay, S.A.; Boyd, J.; Krockenberger, M.B. Severe Subacute Necrotizing Encephalopathy (Leigh-like Syndrome) in American Staffordshire Bull Terrier Dogs. *J. Comp. Pathol.* **2013**, *148*, 345–353. [CrossRef] [PubMed]

12. Vernau, K.M.; Runstadler, J.A.; Brown, E.A.; Cameron, J.M.; Huson, H.J.; Higgins, R.J.; Ackerley, C.; Sturges, B.K.; Dickinson, P.J.; Puschner, B.; et al. Genome-Wide Association Analysis Identifies a Mutation in the Thiamine Transporter 2 (SLC19A3) Gene Associated with Alaskan Husky Encephalopathy. *PLoS ONE* **2013**, *8*, e57195. [CrossRef] [PubMed]

13. Vernau, K.; Napoli, E.; Wong, S.; Ross-Inta, C.; Cameron, J.; Bannasch, D.; Bollen, A.; Dickinson, P.; Giulivi, C. Thiamine Deficiency-Mediated Brain Mitochondrial Pathology in Alaskan Huskies with Mutation in SLC19A3.1. *Brain Pathol.* **2015**, *25*, 441–453. [CrossRef] [PubMed]

14. Marcé-Grau, A.; Martí-Sánchez, L.; Baide-Mairena, H.; Ortigoza-Escobar, J.D.; Pérez-Dueñas, B. Genetic defects of thiamine transport and metabolism: A review of clinical phenotypes, genetics and functional studies. *J. Inherit. Metab. Dis.* **2019**, *42*, 581–597. [CrossRef] [PubMed]

15. Chang, C.C.; Chow, C.C.; Tellier, L.C.A.M.; Vattikuti, S.; Purcell, S.M.; Lee, J.J. Second-generation PLINK: Rising to the challenge of larger and richer datasets. *Gigascience* **2015**, *4*, 1–16. [CrossRef] [PubMed]

16. Jagannathan, V.; Drögemüller, C.; Leeb, T.; Aguirre, G.; André, C.; Bannasch, D.; Becker, D.; Davis, B.; Ekenstedt, K.; Faller, K.; et al. A comprehensive biomedical variant catalogue based on whole genome sequences of 582 dogs and eight wolves. *Anim. Genet.* **2019**, *50*, 695–704. [CrossRef] [PubMed]

17. Thorvaldsdóttir, H.; Robinson, J.T.; Mesirov, J.P. Integrative Genomics Viewer (IGV): High-performance genomics data visualization and exploration. *Brief. Bioinform.* **2013**, *14*, 178–192. [CrossRef] [PubMed]

18. Rozen, S.; Skaletsky, H. Primer3 on the WWW for General Users and for Biologist Programmers. In *Bioinformatics Methods and Protocols*; Humana Press: Totowa, NJ, USA, 2000; Volume 132, pp. 365–386. ISBN 978-0-89603-732-8. [CrossRef]

19. Whitford, W.; Hawkins, I.; Glamuzina, E.; Wilson, F.; Marshall, A.; Ashton, F.; Love, D.R.; Taylor, J.; Hill, R.; Lehnert, K.; et al. Compound heterozygous SLC19A3 mutations further refine the critical promoter region for biotin-thiamine-responsive basal ganglia disease. *Mol. Case Stud.* **2017**, *3*, a001909. [CrossRef] [PubMed]

20. Eudy, J.D.; Spiegelstein, O.; Barber, R.C.; Wlodarczyk, B.J.; Talbot, J.; Finnell, R.H. Identification and characterization of the human and mouse SLC19A3 gene: A novel member of the reduced folate family of micronutrient transporter genes. *Mol. Genet. Metab.* **2000**, *71*, 581–590. [CrossRef] [PubMed]

21. Reidling, J.C.; Lambrecht, N.; Kassir, M.; Said, H.M. Impaired Intestinal Vitamin B1 (Thiamin) Uptake in Thiamin Transporter-2–Deficient Mice. *Gastroenterology* **2010**, *138*, 1802–1809. [CrossRef]

22. Karczewski, K.J.; Francioli, L.C.; Tiao, G.; Cummings, B.B.; Alföldi, J.; Wang, Q.; Collins, R.L.; Laricchia, K.M.; Ganna, A.; Birnbaum, D.P.; et al. The mutational constraint spectrum quantified from variation in 141,456 humans. *Nature* **2020**, *581*, 434–443. [CrossRef]

ATP2A2 SINE Insertion in an Irish Terrier with Darier Disease and Associated Infundibular Cyst Formation

Monika Linek [1,†], Maren Doelle [1,†], Tosso Leeb [2,3,*,†], Anina Bauer [2,3], Fabienne Leuthard [2,3], Jan Henkel [2,3], Danika Bannasch [2,4], Vidhya Jagannathan [2,3] and Monika M. Welle [3,5]

[1] AniCura Tierärztliche Spezialisten, 22043 Hamburg, Germany; monikalinek@gmail.com (M.L.); marendoelle@gmx.net (M.D.)

[2] Institute of Genetics, Vetsuisse Faculty, University of Bern, 3001 Bern, Switzerland; anina.bauer@hotmail.com (A.B.); Fabienne.Leuthard@vetmeduni.ac.at (F.L.); jan.henkel@vetsuisse.unibe.ch (J.H.); dlbannasch@ucdavis.edu (D.B.); vidhya.jagannathan@vetsuisse.unibe.ch (V.J.)

[3] Dermfocus, University of Bern, 3001 Bern, Switzerland; monika.welle@vetsuisse.unibe.ch

[4] Department of Population Health and Reproduction, School of Veterinary Medicine, University of California, Davis, CA 95616, USA

[5] Institute of Animal Pathology, Vetsuisse Faculty, University of Bern, 3001 Bern, Switzerland

* Correspondence: tosso.leeb@vetsuisse.unibe.ch;

† These three authors contributed equally to the paper.

Abstract: A 4-month-old female Irish Terrier presented with a well demarcated ulcerative and crusting lesion in the right ear canal. Histological analysis revealed epidermal hyperplasia with severe acantholysis affecting all suprabasal layers of the epidermis, which prompted a presumptive diagnosis of canine Darier disease. The lesion was successfully treated by repeated laser ablation of the affected epidermis. Over the course of three years, the dog additionally developed three dermal nodules of up to 4 cm in diameter that were excised and healed without complications. Histology of the excised tissue revealed multiple infundibular cysts extending from the upper dermis to the subcutis. The cysts were lined by squamous epithelium, which presented with abundant acantholysis of suprabasal keratinocytes. Infundibular cysts represent a novel finding not previously reported in Darier patients. Whole genome sequencing of the affected dog was performed, and the functional candidate genes for Darier disease (*ATP2A2*) and Hailey-Hailey disease (*ATP2C1*) were investigated. The analysis revealed a heterozygous SINE insertion into the *ATP2A2* gene, at the end of intron 14, close to the boundary of exon 15. Analysis of the *ATP2A2* mRNA from skin of the affected dog demonstrated a splicing defect and marked allelic imbalance, suggesting nonsense-mediated decay of the resulting aberrant transcripts. As Darier disease in humans is caused by haploinsufficiency of *ATP2A2*, our genetic findings are in agreement with the clinical and histopathological data and support the diagnosis of canine Darier disease.

Keywords: *Canis lupus familiaris*; dog; dermatology; skin; desmosome; acantholysis; calcium; animal model; veterinary medicine; precision medicine

1. Introduction

The skin is the largest organ of the human body and forms an essential barrier to protect the body from fluid loss and harmful agents of the environment. The epidermis representing the outermost layer of the skin consists of a stratified epithelium with keratinocytes as its major cell type. Keratinocytes proliferate in the basal layer and subsequently undergo a highly coordinated differentiation program while they move upwards through the spinous and granular layers until they finally reach the stratum corneum, from which they are continuously shed [1]. The barrier function of the epidermis requires tight adhesion between keratinocytes, which is mainly mediated by desmosomes. Ca^{2+} signaling is essential for epidermal differentiation and intraepidermal cohesion [2–5]. Several inherited disorders of the skin involving variants in calcium pumps have been recognized [6].

In humans, Darier disease (MIM #124200), also called Darier-White disease or keratosis follicularis, is inherited as an autosomal dominant trait and caused by heterozygous variants in the *ATP2A2* gene encoding the endoplasmic/sarcoplasmic reticulum Ca^{2+}-ATPase 2 (SERCA2) [7,8]. Darier disease typically starts before the third decade and is clinically characterized by warty papules and plaques in seborrheic areas (central trunk, flexures, scalp, and forehead), palmoplantar pits, and distinctive nail abnormalities [7,9]. Secondary infection is common. Neuropsychiatric abnormalities have been described in a small fraction of the patients with Darier disease [9].

Hailey-Hailey disease (OMIM #169600), also called benign chronic pemphigus, is another autosomal dominant skin disorder caused by heterozygous variants in the *ATP2C1* gene encoding a Ca^{2+}-ATPase expressed in the membrane of the Golgi apparatus [10]. Hailey-Hailey disease usually becomes manifest in the third or fourth decade of life with erythema, vesicles, and painful erosions involving the body folds, particularly the groin and axillary regions [11]. Both diseases are characterized histologically by the breakdown of intercellular contacts between suprabasal keratinocytes (acantholysis) with variable dyskeratosis. Differential diagnosis is based on the skin lesion types, their distribution on the body, and subtle histological differences [9,11,12].

Many independent genetic variants in *ATP2A2* and *ATP2C1* in human patients with Darier disease or Hailey-Hailey disease have been described. Variations in the clinical and histological phenotypes may at least partly correlate with the different specific genetic variants [8]. Nonetheless, both diseases are inherited as autosomal dominant traits and are due to haploinsufficiency of the encoded calcium pumps [6].

Dermatoses affecting desmosomes in domestic animals have been summarized in a comprehensive review [13]. In one report, clinical, histological, immunohistological, and ultrastructural findings in a male English Setter and two of its female offspring were initially reported as Hailey-Hailey disease [14,15]. A subsequent study found depletion of the ATP2A2-gated stores in cultured keratinocytes from one of these dogs and suggested that these dogs had Darier disease and not Hailey-Hailey disease as previously reported [16]. To the best of our knowledge, the underlying causative genetic variant was not reported in these cases and no further cases in dogs have been reported in the scientific literature.

In the present study, we describe the clinical and histological phenotype and the genetic analysis of an Irish Terrier, which all together enabled the diagnosis of canine Darier disease. In addition to the epidermal lesions, this dog presented with multifocal infundibular cysts with suprabasal acantholysis, a feature that has never been described with Darier disease, neither in humans nor in dogs. The successful management of the skin lesions with repeated diode laser ablation is outlined.

2. Materials and Methods

2.1. Ethics Statement

All dogs in this study were privately owned and samples were collected with the consent of their owners. The collection of blood samples from control dogs was approved by the "Cantonal Committee For Animal Experiments" (Canton of Bern; permit 75/16; Approval date: 11 July 2016). The collection of samples from the affected dog was performed for diagnostic or therapeutic reasons and did not constitute an animal experiment in the legal sense.

2.2. Clinical Examinations and Management

A 4-month-old, intact female Irish Terrier with 9.5 kg body weight was initially presented with skin lesions in the outer ear canal in August 2016. The dog was clinically monitored for general growth, general health and skin lesion development over a period of three years. Cytology swabs were taken from crusting lesions and fine needle aspirates from nodules, respectively. Skin lesions in the outer ear canal were visualized and punch biopsies were taken via video otoscopy (Tele Pack Vet X Led, Carl Zeiss, Germany, Tuttlingen) under general anesthesia with endotracheal intubation. Nodules were excised in toto. Tissue samples for histological evaluation were fixed in 10% buffered formalin immediately.

Blood was taken twice for complete blood count and genetic testing. Tear production was assessed by Schirmer's tear test, as recommended during vitamin A therapy. For laser ablation, an MLT Type 109 classic diode laser (Medizinische Laser Technologie GmbH, Ingelheim, Germany) with 4.0 W wave mode in continuous contact mode was used.

2.3. Histopathology

Biopsies were evaluated from the two plaque-like, partially eroded lesions of the external ear canal, one nodular lesion from the hind leg, and two large nodules from the neck. Tissue was processed routinely and stained with hematoxylin and eosin.

2.4. Whole Genome Sequencing

Genomic DNA was isolated from EDTA blood of the affected dog with the Maxwell RSC Whole Blood Kit using a Maxwell RSC 48 instrument (Promega, Madison, WI, USA). An Illumina TruSeq PCR-free DNA library (Illumina, San Diego, CA, USA) with ~350 bp insert size of the affected dog (IT390) was prepared. We collected 269 million 2 × 150 bp paired-end reads on a HiSeq 3000 instrument (32 × coverage). Mapping and alignment were performed as described [17]. The sequence data were deposited under the study accession PRJEB16012 and the sample accession SAMEA104283467 at the European Nucleotide Archive.

2.5. Variant Calling

Variant calling was performed using the Genome Analysis Toolkit (GATK) HaplotypeCaller [18] in gVCF mode as described [17]. To predict the functional effects of the called variants, SnpEff [19] software, together with NCBI annotation release 105 for the CanFam 3.1 genome reference assembly, was used. For variant filtering we used 655 control genomes, which were either publicly available [20,21] or produced during other projects of our group [17] (Table S1). Structural variants were identified by visual inspection of the Illumina short read alignments in the Integrated Genome Viewer (IGV) [22]. The genotypes at the ATP2A2 SINE insertion (Chr26:8,200,944_8,200,945ins205) were also derived by visual inspection of the short read alignments in IGV. Samples were genotyped as homozygous ref/ref, if they did not show any signs of a structural variant at this position and had at least 4 reads aligning from Chr26:8,200,929-8,200,945, thus spanning the 15 nucleotide duplication at the insertion site.

2.6. Gene Analysis

We used the CanFam 3.1 dog reference genome assembly and NCBI annotation release 105. Numbering within the canine ATP2A2 gene corresponds to the NCBI RefSeq accession numbers NM_001003214.1 (mRNA) and NP_001003214.1 (protein).

2.7. RT-PCR and Sanger Sequencing

Total RNA was extracted from skin tissues using the RNeasy mini kit (Qiagen, Hilden, Germany). The tissue was first finely crushed in TRIZOL (Thermo Fisher Scientific, Waltham, MA, USA) using mechanical means, chloroform was then added and the RNA was separated by centrifugation. The RNA was cleared of genomic DNA contamination using the Quantitect Reverse Transcription Kit (Qiagen). The same kit was used to synthetize cDNA, as described by the manufacturer. RT-PCR was carried out using primer ATP2A2_Ex14_F, TCCTCCAAGGATTGAAGTGG, located in exon 14 and primer ATP2A2_Ex16_R, TGTCACCAGATTGACCCAGA, located in exon 16 of the ATP2A2 gene.

After treatment with exonuclease I and alkaline phosphatase, cDNA amplicons were sequenced on an ABI 3730 DNA Analyzer (Thermo Fisher Scientific) using the forward primer ATP2A2_Ex14_F as sequencing primer. Sanger sequences were analyzed using the Sequencher 5.1 software (GeneCodes, Ann Arbor, MI, USA).

PCR on genomic DNA was performed using AmpliTaqGold360Mastermix (Thermo Fisher Scientific) and primers ATP2A2_Ex14_F (same as above) and ATP2A2_Ex15_R, TCAGGGCAGGAG CATCATTC. Genomic PCR products were also sequenced using the forward primer ATP2A2_Ex14_F as sequencing primer.

2.8. Whole Transcriptome Analysis (RNA-seq)

RNA libraries were prepared from total RNA of lesional and non-lesional skin of the affected Irish Terrier using the Illumina TruSeq Stranded mRNA Library Kit according to the manufacturer's instructions. The libraries were sequenced with 2 × 50 bp paired-end sequencing chemistry on an Illumina NovaSeq 6000 instrument. The reads were mapped with STAR aligner version 2.6.0 [23] to the CanFam3.1 reference genome assembly. The sequence data were deposited under the study accession PRJEB33508 and sample accessions SAMEA6800286 and SAMEA6800287 at the European Nucleotide Archive. The read alignments of the affected Irish Terrier were visually compared to a skin RNA-seq dataset from a healthy control dog (ENA project accession PRJEB33508, sample accession SAMEA6800283).

3. Results

3.1. Clinical Examination and Management

During the first consult in August 2016, a 4-month old intact female Irish Terrier presented with several confluent, well demarcated, proliferative, crusted, and partially eroded to ulcerated plaques at the concave pinnae of the right ear extending into the medial aspect of the vertical ear canal (Figure 1A). These lesions had been present since at least 4 weeks prior to the examination. Culture swabs taken by the referring veterinarian revealed *Staphylococcus pseudintermedius* sensible to most antibiotics. The presence of a foreign body had been excluded by an ear flush. At the time of presentation, the dog received amoxicillin/clavulanic acid at a dosage of 26 mg/kg body weight (BW) twice daily (Synulox®, Zoetis, Berlin, Germany) and prednisolone 5 mg/kg BW once daily (Prednisolon 5 mg®, CP Pharma mbH, Burgdorf, Germany). Several commercially available ear cleansers and eardrops had been applied before without any improvement.

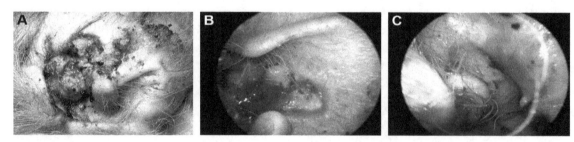

Figure 1. Clinical phenotype. (**A**) Concave pinnae of the right ear showing well demarcated crusting, eroded and ulcerated skin plaques. (**B**) Medial aspect of the right ear canal with well demarcated ulcerated lesions visualized via video otoscopy after crusts had been flushed away. (**C**) Same aspect of the ear canal: Intact, slightly erythematous skin after repeated laser ablation.

The general and dermatological examination did not reveal any abnormalities except the moderately painful and mildly pruritic lesions of the right pinna and ear canal. Cytology showed clusters of acantholytic keratinocytes, non-degenerated neutrophils, and numerous cocci.

Video otoscopy showed intact eardrums and normal horizontal ear canals in both ears. The medial aspect of the right vertical ear canal revealed well demarcated, ulcerated lesions covered with thick crusts confluent with the lesions of the concave pinna (Figure 1B). Waiting for the biopsy results, the dog was treated with squalene ear cleanser every other day, twice daily topically with Triamcinolone Acetonide cream (Volon®A Haftsalbe 1 mg/g, Dermapharm AG) and sulfadiazine creme (Flammizine®, Alliance Pharmaceuticals Limited, Chippenham, UK), changed to customized eardrops of 1% fluoroquinolone in saline solution (Baytril®5%, Bayer AnimalHealth GmbH, Leverkusen, Germany) for easier handling. After the preliminary diagnosis of canine Darier disease, treatment with vitamin A 10,000 IU (Vitamin-A-saar®, Cephasaar, Ingbert, Germany) orally for two weeks daily; then, every other day was initiated and maintained for 3 months.

As no improvement was noticed after 3 months, we decided to ablate the lesional epidermis with a diode laser to remove the defect skin and provoke secondary healing from the periphery. This procedure was partially successful the first time. All lesions healed without crusts after repeated laser ablation of the affected tissue another three times, two, five, and 12 months apart (Figure 1C). On the pinna, small nodules of 1–2 mm remained. They were clinically and cytologically diagnosed as comedones.

In the following three years after the first presentation, the dog developed three well-demarcated, dermal nodules ranging from 2.5 cm to 4 cm in diameter on the dorsal neck, the left side of the neck, and on the right knee. Fine needle aspirates of all nodules revealed clusters of nucleated round to oval keratinocytes with mild anisocytosis and anisocaryosis and two to three nucleoli in the nucleus. These nodules were fully excised and submitted for histopathology. At the time of writing, no further lesions or nodules had developed.

3.2. Histopathology

Biopsies from the external ear canal revealed focally extensive epidermal hyperplasia with severe acantholysis affecting all suprabasal layers of the epidermis and resulting in in the formation of multiple small clefts and lacunae (Figure 2). Acantholytic keratinocytes were frequently dyskeratotic forming "corps ronds" (e.g., round bodies characterized by small pyknotic nuclei, a perinuclear clear halo and eosinophilic cytoplasm) or "grains" (cells with elongated nuclei present mainly in the stratum corneum and the granular layer). The epidermis was covered by compact orthokeratotic or parakeratotic keratin intermingled with dyskeratotic acantholytic cells. In areas of abundant acantholyisis, keratin extended as prominent focal plugs into the epidermis.

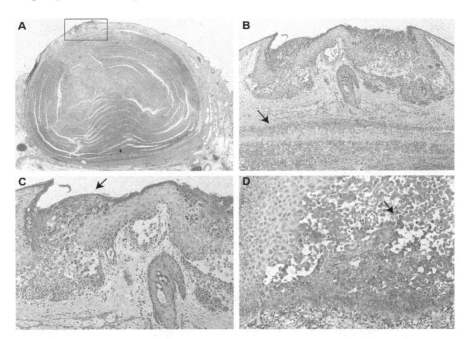

Figure 2. Histopathology. (**A**) Infundibular cyst underneath a focal area of hyperplastic epidermis with abundant suprabasal acantholyisis (rectangle). (**B**) Higher magnification of the focal area of hyperplastic

epidermis with suprabasal acantholysis overlying the cyst wall (arrow). The epidermal plaque is characterized by severely irregularly hyperplastic epidermis with abundant suprabasal acantholytic and dyskeratotic keratinocytes forming the "corps ronds" typical for Darier disease. Keratotic plugs composed of parakeratotic keratin and grains extend into the clefts resulting from abundant acantholysis. The hyperplastic plaque is overlying an infundibular cyst composed of squamous epithelium with abundant suprabasal acantholysis. The cyst is filled with parakeratotic keratin and numerous "corps ronds". (C) Higher magnification of the lesions already presented in (A,B). Note the abundant suprabasal acantholyis of dyskeratotic keratinocytes forming "corps ronds", "grains" and parakeratotic keratin (arrow). (D) Hyperplastic plaque from the outer ear canal. Within the severely hyperplastic epidermis, numerous acantholytic and dyskeratotic keratinocytes forming "corps ronds" (arrow) and causing small clefts are present.

In all biopsies from haired skin, one or multiple infundibular cysts measuring between 0.8 × 0.5 × 0.5 cm up to 3.5 × 3.0 × 1.2 cm were extending from the upper dermis to the subcutis. The cysts were lined by squamous epithelium, which presented with abundant acantholysis of suprabasal keratinocytes. The cysts were filled with parakeratotic keratin and numerous acantholytic and dyskeratotic cells. In one biopsy from the neck, the epidermis overlying the cyst presented with severe hyperplasia and suprabasal acantholysis comparable to the findings described for the outer ear canal. Similar findings were also present in the infundibular epithelium of some hair follicles.

3.3. Identification of a Candidate Causative Variant

We sequenced the genome of the affected dog at 32 × coverage and called single nucleotide and small indel variants with respect to the reference genome. The variants were compared to whole genome sequence data of 8 wolves and 647 control dogs from genetically diverse breeds and searched for private protein-changing variants in the two functional candidate genes ATP2A2 and ATP2C1. This analysis of small variants did not identify any likely candidate causative variants for the phenotype (Table S2).

We then visually inspected the short read alignments in ATP2A2 and ATP2C1 to search for structural variants that would have been missed by our automated variant detection pipeline. Several truncated read alignments at the end of intron 14 of the ATP2A2 gene indicated a potential insertion event including the duplication of 15 nucleotides flanking the insertion site. The inserted sequence represented a tRNA derived SINE (Figure 3A,B).

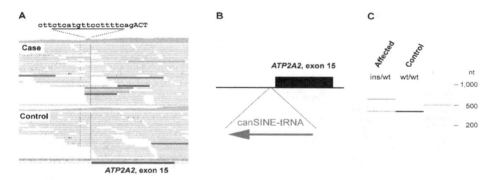

Figure 3. SINE insertion into intron 14 of the ATP2A2 gene. (A) IGV screenshot illustrating the structural variant. The case shows an increased coverage over 15 nucleotides spanning from Chr26:8,200,930-8,200,944 (CanFam3.1 assembly). The sequence at the intron/exon boundary is given with the duplicated bases underlined. Capital letters represent the first 3 bases of exon 15. Several read alignments are soft-clipped at the left or right boundary of the duplicated 15 nt region. Colored reads indicate that their mates map to other chromosomes. These features are characteristic for an insertion of a repetitive element into the genome of the affected dog. (B) Schematic representation of the SINE insertion. A ~205 bp canine SINE-tRNA insertion was found in heterozygous state in the affected Irish Terrier. (C) Experimental genotyping of the SINE insertion by fragment size analysis. We amplified the intron 14/exon 15 boundary of the ATP2A2 gene by PCR in the affected dog and a control and separated the products by capillary gel electrophoresis.

The genotypes at the SINE insertion site were investigated in the 655 control genomes. A total of 592 genomes had at least four reads spanning the insertion site and were genotyped as homozygous wildtype. In the remaining 63 control genomes, we did not see any indication for an insertion event. However, due to low coverage and/or short read lengths, the genotypes in these samples could not be reliably determined (Table S1). PCR amplification with flanking primers on a genomic DNA sample from the affected dog provided independent confirmation of the presence of a ~205 bp insertion in heterozygous state (Figure 3C).

3.4. Analysis of the ATP2A2 mRNA

We next investigated whether the SINE insertion into intron 14 had any effect on the expressed *ATP2A2* mRNA. Initial RT-PCR experiments on RNA from skin of the affected dog with different primer combinations yielded products of the expected size and sequence and did not indicate any obvious qualitative defects in mRNA splicing.

As the genomic insertion was only present in a heterozygous state, the wildtype allele was still expected to give rise to the normal *ATP2A2* transcript. Consequently, a potential splicing defect leading to nonsense mediated decay in transcripts from the mutant allele or transcriptional silencing of the mutant allele would not have been detected by our qualitative analysis of RT-PCR bands. We therefore additionally investigated the allele-specific expression of *ATP2A2* transcripts. This analysis demonstrated that ~85% of the detected transcripts were derived from the wildtype allele with an almost complete absence of transcripts from the mutant allele (Figure 4A,B).

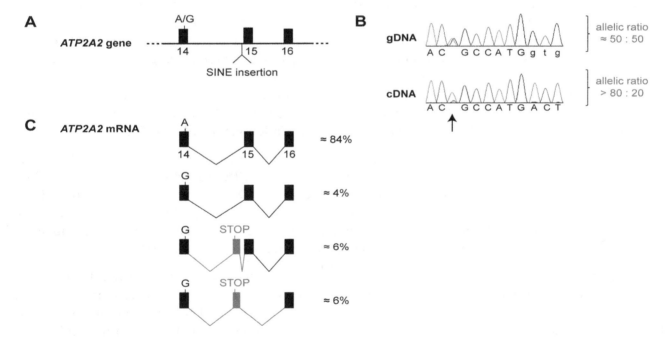

Figure 4. Splicing defect and allele-specific expression of the *ATP2A2* mRNA. (**A**) Genomic organization of the *ATP2A2* gene. The affected dog was heterozygous at the silent c.2091A>G variant located at the end of exon 14 and heterozygous for the SINE insertion in intron 14. (**B**) A Sanger electropherogram obtained from a genomic PCR product shows the expected equal ratio of the two alleles at c.2091A>G. In contrast, a Sanger electropherogram obtained with the same sequencing primer from a cDNA amplicon showed a strong bias towards the A-allele (arrow). This semi-quantitative analysis suggests that the transcripts from the mutant *ATP2A2* allele are degraded, possibly by nonsense mediated decay or another mechanism of the cellular quality control. (**C**) RNA-seq analysis from skin of the affected dog confirmed the strong allelic bias in the transcripts. Only very little functional transcripts are produced from the G-allele. The majority of the transcripts from the G-allele contain an aberrant exon and a premature stop codon. Further details of the RNA-seq analysis are shown in Figure S1.

To gain further insights into possible splicing defects, we performed an RNA-seq experiment and whole transcriptome analysis in skin of the affected dog. Visual inspection of the short-read alignments in the region of the *ATP2A2* gene confirmed the strong allelic bias of the transcripts. Furthermore, this experiment revealed the presence of rare transcripts containing an additional, aberrantly spliced exon. This 139 nt exon was derived from genomic sequence a short distance upstream of the SINE insertion (Chr26:8,200,774-8,200,912). The aberrant exon contained an early premature stop codon. The variant designation of the predicted protein from transcripts containing the aberrant exon is NP_001003214.1:p.(Thr700Valfs*6). Only a small proportion of the transcripts from the mutant allele was correctly spliced and had the correct coding sequence (Figure 4C and Figure S1).

4. Discussion

In this study, we describe the clinical and histological phenotype and the genetic analysis of an Irish Terrier with canine Darier disease. The dog developed two different types of clinical lesions over a follow up time of 3 years. One lesion type presented as demarcated, proliferative, crusted and eroded to ulcerated and was present on the right concave pinna and in the ear canal. This lesion type was overlying an infundibular cyst, which represented the second type of lesion.

The crusted lesions were more severe, painful, and pruritic than the lesions described in the previously published cases [14,15]. Essentially the published cases describe one seven-month-old, male, intact English Setter that exhibited a peculiar crusting lesion on the ventral chest and two of his six living offspring that were intentionally bred by mating the affected English Setter to a normal laboratory Beagle. The two Setter-Beagle crossbred dogs developed similar lesions as the sire with alopecia, erythema, and hyperplasia on the lateral knee (one dog) or dorsal head (second dog) at the age of four and seven weeks, respectively. The lesions slightly enlarged and worsened during adolescence but remained static thereafter and did not require therapy. The histopathology and ultrastructural findings were similar in all three dogs and initially considered to represent Hailey-Hailey disease (benign familiar chronic pemphigus) [14,15]. In a subsequent study, cultured keratinocytes from one of these dogs were investigated and a depletion of ATP2A2-gated Ca^{2+} stores was found. This finding suggested that these dogs had Darier disease rather than Hailey-Hailey disease [16].

Considering the clinical presentation of focal hyperplastic skin lesions in these dogs [14,15], their early age of onset, and the histology with severe acantholysis with prominent dyskeratosis and the formation of corps ronds and grains also suggests that they had Darier disease and not Hailey-Hailey disease as previously reported. In Hailey-Hailey disease, prominent suprabasal acantholyisis is also a feature, but loss of keratinocyte cohesion is not as complete as in Darier disease and detached keratinocytes still form clusters. Dyskeratosis is milder than in Darier disease [12].

The specific molecular mechanisms that lead to the multifocal hyperproliferation, dyskeratosis and acantholysis of epidermal keratinocytes have not yet been identified. It is well known that extracellular calcium plays a crucial role in regulating differentiation and adhesion of cultured keratinocytes [6,16]. Low levels of Ca^{2+} induce keratinocyte proliferation while physiological levels induce cell-to-cell adhesion and keratinocyte differentiation. It has been shown that changes in the intracellular calcium homeostasis in Darier disease impair processing, transport, and assembly of calcium-dependent desmosomal proteins. Desmosomes provide strong adhesive bonds between neighboring cells by correct assembly of their intercellular and intracellular proteins and disturbance of this process results in acantholysis [6,13,16]. An alternative hypothesis is that the defective calcium homeostasis leads to delayed exit of keratinocytes from the cell cycle, which may promote secondary mutations that lead to acantholysis [16]. Furthermore, Ca^{2+} levels in the endoplasmic reticulum play a key role in post-translational modification of proteins. Disturbances of Ca^{2+} homeostasis may result in an accumulation of unfolded proteins in the endoplasmic reticulum and subsequent apoptosis. It has been suggested that the "corps ronds" in Darier disease may be the result of such an impaired protein folding [6].

In our patient, the crusting lesions did not enlarge, and only one similar lesion developed on other parts of the body. However, over a course of 3 years, the dog developed three infundibular cysts where the Darier specific acantholysis with dyskeratosis was seen within the cyst walls. In the epidermis overlying one cyst on the neck, a similar epidermal lesion as described for the ear developed. To the best of our knowledge, infundibular cysts have not yet been described in humans or dogs with Darier disease. In humans, several clinical variants of Darier disease including vesicobullous, hypopigmented, cornifying, zosteriform or linear, acute, and comedonal subtypes have been described [9]. Comedonal Darier disease is a very rare variant with severe follicular involvement and characterized by open or closed comedones with central keratotic plugs and the presence of greatly elongated epidermal protrusions at the base of the comedones [24,25]. However, in the canine case presented here, no comedones but true infundibular cysts without the described elongated papillary projections at the base of the cysts were present. Thus, this presentation of our case is new and has never been described in humans or dogs.

The dermal nodules were successfully excised and no recurrence was noted at the site of excision. The hyperplastic and ulcerated lesions on the pinna and the ear canal required treatment, as they were painful and prone to secondary infection at any time-point.

In human medicine, numerous therapeutic options have been described, including systemic or topical retinoids, cyclosporine, vitamin A, systemic or topical corticosteroids, topical 5-fluorouracil, keratolytics with urea, or interventional treatment, like dermabrasion, laser ablation, and excision [26–30].

The age of the dog, the difficulty in the application of topical treatments, and financial and psychological restrictions of the owner limited the treatment options in our patient. Systemic and topical glucocorticoids, as well as systemic vitamin A, were not successful. As other medical treatments were denied, we treated the lesions in the ear with a diode laser. Carbon dioxide (CO_2) laser or yttrium aluminum garnet (YAG) laser ablation in Darier disease and Hailey- Hailey disease has been reported as a successful treatment option in human medicine [28–30]. We chose a diode laser, as this device can be used via the working channel of the video otoscope and allowed us to ablate the lesional skin of the medial aspect of the vertical ear canal under visual control. The concept of laser therapy in Darier disease is the ablation of the defective epidermis and the follicular infundibulum, which might be the focus of recurrence. In the described laser-treated human patients, remodeling of normal skin, as well as cicatrization, occurred. In our canine patient, the treatment was very well tolerated and led to full resolution of the lesion after several interventions. The ear canal tissue provides only a thin layer of dermis over the underlying cartilage, which is prone to necrosis if damaged. Therefore, our inventions had most likely not been aggressive enough to completely destroy the affected tissue and the follicular infundibulum in one session. In less vulnerable areas of the skin, a laser treatment might be more favorable.

Darier disease in human patients is caused by heterozygous genetic variants in *ATP2A2*. These include missense, nonsense, frameshift, and splice site variants [7,8,31]. An intronic 18 bp insertion, 12 nucleotides upstream of exon 3, caused Darier disease in one human family. This insertion altered splicing and resulted in an aberrant transcript with 6 additional codons, which could be detected as in-frame insertion that did not lead to nonsense mediated decay [31].

Our genetic analysis revealed a heterozygous SINE insertion in intron 14 of the *ATP2A2* gene, which was exclusively found in the affected dog, but not in 592 controls. The functional analysis at the mRNA level indicated nearly mono-allelic expression of *ATP2A2* transcripts in skin of the affected dog. RNA-seq showed that the SINE insertion led to the activation of cryptic splice sites in intron 14 and the inclusion of an aberrant exon containing a premature stop codon. The observed allelic imbalance of the transcripts can be plausibly explained by nonsense-mediated decay [32] of the transcripts with the premature stop codon.

A limitation of our genetic analysis is the lack of family data. We hypothesize that the SINE insertion in the affected dog is the consequence of a *de novo* mutation event. Thus, the parents of the dog are assumed to be phenotypically and genotypically wildtype. If the homozygous wildtype genotype were confirmed in both parents, this would provide proof for the hypothetical *de novo* mutation event and another strong supporting argument for the pathogenicity of the SINE insertion. Unfortunately, we did not have access to the parents of the affected dog.

Given the extensive functional knowledge on *ATP2A2* and the role of *ATP2A2* variants in human Darier disease, we nonetheless think that our data strongly suggest that the SINE insertion may be considered a candidate causative variant for the phenotype in the affected dog.

5. Conclusions

We provided a comprehensive clinical, histopathological and genetic characterization of an Irish Terrier with Darier disease. The genetic analysis revealed an intronic SINE insertion into *ATP2A2* as a candidate causative genetic variant leading to aberrant splicing and degradation of aberrant transcripts.

Author Contributions: Conceptualization, M.L., T.L., M.M.W.; Data curation, V.J.; Investigation, M.L., M.D., T.L., A.B., F.L., J.H.; Supervision, M.L., T.L.; Visualization, M.L., M.D., T.L., M.M.W.; Writing—original draft, M.L., T.L., M.M.W.; Writing—review & editing, M.L., M.D., T.L., A.B., F.L., J.H., D.B., V.J., M.M.W. All authors have read and agreed to the published version of the manuscript.

Acknowledgments: The authors are grateful to all dog owners who donated samples and shared health and pedigree data of their dogs. We thank Eva Andrist, Nathalie Besuchet Schmutz, and Sabrina Schenk for expert technical assistance, the Next Generation Sequencing Platform of the University of Bern for performing the high-throughput sequencing experiments, and the Interfaculty Bioinformatics Unit of the University of Bern for providing high performance computing infrastructure. We thank the Dog Biomedical Variant Database Consortium (Gus Aguirre, Catherine André, Danika Bannasch, Doreen Becker, Brian Davis, Cord Drögemüller, Kari Ekenstedt, Kiterie Faller, Oliver Forman, Steve Friedenberg, Eva Furrow, Urs Giger, Christophe Hitte, Marjo Hytönen, Vidhya Jagannathan, Tosso Leeb, Hannes Lohi, Cathryn Mellersh, Jim Mickelson, Leonardo Murgiano, Anita Oberbauer, Sheila Schmutz, Jeffrey Schoenebeck, Kim Summers, Frank van Steenbeek, Claire Wade) for sharing whole genome sequencing data from control dogs. We also acknowledge all researchers who deposited dog or wolf whole genome sequencing data into public databases.

References

1. Koster, M.I. Making an epidermis. *Ann. N. Y. Acad. Sci.* **2009**, *1170*, 7–10. [CrossRef] [PubMed]

2. Green, K.J.; Simpson, C.L. Desmosomes: New perspectives on a classic. *J. Investig. Dermatol.* **2007**, *127*, 2499–2515. [CrossRef]

3. Müller, E.J.; Williamson, L.; Kolly, C.; Suter, M.M. Outside-in signaling through integrins and cadherins: A central mechanism to control epidermal growth and differentiation? *J. Investig. Dermatol.* **2008**, *128*, 501–516. [CrossRef] [PubMed]

4. Burdett, I.D.; Sullivan, K.H. Desmosome assembly in MDCK cells: Transport of precursors to the cell surface occurs by two phases of vesicular traffic and involves major changes in centrosome and Golgi location during a Ca^{2+} shift. *Exp. Cell Res.* **2002**, *276*, 296–309. [CrossRef] [PubMed]

5. Elias, P.M.; Ahn, S.K.; Denda, M.; Brown, B.E.; Crumrine, D.; Kimutai, L.K.; Kömüves, L.; Lee, S.H.; Feingold, K.R. Modulations in epidermal calcium regulate the expression of differentiation-specific markers. *J. Investig. Dermatol.* **2002**, *119*, 1128–1136. [CrossRef]

6. Foggia, L.; Hovnanian, A. Calcium pump disorders of the skin. *Am. J. Med. Genet. C Semin. Med. Genet.* **2004**, *131*, 20–31.

7. Sakuntabhai, A.; Ruiz-Perez, V.; Carter, S.; Jacobsen, N.; Burge, S.; Monk, S.; Smith, M.; Munro, C.S.; O'Donovan, M.; Craddock, N.; et al. Mutations in *ATP2A2*, encoding a Ca^{2+} pump, cause Darier disease. *Nat. Genet.* **1999**, *21*, 271–277. [CrossRef]

8. Nellen, R.G.; Steijlen, P.M.; van Steensel, M.A.; Vreeburg, M.; European Professional Contributors; Frank, J.; van Geel, M. Mendelian disorders of cornification caused by defects in intracellular calcium pumps: Mutation update and database for variants in *ATP2A2* and *ATP2C1* associated with Darier disease and Hailey-Hailey disease. *Hum. Mutat.* **2017**, *38*, 343–356.

9. Burge, S.M.; Wilkinson, J.D. Darier-White disease: A review of the clinical features in 163 patients. *J. Am. Acad. Dermatol.* **1992**, *27*, 40–50. [CrossRef]

10. Hu, Z.; Bonifas, J.M.; Beech, J.; Bench, G.; Shigihara, T.; Ogawa, H.; Ikeda, S.; Mauro, T.; Epstein, E.H., Jr. Mutations in *ATP2C1*, encoding a calcium pump, cause Hailey-Hailey disease. *Nat. Genet.* **2000**, *24*, 61–65.

11. Poblete-Gutierrez, P.; Wiederholt, T.; Konig, A.; Jugert, F.K.; Marquardt, Y.; Rubben, A.; Merk, H.F.; Happle, R.; Frank, J. Allelic loss underlies type 2 segmental Hailey-Hailey disease, providing molecular confirmation of a novel genetic concept. *J. Clin. Investig.* **2004**, *114*, 1467–1474. [CrossRef] [PubMed]

12. See, S.H.C.; Peternel, S.; Adams, D.; North, J.P. Distinguishing histopathologic features of acantholytic dermatoses and the pattern of acantholytic hypergranulosis. *J. Cutan. Pathol.* **2019**, *46*, 6–15. [CrossRef] [PubMed]

13. Olivry, T.; Linder, K.E. Dermatoses affecting desmosomes in animals: A mechanistic review of acantholytic blistering skin diseases. *Vet. Dermatol.* **2009**, *20*, 313–326. [CrossRef] [PubMed]

14. Shanley, K.J.; Goldschmidt, M.H.; Sueki, H.; Lazarus, G.; George, M. Canine Benign Familial Chronic Pemphigus. In *Advances in Veterinary Dermatology*; Ihrke, P.J., Mason, I.S., White, S.D., Eds.; Pergamon Press: Oxford, UK, 1993; Volume 2, pp. 353–365.

15. Sueki, H.; Shanley, K.; Goldschmidt, M.H.; Lazarus, G.S.; Murphy, G.F. Dominantly inherited epidermal acantholysis in dogs, simulating human benign familial chronic pemphigus (Hailey Hailey disease). *Br. J. Dermatol.* **1997**, *136*, 190–196. [CrossRef]

16. Müller, E.J.; Caldelari, R.; Kolly, C.; Williamson, L.; Baumann, D.; Richard, G.; Jensen, P.; Girling, P.; Delprincipe, F.; Wyder, M.; et al. Consequences of depleted SERCA2-gated calcium stores in the skin. *J. Investig. Dermatol.* **2006**, *126*, 721–731. [CrossRef]

17. Jagannathan, V.; Drögemüller, C.; Leeb, T.; Dog Biomedical Variant Database Consortium (DBVDC). A comprehensive biomedical variant catalogue based on whole genome sequences of 582 dogs and eight wolves. *Anim. Genet.* **2019**, *50*, 695–704. [CrossRef]

18. McKenna, A.; Hanna, M.; Banks, E.; Sivachenko, A.; Cibulskis, K.; Kernytsky, A.; Garimella, K.; Altshuler, D.; Gabriel, S.; Daly, M.; et al. The Genome Analysis Toolkit: A MapReduce framework for analyzing next-generation DNA sequencing data. *Genome Res.* **2010**, *20*, 1297–1303. [CrossRef]

19. Cingolani, P.; Platts, A.; Wangle, L.; Coon, M.; Nguyen, T.; Wang, L.; Land, S.J.; Lu, X.; Ruden, D.M. A program for annotating and predicting the effects of single nucleotide polymorphisms, SnpEff: SNPs in the genome of Drosophila melanogaster strain w1118; iso-2; iso-3. *Fly* **2012**, *6*, 80–92. [CrossRef]

20. Bai, B.; Zhao, W.M.; Tang, B.X.; Wang, Y.Q.; Wang, L.; Zhang, Z.; Yang, H.C.; Liu, Y.H.; Zhu, J.W.; Irwin, D.M.; et al. DoGSD: The dog and wolf genome SNP database. *Nucleic Acids Res.* **2015**, *43*, 777–783. [CrossRef]

21. Plassais, J.; Kim, J.; Davis, B.W.; Karyadi, D.M.; Hogan, A.N.; Harris, A.C.; Decker, B.; Parker, H.G.; Ostrander, E.A. Whole genome sequencing of canids reveals genomic regions under selection and variants influencing morphology. *Nat. Commun.* **2019**, *10*, 1489. [CrossRef]

22. Robinson, J.T.; Thorvaldsdóttir, H.; Winckler, W.; Guttman, M.; Lander, E.S.; Getz, G.; Mesirov, J.P. Integrative genomics viewer. *Nat. Biotechnol.* **2011**, *29*, 24–26. [CrossRef] [PubMed]

23. Dobin, A.; Davis, C.A.; Schlesinger, F.; Drenkow, J.; Zaleski, C.; Jha, S.; Batut, P.; Chaisson, M.; Gingeras, T.R. STAR: Ultrafast universal RNA-seq aligner. *Bioinformatics* **2013**, *29*, 15–21. [CrossRef] [PubMed]

24. Derrick, E.K.; Darley, C.R.; Burge, S. Comedonal Darier's disease. *Br. J. Dermatol.* **1995**, *132*, 453–455. [CrossRef]

25. Lora, V.; Cota, C.; Grammatico, P.; Pedace, L.; Kerl, H.; Cerroni, L. Comedonal Darier disease: Report of 2 cases. *J. Am. Acad. Dermatol.* **2013**, *69*, e307–e309. [CrossRef] [PubMed]

26. Cooper, S.M.; Burge, S.M. Darier's disease: Epidemiology, pathophysiology, and management. *Am. J. Clin. Dermatol.* **2003**, *4*, 97–105. [CrossRef]

27. Letulé, V.; Herzinger, T.; Ruzicka, T.; Molin, S. Treatment of Darier disease with oral alitretinoin. *Clin. Exp. Dermatol.* **2013**, *38*, 523–525. [CrossRef]

28. McElroy, J.A.; Mehregan, D.A.; Roenigk, R.K. Carbon dioxide laser vaporization of recalcitrant symptomatic plaques of Hailey-Hailey disease and Darier's disease. *J. Am. Acad. Dermatol.* **1990**, *23*, 893–897. [CrossRef]

29. Beier, C.; Kaufmann, R. Efficacy of erbium:YAG laser ablation in Darier disease and Hailey-Hailey disease. *Arch. Dermatol.* **1999**, *135*, 423–427. [CrossRef]

30. Benmously, R.; Litaiem, N.; Hammami, H.; Badri, T.; Fenniche, S. Significant alleviation of Darier's disease with fractional CO_2 laser. *J. Cosmet. Laser Ther.* **2015**, *17*, 77–79. [CrossRef]

31. Sakuntabhai, A.; Burge, S.; Monk, S.; Hovnanian, A. Spectrum of novel *ATP2A2* mutations in patients with Darier's disease. *Hum. Mol. Genet.* **1999**, *8*, 1611–1619. [CrossRef] [PubMed]

32. Kishor, A.; Fritz, S.E.; Hogg, J.R. Nonsense-mediated mRNA decay: The challenge of telling right from wrong in a complex transcriptome. *Wiley Interdiscip. Rev. RNA* **2019**, *10*, e1548. [CrossRef] [PubMed]

16

The Genetic Basis of Obesity and Related Metabolic Diseases in Humans and Companion Animals

Natalie Wallis and Eleanor Raffan *

Anatomy Building, Department of Physiology, Development and Neuroscience, University of Cambridge, Downing Street, Cambridge CB2 3DY, UK; njw64@cam.ac.uk
* Correspondence: er311@cam.ac.uk

Abstract: Obesity is one of the most prevalent health conditions in humans and companion animals globally. It is associated with premature mortality, metabolic dysfunction, and multiple health conditions across species. Obesity is, therefore, of importance in the fields of medicine and veterinary medicine. The regulation of adiposity is a homeostatic process vulnerable to disruption by a multitude of genetic and environmental factors. It is well established that the heritability of obesity is high in humans and laboratory animals, with ample evidence that the same is true in companion animals. In this review, we provide an overview of how genes link to obesity in humans, drawing on a wealth of information from laboratory animal models, and summarise the mechanisms by which obesity causes related disease. Throughout, we focus on how large-scale human studies and niche investigations of rare mutations in severely affected patients have improved our understanding of obesity biology and can inform our ability to interpret results of animal studies. For dogs, cats, and horses, we compare the similarities in obesity pathophysiology to humans and review the genetic studies that have been previously reported in those species. Finally, we discuss how veterinary genetics may learn from humans about studying precise, nuanced phenotypes and implementing large-scale studies, but also how veterinary studies may be able to look past clinical findings to mechanistic ones and demonstrate translational benefits to human research.

Keywords: obesity; genetics; companion animals; metabolic disease; comparative genomics; dogs; cats; horses

1. Introduction

Obesity presents a major health problem in humans and companion animals alike. An estimated 39% of people were overweight or obese in 2016, a value nearly triple that recorded in 1975 and equating to over 2 billion adults [1]. Mirroring that trend are increases in pet obesity, with as many as 63% of cats [2] and 59% of dogs [3] reported to be overweight or obese. Obesity was declared an epidemic by the World Health Organisation (WHO) in 1997 [4] and similarly identified as a major threat to pet health by BSAVA and WSAVA [5].

Precise definitions of obesity are debated, but it is generally accepted that obesity is the unhealthy accumulation of body fat. What is not controversial is that obesity is a consequence of energy intake chronically exceeding energy output. Consequently, obesity has commonly been considered a ramification of poor self-control in people or of inept management by animal owners. However, considerable evidence now shows obesity is better regarded as a disease of disordered energy homeostasis in which a multitude of genetic and environmental factors can contribute to increasing body fat.

This review first examines the pathophysiology of obesity and the role of genetics in the disease, focussing on the wealth of evidence from human and rodent studies. We then review the genetics of obesity and related metabolic disease in companion animals. Finally, we consider opportunities for future research in companion animals that may improve understanding of both animal and human obesity.

2. Factors Contributing to Obesity

Recent, rapid increases in the prevalence of obesity have been caused by changes in activity and diet in the human population, and the same is likely true in animal populations [6,7]. However, it is clear that, although much of the human population is exposed to an "obesogenic environment" (with ready access to high calorie food and increasingly sedentary lifestyles), only a subset become overweight or obese. It is now well established that multiple factors including socioeconomic status, education level, and genetics are associated with whether a person is likely to develop obesity [8]. In companion animals, similarly diverse risk factors have been identified, with biological factors such as age, sex, and breed recognised alongside owner management factors in dog, cat, and horse obesity [9–12].

Acknowledgement of the multiple obesity risk factors is important, because it informs efforts to reduce obesity. Stigma against overweight people and parents of overweight children is well recognised [13,14], and the same is true for owners of overweight companion animals [15,16]. Such stigmas arise from the widespread view that weight gain is due to lax efforts to regulate food intake and exercise, either by a person, parent, or animal owner. It is important to acknowledge the risk factors beyond an individual's control (such as genetics) in order to improve the effectiveness of obesity prevention and treatment programmes.

Obesity Susceptibility Is Highly Heritable

Humans within the same environment, be that energy surplus or energy scarcity, display a highly heritable variance in body condition [17]. A wealth of data from twin and adoption studies, bolstered by later estimates of chip heritability in the era of high-density genotyping, supports that human obesity, indicated by body mass index (BMI), is a highly heritable trait. Heritability estimates range from 71–81% [17–19]. However, despite intensive efforts, the genes and mutations responsible for the majority of this heritability remains to be elucidated.

3. Studies of Monogenic Obesity Have Been Highly Informative

Obesity is usually a complex trait, with many genomic loci contributing incrementally to modulate an individual's susceptibility. However, monogenic forms of obesity also exist with patients usually coming to attention, because they develop severe obesity early in life. Interrogating the genetics of these rare patients, in combination with research in rodent and cellular models, has been hugely informative in elucidating the molecular basis of the regulation of energy homeostasis and body weight. Early studies of patients with monogenic forms of obesity focussed on candidate genes chosen based on information from rodent models of obesity [6].

3.1. The Discovery of Leptin

In 1950, a rodent model demonstrating severe obesity was identified, and the gene responsible named the obesity (*ob*) gene [20]. A similar obesity phenotype due to a different gene was discovered in diabetic mice, named the diabetes (*db*) gene [21,22]. Subsequent parabiosis experiments in which mice of contrasting genotype were surgically joined to share a circulation led to the conclusion that *ob/ob* mice lacked a circulating factor that controls eating behaviour, whereas *db/db* mice possessed such a factor but were not able to respond to it [23,24]. In 1994, the circulating factor was pinpointed and its function delineated; a hormone called leptin, which is secreted from fat cells [25]. The *ob* and *db* genes were subsequently identified as the genes for leptin (*Lep*) and its receptor (*Lepr*), respectively.

Shortly afterwards, a frameshift mutation in the human leptin gene (*LEP*) [26] was identified in children with severe, early-onset obesity. The mutation caused congenital leptin deficiency that was successfully treated with recombinant leptin therapy (See Figure 1). Since this, many more severely obese individuals have been identified with mutations in *LEP* [27–29] and provided help with recombinant leptin. Such studies clearly justify the importance of genetic research and its translational significance for prevention and treatment of disease.

Patients with mutation in the human leptin receptor gene (*LEPR*) [30–32] who display extreme obesity have also been identified. However, recombinant leptin treatment in these patients is entirely ineffective, since they suffer from leptin resistance as opposed to leptin deficiency [33–35].

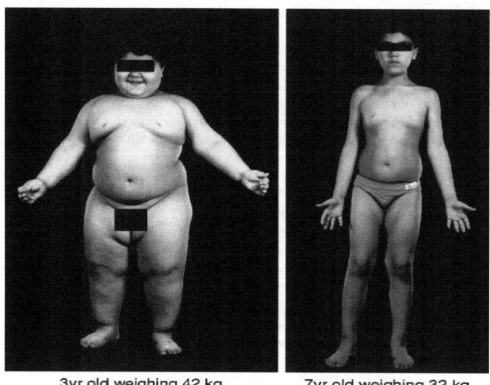

Figure 1. Effect of recombinant leptin treatment on child with congenital leptin deficiency. Photographs of a 3-year-old child before leptin treatment weighing 42 kg (**left**) and the same child weighing 32 kg (**right**) after 4 years of treatment with recombinant leptin therapy. Figure from Farooqi et al. [36].

3.2. The Leptin–Melanocortin Pathway

We now understand that the primary effector mechanism for leptin's action is in the central nervous system (CNS), where it activates the hypothalamic leptin–melanocortin pathway [37], a neuroendocrine signalling mechanism, which transmits a signal about the status of the body's energy reserves to the brain and translates it into effector signals to promote optimal energy balance. In summary (See Figure 2), the hormone leptin is produced and released from adipose tissue. In the insulin-dependent fed state, insulin stimulates leptin release, and in greater amounts when energy reserves (in the form of fat stored in adipocytes) are larger [38,39]. In the brain, leptin acts on receptors in the arcuate nucleus (ARC) of the hypothalamus to activate proopiomelanocortin (POMC) neurons to produce the pre-pro-protein proopiomelanocortin (POMC). POMC undergoes proteolytic cleavage to produce a number of neuroactive peptides, the most important of which in regulating energy homeostasis are α- and β- melanocyte stimulating hormone (α-MSH, β-MSH). MSH peptides act on melanocortin receptor 4 (MC4R) expressed on second-order neurons of the paraventricular nucleus (PVN) of the hypothalamus, resulting in reduction in food intake and modified energy metabolism by interaction with multiple other pathways [17,40].

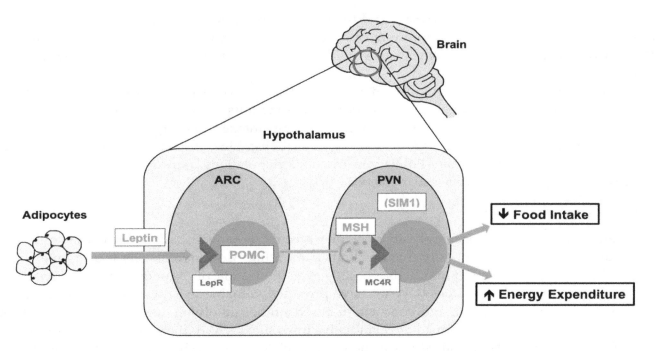

Figure 2. The leptin–melanocortin pathway. Simplified schematic of the leptin–melanocortin signalling pathway, which has a critical role in energy homeostasis by acting as a nexus through which information about energy status in the periphery can be relayed to the central nervous system (CNS) and integrated to control food intake and energy expenditure. ARC, arcuate nucleus of the hypothalamus; POMC, proopiomelanocortin; LepR, leptin receptor; PVN, paraventricular nucleus of the hypothalamus; MSH, melanocyte-stimulating hormone (α-MSH, β-MSH, γ-MSH); MC4R, melanocortin-4 receptor; SIM1, single-minded 1.

3.3. Disruption of Leptin–Melanocortin Signalling Leads to Obesity

Mutations that disrupt the leptin–melanocortin pathway are associated with severe obesity in both rodents and humans [41,42]. Dominant mutations in the proopiomelanocortin gene (*POMC*) are reported to cause severe, early-onset obesity in affected patients, often with other neuroendocrine features consistent with the diverse physiological roles of the multiple POMC-derived peptides [43–46]. Similarly, obesity has been reported due to mutations affecting prohormone convertase 1 gene (*PCSK1*), one of the enzymes responsible for proteolytic cleavage of POMC to its neuroactive derivatives, either singly or as part the more complex genetic condition Prader–Willi Syndrome [47].

Variants residing in the gene *SIM1* have also been associated with severe obesity and Prader–Willi-like syndromes [48,49], an effect attributed to this transcription factor's integral role in development of the PVN, a hypothalamic nucleus, which is most notable as the major site of MC4R expression [48].

More common are mutations in the *MC4R* gene, which have been shown to cause both dominant and recessive forms of monogenic obesity [50–53] and are responsible for up to 6% of severe, early-onset obesity cases [46,54–56]. More recently, *MC4R* variants with less severe effects on receptor function have been shown to be major modifiers of obesity risk in the wider human population [57–59]. Notably, those data show that the genetic background against which the *MC4R* mutation occurs has a large influence on the penetrance of the obesity phenotype.

3.4. Other Causes of Monogenic Obesity

Variants affecting other biological pathways have also been identified as monogenic causes of obesity, with the majority related to CNS regulation of energy metabolism. Semaphorin 3 gene (*SEMA3*) variants are rare causes of severe early-onset obesity and affect energy balance through their role in melanocortin neuron development [60]. Brain-derived neurotrophic factor (BDNF) acts on its receptor tropomyosin receptor kinase B (TRKB), and there is increasing evidence that this signalling plays a significant role in sustaining equilibrium of energy balance in the brain [61]. Mutations affecting the concordant protein-coding genes (*BDNF/TRKB*) have been reported as causes of monogenic human obesity.

It is noteworthy that all the aforementioned variants primarily modify eating behaviour. The exception to this came with the discovery that rare variants in the Kinase suppressor of Ras 2 gene (*KSR2*) appear to cause obesity by affecting both energy intake and energy expenditure (although primarily via affecting the central control of energy metabolism) [62]. Reminiscent of this, a *CREBRF* variant that is common in Samoans but very rare in other populations, appears to be a major modifier of obesity risk by altering energy use in the body [63].

4. Common Human Obesity

Although cases of monogenic obesity exist, they account for only 5–7% of severe obesity cases [17, 54,64] and much less of the obesity that develops later in life. Common obesity is a complex trait, caused by the additive effect of hundreds, possibly even thousands, of common genetic variants [65]. Genome-wide association studies (GWAS) have provided valuable insight into which loci, genes, and variants are responsible. Large, consortium-based studies involving hundreds of thousands of human subjects have been performed on quantitative traits such as BMI (the best available indicator of body fat percentage for large scale studies) and obesity-related traits such as waist-to-hip ratio (WHR, an indicator of where an individual's body fat is stored) and measures of insulin resistance (and related metabolites), leading to identification of hundreds of quantitative trait loci [66] for obesity and related traits across the genome [66–71].

Despite those successes, just 3–5% of obesity heritability is explained by existing GWAS data [72]. The "missing heritability" of obesity [72,73] is hypothesised to be due to large effect rare variants yet to be identified: many loci of small/moderate effect too common to find with GWAS; non-additive genetic effects; and copy number variants (CNVs); among others [73–76]. Of those, the large-effect rare variant is particularly relevant to those studying veterinary species—selective breeding may lead to enrichment of variants of large effect within a breed, which are otherwise rare across the species overall [77]. Notably, an expanding body of evidence implicates the microbiome in obesity pathophysiology, and obesity-associated gut microbiota populations have been shown to be heritable [78]. Thus, an individual's microbiome may also account for a fraction of the heritable component.

Nonetheless, identified obesity-associated loci can be used to generate estimates of individuals' risk of developing obesity, known as polygenic risk scores (PRS), whereby a weighted effect score is generated as the product of allele count and effect score for risk variants. PRS have been proposed as clinical tools although their application is currently limited [79,80], in part because there is evidence that their validity may be limited in ethnic groups other than that in which they were originally derived. Nonetheless, PRS have been shown to be effective measures with which to stratify genetic obesity risk across a population, as in Figure 3. They have also improved our understanding of how background polygenic risk can alter trait penetrance in the presence of mutations with moderate–large effect on the trait, such as in *MC4R* [57], mentioned above.

From GWAS to Function

Notably, a large proportion of genes implicated by human obesity GWAS are preferentially expressed in the CNS [67,81], providing further evidence for the critical role of the brain in controlling energy homeostasis. Many genes implicated in monogenic obesity have also been flagged in these large-scale obesity GWAS, including *LEPR*, *MC4R*, and *POMC*, although they are usually not the most prominent findings [67,82].

Moving from GWAS-associated locus to identify causative variants and their mechanisms of action is difficult. Some of the most common obesity-associated loci identified lack clear mechanisms by which variants exert their effects. A notorious example of this is the repeated and robust association of

BMI with genetic variants lying within an intron of FTO α-ketoglutarate-dependent dioxygenase gene (*FTO*) also known as fat-mass- and obesity-associated gene (in mice). Those findings led to extensive efforts to characterise the role of this gene and provide evidence that *FTO* plays a part in regulating food intake. However, it later transpired that the focus on the closest gene was inappropriate and that obesity association for this locus is, at least in large part, due to altered regulation of a neighbouring gene, iroquois homeobox 3 (*IRX3*), which has an impact on peripheral adipocyte metabolism [83]. Although those findings have been challenged [84,85], it remains an example of how complex it has been to move from BMI locus to novel obesity biology.

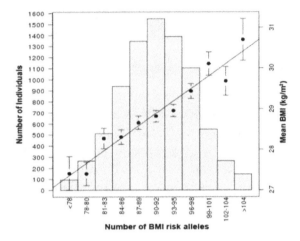

Figure 3. Histogram of cumulative effect of BMI risk alleles in a large human GWAS. Mean BMI for each bin is shown by the black dots (with standard deviation), corresponding to the right-hand y axis and is compared to simple PRS, based on unweighted risk allele counts. These data demonstrate how the cumulative effect of multiple polygenic risk alleles is strongly associated with BMI across the human population. Figure from Locke et al. [67].

5. Genetic Insight into Obesity Comorbidities and Metabolic Syndrome

Obesity exerts a huge toll on human health due to its attendant comorbidities including type 2 diabetes mellitus (T2D), cardiovascular disease (CVD), stroke, and non-alcoholic fatty liver disease (NAFLD), among others [86–88]. Development of these comorbidities is largely mediated by a constellation of clinical features commonly referred to as "metabolic syndrome" that include raised blood pressure, dyslipidaemia, increased triglycerides, and insulin resistance [89,90].

However, it is recognised that the severity of obesity does not necessarily correlate with the onset or severity of metabolic syndrome, and that some people remain metabolically healthy despite severe obesity [91–93]. Those differences occur not just between individuals but also between ethnic groups, leading to different recommended cut-offs for what is regarded as a "healthy" BMI in different populations. For example, a WHO expert consultation considered alternative BMI "cut-offs" in Asian populations given their high risk of T2D and CVD at BMIs considerably lower than previously recommended [94].

How obesity leads to its comorbidities has been intensively studied in humans and model organisms, informed by genetics. For instance, the relationship between obesity and T2D is reinforced by the presence of vertical pleiotropy with shared loci implicated in GWAS for both T2D and BMI. The causal relationship between obesity and its complications has been confirmed by Mendelian randomisation studies [95]. Similar suggestions and confirmation of cause and effect come from GWAS and Mendelian randomisation studies of BMI/insulin resistance and NAFLD [96].

More nuanced mechanistic insight has come from the study of rare patients with severe, early-onset, monogenic forms of insulin resistance. Studies of rare patients with mutations affecting the insulin receptor (INSR) or which interrupt signalling downstream of it have provided insight into the pathogenesis of insulin resistance and consequent dyslipidaemia or hepatic lipid accumulation in common obesity [93]. For instance, common variants in the gene encoding insulin receptor substrate 1 (*IRS1*), an important component of the intracellular signalling pathway, are associated with T2D, most likely by making affected individuals more susceptible to developing obesity-associated insulin resistance [97].

Similar value came from the study of patients with lipodystrophy, a rare condition in which there is complete or partial absence of adipose tissue. Recognition that the absence of fat was associated with early and severe insulin resistance and features of metabolic syndrome was central to establishing that the ability to store fat is critical to maintenance of normal metabolic function [98]. Those conclusions were later supported by analysis of genetic determinants of insulin resistance in the wider population, which provided evidence that variation in susceptibility to obesity co-morbidities are in part due to variation in individuals' ability to develop and maintain healthy fat storage depots [70].

Overview—Molecular Mechanisms Underlying Obesity Co-Morbidities

Together, human genetic studies and those in cell and animal models mean we now understand much more about how obesity causes disease. Much of those data support the theory of "limited adipose expandability". In brief summary, it appears that the body can accumulate fat in a healthy manner only until it reaches the limit of adipose tissue's ability to expand. Subsequently, adipose tissue dysfunction leads to inflammation and increased lipid flux, which in turn leads to ectopic lipid accumulation in non-adipose organs such as the liver and muscles. Combined with local and systemic inflammation, this leads to widespread insulin resistance, which in turn, results in increased insulin demand as the body attempts to maintain glucose homeostasis. Initially, insulin-producing β cells in the pancreas meet this demand but ongoing insulin resistance and ectopic lipid deposition in the pancreas itself can ultimately lead to β cell failure, hyperglycaemia, and T2D. Simultaneously, the altered lipid flux leads to dyslipidaemia and multiple mechanisms converge to cause hypertension [99,100].

Whether an individual develops obesity-associated co-morbidities may therefore be influenced by genes at many levels: a genetic predisposition to weight gain increases the chance of obesity developing; the ability to develop and maintain healthy fat stores appears to differ between individuals and across ethnic groups; if variants that perturb insulin signalling are present, they may promote the development of insulin resistance; and genes may also influence the ability of β cells to respond with adequate insulin where resistance develops. Consequently, in common disease, it is the net effect of many variants affecting such systems, combined with environmental influences, which determines whether obesity-related comorbidities develop.

6. Applying Current Knowledge to Study Companion Animal Disease

It is well established that obesity and its sequelae are heritable traits in humans and laboratory animals. The majority of obesity genes affect central regulation of food intake but notable examples whereby genes affect energy expenditure do exist. Genetic variance in susceptibility to obesity co-morbidities is well established and can be due to effects on a variety of body systems and processes.

Importantly, this wealth of information is available to inform investigations into companion animal disease. However, there is much yet to learn, and it is equally true that study of spontaneously occurring, companion animal models of obesity is a potentially valuable way to learn new biology relevant to all species. To date, studies of the molecular basis of obesity and associated disease remain limited in companion animals, with the predominance of small-scale and candidate genes studies somewhat limiting their value.

Available evidence suggests much commonality in the pathophysiology of obesity between humans, dogs, cats, and horses, but there are important differences in the incidence and severity of obesity-related co-morbidities between companion animal species, which likely reflect fundamental differences in physiology. Below, we consider in sequence the studies performed in dogs, cats, and horses to investigate the genetic basis of weight gain and, where relevant, obesity-related disease.

7. Canine Obesity Genetics

An estimated 34–59% of pet dogs in developed countries are overweight or obese [3,9,101–104]. Multiple comorbidities are associated with canine obesity, most notably: orthopaedic disease, exacerbation of breathing difficulties, and urinary incontinence, along with significantly decreased life expectancy [105–108]. Canine obesity is associated with increased blood pressure, dyslipidaemia, and insulin resistance, and this has been characterised as "obesity-related metabolic dysfunction" [109,110]. There is also some epidemiological evidence that obesity is a risk factor for developing canine, but this is not a recognised problem in clinical practice diabetes [111]. Other human obesity-related complications such as CVD and NAFLD do not have equivalent recognised presentations in canine practice. As with humans, studies suggest that weight loss leads to normalisation of many of the associated metabolic perturbations in dogs [109].

Evidence for the role of genetics in governing canine obesity susceptibility comes from the fact that obesity prevalence differs dependent on breed, with some breeds predisposed (e.g., Labrador retrievers, pugs, golden retrievers) and others resistant (e.g., greyhounds, whippets) [10,112,113]. Concordantly, differences in eating behaviour and food preference between breeds have been shown [114,115].

Although some of the variation in obesity susceptibility between breeds could be down to differences in "fashion" for each breed, the repeated finding of breed as a risk factor for obesity means genetic determinants are more likely the cause. Such variation in trait susceptibility between breeds is common in dogs due to the species' unusual population architecture in which there is high diversity as a whole combined with high homogeneity within breeds, the product of population bottlenecks at breed formation and subsequent intensive selection for breed-specific traits [116–118]. Heritability of canine obesity is yet to be determined, but some have speculated that it will be reminiscent of high estimates in humans and other animal species [119–122].

The genetic basis of body mass has been investigated using GWAS in dogs, but those results cannot be regarded as indicative of obesity because of the wide variability in body morphology breeds. Instead, those study results likely better reflect the combination of height, length, musculature, and limb: trunk ratio [123].

To date, no GWAS of canine fat mass or related traits have been reported. In part, this may be related to the difficulty of accurately phenotyping obesity in dogs; the aforementioned wide variety of skeletal size and shape in dogs precludes using simple and commonly available measures such as weight to estimate fat mass. Quantification of adiposity can be done using sophisticated imaging or biochemical techniques, electrical impedance or ultrasound measurement of fat deposits, but those cannot practically be applied in large cohorts [124]. The clinically widely used and well-validated alternative is to assign dogs a "body condition score" (BCS). This should be performed by a veterinary professional who uses a variety of haptic and visual clues to assign dogs to one of a series of ordinal scores. The most widely used 9-point scale [125] has been thoroughly validated [124,126] such that each one point increase in BCS above "normal" equates to approximately 10% increase in fat mass. A 5-point scale is also available and has been reported in some of the studies below.

7.1. Genes Investigated in Canine Obesity

Several candidate gene studies have been performed in domestic dogs and closely related, farmed *Canidae* species. The merit of looking at genetic factors in other *Canidae* species is arguable, but they are reported here, since previous studies have found them relevant. The best characterised of the later mentioned studies are the ones that have considered genes implicated in the leptin–melanocortin signalling pathway. All gene variants discussed can be found in Supplementary Table S1.

7.1.1. POMC

As discussed above, POMC has an integral role in leptin–melanocortin signalling, a neuroendocrine pathway highly conserved across species. Raffan et al. [7] identified various canine *POMC* variants including a 14 bp deletion at position 17:19431807-19431821, present in Labrador retrievers and flat-coated retrievers (FCRs) but absent from a wide variety of other breeds tested. The deletion was shown to be a major modifier of weight, adiposity (measured as BCS on a 9-point scale), and appetite (measured using a validated, owner-reported measure of eating behaviour [114]) in ≥210 Labrador retrievers, with findings for weight and appetite replicated in ≥196 FCRs. Appropriate confounders were accounted for by adjustment for age, sex, neuter status, and colour, thus association results can be confirmed with high confidence. Notably, the mutation was more common in Labrador retrievers working as assistance dogs compared to the pet population. For each additional allele carried by either breed, there was an approximately 0.5 BCS/2 kg increase in adiposity/body mass, and a similar incremental increase in food motivation.

The authors showed the *POMC* deletion results in altered production of β-MSH and β-endorphin, two neuroactive peptides derived from *POMC*, and confirmed that canine MC4R receptors have similar affinity for and response to α-MSH and β-MSH as the equivalent human pairings. Whilst the reduced action of β-MSH on MC4R in the leptin–melanocortin signalling pathway is the most likely mechanism resulting in this phenotype, β-endorphin may also be implicated.

Subsequent studies have confirmed the presence of this mutation [120,127,128]. In the British Labrador retriever population, Davison et al. [127] found there was no association for the deletion with occurrence of diabetes mellitus (DM) in the breed (a finding that is not surprising given that obesity-associated insulin resistance is not clinically recognised as predisposing dogs to diabetes, despite there being some epidemiological evidence that it may play a role population-wide).

The data had relevance to those studying human obesity biology, because canine *POMC* is highly homologous to human *POMC*. The same cannot be said for rodents that lack a proteolytic cleavage site in the pro-protein and so do not produce β-MSH. Since humans with mutations causing β-MSH absence are very rare [129,130], the canine model in this case provided important insight into the role of this particular peptide in energy homeostasis, as well as establishing a clear role for genetics in governing obesity susceptibility in dogs.

7.1.2. MC4R

Canine *MC4R* gene polymorphisms have been identified in several studies, with some attempting to analyse their effects on obesity-related phenotypes. *MC4R* is a suitable candidate gene due to MC4R's central position in the leptin–melanocortin pathway and given *MC4R* variants are among the most common cause of monogenic human obesity. Humans with *MC4R* mutations are also modestly taller than unaffected individuals of the same age and sex, or similarly obese unrelated subjects without *MC4R* mutations [53,131]. The majority of the identified variants lack functional data for characterisation of their consequences, but Yan et al. [132] reported that the missense variant c.637G>T (p.Val213Phe, rs852614811) had no significant effect on cAMP-mediated signalling downstream of the receptor.

Skorczyk et al. [133] conducted a study on canid *MC4R*, mapping and characterising it for the first time. The study cohort incorporated 31 dogs of 19 breeds and 35 farmed red foxes (*Vulpes vulpes*). They identified three polymorphic sites in the canine *MC4R* gene and four in the red fox. The three canine *MC4R* polymorphisms identified were a non-synonymous variant (c.637G>T, p.Val213Phe, rs852614811); a synonymous coding variant (c.777T>C, p.Ala259Ala, rs851987283); and a 3'UTR variant (c.*33C>G, rs851539399). No association testing was conducted.

Van den Berg et al. [134] studied *MC4R* in 32 golden retrievers. They identified the same polymorphic sites as Skorczyk et al. [133] (c.637G>T, p.Val213Phe, rs852614811; c.777T>C, p.Ala259Ala, rs851987283; c.*33C>G, rs851539399), plus an additional synonymous coding variant (c.868C>T, p.Leu290Leu, rs851062983). After linkage disequilibrium (LD) filtering, they performed an association study for the three remaining polymorphisms (c.637G>T, c.777T>C, c.868C>T) in a larger cohort of golden retrievers ($n = 187$). Several morphological measures were tested: weight, length, height, and body index score (BIS), but not BCS. For the association, they appropriately corrected for sex, age, and polygenic effects. However, they do not mention any account for neuter status (a well-recognised risk factor), and there was no measure of relatedness in the sample. No statistically significant association was found for any of the phenotypes. Whilst this may be genuine, the study was underpowered to find a small effect size, and these variants may warrant further investigation.

Zeng et al. [135] conducted an *MC4R* candidate gene study in beagles from a research colony. By sequencing two beagle dogs, they identified the previously reported synonymous coding mutation (c.777T>C, p.Ala259Ala, rs851987283) and a novel missense substitution (c.302C>A, p.Thr101Asn). (Note that the way this mutation is referred to in the original paper and a subsequent review article is somewhat confused. Zeng et al. [135] mis-name the mutations as C895T (for c.777T>C) and A420C (for c.302C>A). The missense mutation (c.302C>A) results in an amino acid substitution from threonine to asparagine (p.Thr101Asn = T101N), which can be clarified by figures within the paper. However, they misname this as N101T. Mankowska et al. [136], in a subsequent review, note the mistake but further misname it c.301A>C (p.Asn101Thr). The authors' (unpublished) capillary sequencing data means we can confirm the correct annotation as c.302C>A, p.Asn101Thr. Variant nomenclature corrections can be found in Supplementary Table S1). In 120 beagles, c.302C>A was significantly associated with body weight ($p < 0.05$). In contrast, c.777T>C was only significantly associated with body weight in the heterozygous (but not homozygous) state and in bitches only. Whilst it is plausible at least one of the single nucleotide polymorphisms (SNP) are associated with adiposity, there are important limitations to the study. Specifically, weight does not equate to adiposity but could indicate changes in height, length, or muscle mass. There was no adjustment for confounding factors such as age, sex, or neuter status, and no assessment of whether the variants were in LD and therefore whether these associations constitute independent signals.

Raffan et al. [7] sequenced the *MC4R* region in 33 Labrador retrievers of which 15 were obese and 18 were lean. Two novel *MC4R* variants were identified (c.989G>T, p.Ser330Ile; c.*227C>T) plus three previously reported variants (c.637G>T, p.Val213Phe, rs852614811; c.*33C>G, rs851539399; c.777T>C, p.Ala259Ala, rs851987283). None were distributed differently between the small lean and obese groups, and the variants were not pursued further. This group also sequenced *AGRP* in this cohort, another valid candidate gene which codes for agouti-related protein—a neuropeptide known to modulate food intake in the ARC [137]. No *AGRP* variants were identified.

Mankowska et al. [136] investigated *MC4R* variants in 270 dogs of four breeds in which they identified six known polymorphic sites (c.637G>T, p.Val213Phe, rs852614811; c.777T>C, p.Ala259Ala, rs851987283; c.868C>T, p.Leu290Leu, rs851062983; c.*33C>G, rs851539399; c.*227C>T; and c.-435T>C, rs852471376). Of the 270 dogs, they had full phenotypic data for 164. They concluded that none of the identified variants displayed differential association with BCS (5-point scale) or body weight. The study population was dominated by Labrador retrievers ($n = 187$) and no potential confounding factors were accounted for.

7.1.3. FTO

The top association signal on most human GWAS for BMI, *FTO*, is of debatable merit as a candidate gene for canine obesity, due to the controversy as to whether *FTO* itself or neighbouring genes are the true effector pathway causing the association signal (see above). Grzes et al. [138] investigated *FTO* SNPs in four *Canidae* species including the dog. In 39 dogs of 14 breeds, sequencing identified six polymorphic sites in *FTO*: one missense variant (c.23C>T, p.Thr8Met, rs852870212 described as "23 C/T, Thr1Met"), two intronic variants, and three 3′ flanking variants. Presence of the missense mutation differed by dog breed, but the small number of dogs genotyped meant association tests were (appropriately) not performed. However, of seven *FTO* polymorphisms in the red fox, one (a 5′ flanking region variant) was tested for association with body weight and pelt weight (which the authors report is affected by subcutaneous fat mass) in a larger cohort of 390 red foxes. No significant association was identified.

Grzemski et al. [139] used targeted next generation sequencing (NGS) in 32 Labrador retrievers in a region incorporating *FTO* and *IRX3*. Several polymorphisms were identified and tested for association with BCS (5-point scale) in a larger Labrador retriever cohort (*n* = 165), suitably adjusted for sex, age, and multiple testing. No association was found. The authors reported 56% nucleotide identity between human and canine *FTO* and 72% for *IRX3*. Additionally, they compared methylation status of CpG islands between lean and obese dogs in a smaller cohort (*n* = 28)—no differences were found.

7.1.4. MC3R

Skorczyk et al. [140] conducted a candidate gene study on the gene encoding melanocortin receptor 3 (*MC3R*). The *MC3R* gene is a reasonable candidate, although it is notable that rodent and human phenotypes associated with *MC3R* variants are more subtle than for the related *MC4R*, with *MC3R* most likely affecting the maintenance of body mass within the homeostatically controlled upper and lower limits [141–144].

The study cohort used by Skorczyk et al. [140] consists of four canid species: 31 dogs of 19 breeds, 35 red foxes, 30 arctic foxes (*Vulpes lagopus/Aloplex lagopus*), and 30 Chinese raccoon dogs (*Nyctereutes procyonoides procyonoides*). Multiple polymorphisms were found in *MC3R* in three of the species; no variants were identified in *MC3R* of the arctic fox. Two polymorphic sites were identified in the dog: short tandem repeat (STR) in 5′ flanking region (c.-90delT, rs853092001) and a synonymous substitution (c.142C>T, p.Leu48Leu, rs8916554). Association analysis for *MC3R* variants was then performed in cohort of 376 male red foxes. Two SNPs were in LD and both were associated with a small, statistically significant increase in body mass. There was limited information provided on potential environmental confounders and population stratification, with no apparent adjustment. It therefore cannot be ruled out that any associations observed may be as a result of these factors.

7.1.5. INSIG2

Insulin-induced gene 2 protein (INSIG2) has a role in lipid metabolism and has been linked in human GWAS studies to various measures of circulating blood lipids. Its coding gene (*INSIG2*) has been implicated in human GWAS for BMI [145], but that association has not been reliably replicable [146], so its validity as a candidate obesity gene is somewhat limited. Grzes et al. [138] analysed polymorphic sites in *INSIG2* in four *Canidae* species including the dog. In 32 dogs of 14 breeds, seven polymorphic sites were identified: two 5′ UTR variants referred to as 5′ flanking region variants, (c.-90G>A (referred to as–91 G/A), rs852813691; c.-1C>T, rs852335828), one missense variant (c.40C>A, p.Arg14Ser, rs850773724), and four intronic variants. No association test was conducted in dogs, but one intronic SNP identified in the red fox was significantly associated with pelt weight in 390 red foxes. Skin weight may be influenced by subcutaneous fat mass, but this is not a valid measure of adiposity and such findings in the red fox may not be translatable to dogs.

7.1.6. GPR120/FFAR4

G-protein coupled receptor 120 (GPR120), also known as free fatty acid receptor 4 (FFA4/FFAR4), functions as a receptor for unsaturated long-chain free fatty acids. The gene encoding this protein is known as *GPR120/FFA4/FFAR4* [147,148], and coding mutations in the gene have been associated with human obesity [149]. The following variants are described based on alignment to the canine *FFAR4* gene. Miyabe et al. [150] found nine *FFAR4* polymorphisms in a cohort of 141 dogs of 21 breeds: five synonymous substitutions (c.252C>G, p.Ala84Ala, rs852631320; c.282C>G, p.Pro94Pro (referred to as p.Asp94Asp), rs851850900; c.702A>G, p.Thr234Thr; c.726G>A, p.Thr242Thr; c.984T>C, p.Asn328Asn, rs852472019) and four non-synonymous substitutions (c.287T>G, p.Leu96Arg; c.307G>A, p.Ala103Thr; c.446G>C, p.Gly149Ala; c.595A>C, p.Thr199Pro, rs853030954 (referred to as c.595C>A, p.Thr199Pro)). SNPs were tested for association with BCS, the frequency of c.595A>C (referred to as c.595C>A) was significantly higher in dogs with a higher BCS. However, several confounding factors are unaccounted for and the study failed to correct for population stratification. Therefore, such identified associations may have been due to confounders or, given the unequally represented multi breed cohort, due to unaccounted-for population stratification.

7.1.7. PPARs

Peroxisome proliferator-activated receptors (PPARs) are a group of nuclear receptor proteins that function as transcription factors and have roles in the regulation of cellular differentiation, development, and metabolism [151,152]. Nishii et al. [153] sequenced the genes encoding PPARβ and PPARγ (*PPARB* and *PPARG*) in two dogs and observed tissue-specific expression of various PPARs. They also investigated the presence of polymorphic sites in *PPARG* and identified a single polymorphism. No association test with phenotype was conducted. Since a relatively small canine cohort were genotyped, it is possible that other *PPARB* polymorphisms were missed.

7.1.8. Adipokines

Adipose tissue communicates with the rest of the body in part by release of a range of molecular signals known as adipokines. Adipokines include leptin, pro-inflammatory molecules such as TNFα and IL6, and the much-debated resistin, the latter three of which were investigated in dogs by Mankowska et al. [154]. The choice of these genes is a little surprising in that, although there is evidence that each has a role in the development of insulin resistance secondary to obesity, there is little evidence that variants promoting inflammation are causal in obesity [155] and considerable evidence to the contrary (https://www.ebi.ac.uk/gwas/) [156]. Nevertheless, in 77 dogs of 17 breeds, Mankowska et al. identified multiple variants, including 13 in *TNF*, four in *IL6*, and eight in *RETN*. Three of these variants were missense substitutions: one in *TNF* (c.548A>T, p.Glu183Val) and two in *RETN* (c.19C>T, p.Leu7Phe, rs852470997; c.236C>G, p.Ser79Cys, rs851766760—referred to in the paper as a synonymous coding variant). The five most common variants (*TNF*: c.-40A>C, rs22216187; c.233+14G>A; *IL6*: c.309+215T>C; *RETN*: c.194-69T>A, rs853182485; c.75G>A, p.Glu25Glu, rs852185407) were genotyped in 260 dogs and tested for association with BCS, using breed-specific sub-groups to do the association analysis, including an "others" category for the poorly represented breeds. No association was found for the *IL6* and *RETN* variants with BCS in any breed group. The two *TNF* SNPs (c.-40A>C and c.233+14G>A) were significantly associated with body condition in Labrador retrievers but not in any other breed group. Whilst those associations may be meaningful, the failure to include recognised risk factors such as age, sex, and neuter status or to detect or correct for population stratification in the sample could have affected these results.

8. Feline Obesity and Associated Disease

Estimates suggest 12–63% of pet cats are overweight or obese [2,157–162]. Feline obesity is associated with multiple comorbidities, most notably DM and hepatic lipidosis [12,158,163–167]. This arguably makes human and feline obesity comorbidities closer compared to dogs [168,169]. However, human comorbidities such as hypertension and atherosclerosis are not commonly observed in obese cats [107,170,171].

Obesity's relationship to DM in cats is well characterised with evidence suggesting a similar pathophysiology to human T2D [107,171–173] in which obesity leads to insulin resistance and ultimately β-cell dysfunction and diabetes [166,173–177]. Cats are therefore considered a suitable animal model for study of obesity associated T2D, with translational significance to humans. In contrast, whilst obesity is a well-recognised risk factor for feline hepatic lipidosis, the pathophysiological link between the two is less well characterised and subject to some debate [176,178,179].

8.1. Evidence for the Role of Genetics in Feline Obesity and Related Disease

Multiple studies suggest breed as a risk factor of feline obesity, with certain breeds displaying predisposition to becoming overweight/obese [12,180–182]. Although breed-specific obesity risk differs by study, domestic shorthaired cats (DSH) are consistently found to be at high risk, whilst longhaired breeds are generally at lower risk. Persian cats also have low obesity risk in most studies [12,181,182], but one study found them to be at high risk [180]. Together, these data suggest obesity may be at least in part a heritable trait in cats.

Notably, pet cats are made up of a majority of mixed breed cats (commonly referred to as DSH and domestic long-haired (DLH) breeds but are most commonly outbred and relatively genetically diverse) and a minority of pedigree cats, in which genetic architecture is reminiscent of dogs, with low within-breed diversity and evidence of population bottlenecks and genetic selection [183,184].

Until recently, genetic studies in cats have been stymied by the absence of a well-annotated, complete feline genome and lack of a commercial feline SNP genotyping array. Consequently, there are fewer genetic studies reported in cats overall, and none of the common forms of feline obesity. However, one group has reported candidate gene studies for feline DM [185], a related trait and one that is likely to be subject to similar genetic influences (including overlap with obesity predisposition) as described above for humans.

8.2. Familial Obesity in a Feline Colony

In a population of well-characterised, related research cats, a familial form of obesity has been reported [186]. Some cats displayed a clear predisposition to obesity, and segregation analysis suggested a single major gene was likely responsible. The report is more akin to human monogenic obesity or mutations of large effect against a variably obesogenic polygenic background.

A subsequent study found that the cats predisposed to being obese had a lower energy requirement and higher food intake than cats that did not tend to gain weight [187]. However, the energy requirement measurements were (for the obesity-prone group) performed not long after a period of restricted feeding and weight loss, interventions well recognised to cause reduced energy expenditure irrespective of baseline status [188]. In a subsequent generation of the same cohort, food intake and energy expenditure were investigated [189], and obesity-prone cats had higher food intake early in life but not lower energy expenditure.

In the same feline cohort, Keller et al. [190] investigated metabolic responses to different diets in cats predisposed to obesity vs. lean cats. No difference in metabolic response was found between the two groups. Additionally, in conference proceedings [191] the same group report attempts to map obesity genes were made and identified plausible candidate genes. Further comment is not possible given the scant information reported.

8.3. Genetics of Diabetes Mellitus in Pet Cats

Forcada et al. [185] investigated whether *MC4R* polymorphisms were associated with diabetes in DSH and Burmese cats. For each of a non-diabetic control group and a diabetic case group, there were 60 lean and 60 overweight cats, making 240 in total. The authors report that one *MC4R* polymorphism (c.92 C>T, p.Leu31Pro, rs783632116) was significantly more common in obese diabetic cats than obese non-diabetic cats, a finding not replicated in lean cats. Heterozygous and homozygous carriers in the non-diabetic subgroup were merged (assuming a dominant mode of inheritance). The authors do not report comparison of allele frequencies between lean and overweight cats (irrespective of DM status).

The authors speculate that this variant may act independently of an effect on body weight, but these reviewers suggest that to be a bold statement given the limitations of the data presented and the weight of evidence from other species about the role of MC4R in controlling food intake and obesity predisposition. For example, although *MC4R* is significantly associated with T2D in human GWAS, that association disappears when the analysis model corrects for BMI [192,193]. Consequently, it seems equally or more plausible that the association reported may in fact be a result of vertical pleiotropy rather than a direct effect.

The same group in conference abstracts report the results of a GWAS for feline DM in a cohort of 581 DSH cats [194,195], later adding Burmese cats [196]. However, the data are not reported in sufficient detail to reiterate here.

9. Obesity and Related Metabolic Disease in Horses

As in other companion animal species, equine obesity is common with an estimated 20–70% of horses overweight/obese [11,197–200]. This is a significant clinical problem, because obesity is a risk factor for the development of laminitis, a common, crippling disorder of the equine hoof. That association is thought to be mediated predominantly via a collection of risk factors known as equine metabolic syndrome (EMS). EMS was first described in 2002 [201], and the pathophysiological links between obesity and laminitis have been extensively studied since, although it is acknowledged that the current working understanding requires refinement [202].

EMS is defined by the presence of insulin dysregulation, characterised by clinical features including hyperinsulinaemia (either at baseline or in response to glucose challenge), hyperglycaemia, and/or evidence of peripheral insulin resistance [202]. Insulin resistance is commonly present in EMS, although there has been some debate as to whether that is always true and if alternative routes by which insulin dysregulation may develop exist [203]. Notably, although obesity and EMS are common, it is rare for horses and ponies to become diabetic [202].

Not all overweight equines develop EMS, nor does EMS always cause laminitis. Similarly, not all horses that have clinical features of EMS are overweight. Those paradoxes exist between individuals and across breeds, with some breeds apparently particularly prone to developing laminitis despite only moderate weight gain [198]. This is reminiscent of the situation described above in humans, whereby there is variability between individuals and ethnic groups concerning whether, and at what point, obesity-associated complications occur. It is clear, therefore, that a better understanding of equine obesity and its related conditions is required.

9.1. Genetics Influence Equine Obesity, EMS, and Laminitis

Evidence that genetics influence the development of equine obesity come from recognition that breed and "type" are clear risk factors with ponies at highest risk, followed by cob type breeds [11,204–208]. In Pura Raza Español horses, the heritability of BCS was found to be 14–24% [209]. Importantly, a within-breed study can only estimate the variance due to genetic variation within that (homogeneous) breed, so this heritability figure should not be generalised to the species as a whole. To date, there are no reports of GWAS or candidate gene studies in equine obesity.

The genetics of EMS have been more intensively interrogated. Breed is a well-recognised risk factor and breeds largely overlap with breeds at high obesity risk, unsurprising given the association between the conditions [202]. A similar variability between breeds has been demonstrated for insulin sensitivity and related biochemical parameters [210–213]. A recent study used genome-wide SNP data to estimate heritability of several traits known to be perturbed by EMS (glucose, insulin, measures of insulin sensitivity, and dyslipidaemia) and found they were moderately to highly heritable [214]. Again, such within-breed comparisons are valuable but are likely to underestimate the true heritability in the equine population.

Genetic studies of laminitis are worthy of report, given the common co-segregation of obesity, EMS, and laminitis. In an early study of crossbreed ponies, the authors concluded laminitis was a dominant trait in the pedigree with variable penetrance due to sex, age, and epigenetic-related variables [215]. Subsequent GWAS are mentioned below.

9.2. GWAS for EMS and Related Traits

Lewis et al. [216] performed a GWAS for laminitis and related traits in a population of 64 Arabian horses. A locus on chromosome 14 was associated with laminitis and insulin concentration. In a second cohort of 50 horses of the same breed, the identical phenotypes were not available, but the same region was associated with BCS and an alternative measure of insulin resistance. The closest gene was the poorly characterised *FAM174A*, which the authors sequenced. They found two closely linked variants, present in multiple breeds. The authors suggested an 11-guanine polymorphism near *FAM174A* might have potential as a predictive test for horses at risk of obesity/EMS/laminitis. Subsequently, an Australian group found no association with metabolic traits for that marker in 20 (non-Arabian) ponies [217]. Similarly, a larger study in multiple breeds, including Arabians, failed to replicate the BCS, laminitis, or insulin resistance associations, although assuming a dominant model did identify a significant association with the adipokine adiponectin [218].

Selective breeding can lead to enrichment of alleles within a breed, which are scarce in the wider population, meaning it is plausible that a genetic variant may exist in Arabians at this locus, genetically linked to the 11-guanine allele but which has yet to be identified. Thus, a real finding in Arabians might not be replicated in other breeds. However, replication in a larger, independent cohort of Arabians would be advisable. There is no evidence that this allele would be a suitable genetic test for obesity, EMS, or laminitis predisposition in other breeds.

Norton et al. [219] recently performed a GWAS focussed on EMS in a larger equine cohort (n = 550) representing two high-risk breeds (Welsh ponies and Morgan horses). By collecting rich metabolic data, they were able to test for association with multiple "endophenotypes", more precise biochemical markers of insulin-related traits. Using endophenotypes may be more informative than performing a GWAS for a "convergent" phenotype such as laminitis, which can represent the clinical endpoint of multiple pathophysiological processes. The group appropriately adjusted for relevant confounding factors and for population stratification although not for BCS, meaning the results may identify loci associated with obesity rather than EMS per se. Hundreds of loci were identified across the multiple genome scans and the authors prioritised those which appeared to affect more than one breed.

The authors expressed surprise that there was not more overlap between breeds. That may be because major genetic determinants may be private to individual breeds, but it is perhaps more likely that the study was underpowered to find variants of small effect, or which were rare or invariate in one population. Protein coding genes in prioritised regions were enriched for involvement in pathways of inflammation, glucose metabolism, and lipid metabolism, all plausible as contributing to EMS pathology.

A final equine study considered the gene *HMGA2*, which had previously been identified as associated with short stature in pony breeds. In humans, short stature is a risk factor for insulin resistance. Concordantly, a study found pony breeds (which are smaller than horses) are more likely to get EMS [220]. The authors hypothesised a causal link between *HMGA2* and increased EMS susceptibility in ponies. They found a strong association with height in 264 Welsh ponies and a lesser association with several metabolic traits, which they reported as a pleiotropic effect.

10. From Humans to Animals and Back Again

10.1. Lessons for Animal Genetics

This review has summarised the wealth of research into the genetics of human obesity and its related metabolic perturbations, and the relative paucity of efforts to date in dogs, cats, and horses. Consequently, those studying veterinary species have much to learn from human geneticists and those studying laboratory animal models. By familiarising ourselves with those fields, there is much scope to fast-track animal studies to provide maximum insight into animal disease.

In particular, we note how careful delineation of clinical phenotypes has led to both genetic diagnoses and mechanistic insight in human patients, such as with familial partial lipodystrophy. Historically, such lean patients presenting with metabolic syndrome or T2D were considered inexplicable outliers. By recognising groups with shared clinical features, lipodystrophy has been recognised, patient care has improved, and we have a matured understanding of how healthy fat depots are essential to metabolic health [98]. Might similar clinical groupings exist, unrecognised, as underlying atypical presentations of EMS or determining why only some overweight cats become diabetic?

Human genetic epidemiological studies have, for some time, attempted to address the issue of cause and consequence between obesity and related pathologies. Performing GWAS not only for endpoints such as T2D or NAFLD, but also for those phenotypes corrected for BMI was a start in teasing out causal relationships between them, a process that has been improved with the advent of Mendelian randomisation [95]. Such approaches operate best at scale, which may limit their application in veterinary studies. Even so, an acute awareness that multiple routes can converge on a single phenotype (e.g., obesity, adipose dysfunction, and insulin signalling impairment converge to produce signs of metabolic syndrome) should inform our design and interpretation of veterinary GWAS.

Finally, human genetics also provides a lead in how to maximise the benefit of genetic studies. One notable contrast is that results of human genetic studies are rarely left "hanging"—mapped loci are further investigated, mouse models made to test the function of unknown genes, patients with specific genetic diagnoses are further studied, and precision treatments developed. This reflects a more established, larger, and better-funded research environment but provides a model for veterinary researchers to emulate.

Genetic findings have informed best practice to flag patients with uncommon presentations of common disease who may benefit from precision treatments [98,221]. In common, polygenic human disease, PRS are being used to counsel human patients about disease risk [80] and to stratify patients in research studies to understand better variable penetrance of variants of large effect [57]. In companion animals, there is a genetic test available for the retriever *POMC* mutation that can warn owners they have a dog at high risk of obesity and prompt them to effectively institute appropriate preventative measures [7], but other genetic findings in the field of obesity have yet to reach the veterinary clinic. Might we in future years detect cats with insulin signalling defects as candidates for insulin sensitising drugs in the pre-diabetic stage? Or might genetic profiling identify ponies at highest risk of laminitis? If so, genetic testing might prove a valuable clinical tool although one to be used only after robust validation of their utility in populations (e.g., breeds) different to that in which they were initially proposed.

10.2. Lessons from Animal Genetics

Fortunately, the flow of information between species need not be along a one-way street. Genetic studies of animal disease have already been informative to human research [7,222,223], and there is much potential to discover more. As genomic tools and better-annotated genomes become available, veterinary studies will be better able to provide insight into not just disease-associated loci but particular genes, mutations, and mechanisms too. That will clearly be a benefit to the species studied but also has the potential to benefit human health.

The current quality of genome builds and genomic tools available for companion animal studies vary by species. In dogs, the third-generation genome build (CanFam 3.1) has been available since 2014 [224], based on data from a Boxer dog, Tasha. Sequencing efforts integrating data from long read technologies produced genome sequences from a Great Dane (UMICH_Zoey_3.1, GCA_005444595.1, PacBio RSII) [225] and a basenji, (Basenji_breed-1.1, GCA_004886185.2, Sequel), meaning there are now three potential reference sequences available in the species. Canine geneticists were also the first to drive production of commercial companion animal genotyping arrays, with the earliest containing 49k SNP markers [226], later increasing to 173k, 220k (CanineHD BeadChip, Illumina, San Diego, CA, USA), and 710k densities (CanineHD Array, Thermofisher, Waltham, MA, USA). Today, there are available arrays that cover >1 million genetic markers (Canine Genotyping Array, Thermofisher, Waltham, MA, USA), a subset of which were selected for use on the 460k/670k arrays (Canine Genotyping Array A/B, Thermofisher, Waltham, MA, USA). Additionally, high quality imputation from a lower to higher density SNP array level and to genome sequencing density has been successful in dogs [227,228].

In cats, the newest genome build (Felis_catus_9.0) was made available in 2017 [184], and one relatively low-density genotyping array of 63k SNP markers exists [229] but is not commercially available. No use of imputation software in cats has been reported. In horses, the most recent genome build EquCab3.0 has been available since 2018 [230], and the first equine array was reported in 2014 at a density of 54k (Equine BeadChip, Illumina, San Diego, CA, USA) [231]. Nowadays, two more SNP arrays exist, both of which are commercially available, with marker densities of 65k (Equine BeadChip, Illumina, San Diego, CA, USA) and 670k (MNEc670K, Affymetrix, Santa Clara, CA, USA) [232]. Notably, a test equine array containing 2 million markers (MNEc2M) was created to inform the creation of MNEc670K and used successfully for imputation [232,233]. Imputation has also been performed in an equine population, from 54/65k density up to 670k [234].

Companion animal models of disease have the potential to "add value" to understanding broader biology for many reasons. Our animal companions share our homes and environments, spontaneously develop diseases similar to human conditions, for which they are often diagnosed and treated similarly but over a shorter time course. In some cases, disease processes that occur commonly in companion animals may be hard to study in humans. For instance, the retriever POMC mutation occurs in approximately 25% of Labrador retrievers, but the equivalent human mutations are very rare. The same molecule, β-MSH, is absent in rodents. Hence, in this situation, dogs provide an excellent animal model to shed light on a previously hard-to-illuminate area of human biology [7].

Similarly, cats are arguably more suitable than traditional animal models for the study of obesity associated T2D. Diabetes in cats bares closer resemblance to human T2D than that of the rodent model; it occurs naturally in cats, whereas T2D research in rodents is most often an induced disease state [235]. This means using the feline model of diabetes offers benefits for improved understanding of human T2D development, particularly for polygenic models [236,237].

Notably, there are advantages to studying such inbred populations, particularly dogs. Recent population bottlenecks at breed formation mean dogs have a very different genetic architecture to humans that makes complex trait mapping uniquely tractable in the species [238]. This means complex traits can be mapped in a breed with fewer individuals and fewer markers than in human populations. Dogs are therefore a compelling model for studying human metabolic disease [77,239–241]. Although, trait mapping in such inbred species means mapping to much larger loci than in humans [242,243], making causative variant identification within an associated locus more difficult.

Although cats do not display the same high level of LD as dogs, they have also been selectively bred and are proposed as potentially valuable models of human hereditary disease [183,244,245]. Horse genomes display lower levels of LD than both dogs and cats [183], but breed structure means there is potential for disease alleles being enriched and relatively easily studied within a discrete, definable population, meaning they too have potential to be valuable models of human disease [246].

11. Conclusions

The obesity epidemic is a major health concern in both human and companion animals, and there is a lot more to be discovered regarding the molecular basis of obesity and associated metabolic conditions. Despite clear evidence that obesity and related traits are highly heritable in companion animals, there are only limited studies to date investigating which genes are responsible and how they exert their effect. As this field matures, it promises tangible benefits for animal populations and, where considered as non-traditional animal models of obesity, has the potential to offer translational benefits too.

Author Contributions: N.W.: writing—original draft preparation, writing—review and editing; E.R.: writing—review and editing, funding acquisition, supervision. All authors have read and agreed to the published version of the manuscript.

References

1.   World Health Organization. Obesity and Overweight. Global Health Observatory (GHO) Data. 2020. Available online: https://www.who.int/news-room/fact-sheets/detail/obesity-and-overweight (accessed on 21 June 2020).

2.   Cave, N.J.; Allan, F.J.; Schokkenbroek, S.L.; Metekohy, C.A.; Pfeiffer, D.U. A cross-sectional study to compare changes in the prevalence and risk factors for feline obesity between 1993 and 2007 in New Zealand. *Prev. Vet. Med.* **2012**, *107*, 121–133. [CrossRef]

3. Courcier, E.A.; Thomson, R.M.; Mellor, D.J.; Yam, P.S. An epidemiological study of environmental factors associated with canine obesity. *J. Small Anim. Pract.* **2010**, *51*, 362–367. [CrossRef]

4. World Health Organisation. Obesity: Preventing and managing the global epidemic. *WHO Consult.* **2000**, *894*, 1–253.

5. BSAVA. Obesity. 2019. Available online: https://bit.ly/2Pb9oRa (accessed on 4 September 2020).

6. Farooqi, S.; O'Rahilly, S. Genetics of obesity in humans. *Endocr. Rev.* **2006**, *27*, 710–718. [CrossRef] [PubMed]

7. Raffan, E.; Dennis, R.J.; O'Donovan, C.J.; Becker, J.M.; Scott, R.A.; Smith, S.P.; Withers, D.J.; Wood, C.J.; Conci, E.; Clements, D.N.; et al. A Deletion in the Canine POMC Gene Is Associated with Weight and Appetite in Obesity-Prone Labrador Retriever Dogs. *Cell Metab.* **2016**, *23*, 893–900. [CrossRef] [PubMed]

8. Paeratakul, S.; Lovejoy, J.C.; Ryan, D.H.; Bray, G.A. The relation of gender, race and socioeconomic status to obesity and obesity comorbidities in a sample of US adults. *Int. J. Obes. Relat. Metab. Disord.* **2002**, *26*, 1205–1210. [CrossRef]

9. McGreevy, P.D.; Thomson, P.C.; Pride, C.; Fawcett, A.; Grassi, T.; Jones, B. Prevalence of obesity in dogs examined by Australian veterinary practices and the risk factors involved. *Vet. Rec.* **2005**, *156*, 695–702. [CrossRef]

10. Lund, E.M.; Armstrong, P.J.; Kirk, C.A.; Klausner, J.S. Prevalence and Risk Factors for Obesity in Adult Dogs from Private US Veterinary Practices. *Int. J. Appl. Res. Vet. Med.* **2006**, *4*, 177–186.

11. Robin, C.A.; Ireland, J.L.; Wylie, C.E.; Collins, S.N.; Verheyen, K.L.; Newton, J.R. Prevalence of and risk factors for equine obesity in Great Britain based on owner-reported body condition scores. *Equine Vet. J.* **2015**, *47*, 196–201. [CrossRef]

12. Lund, E.M.; Armstrong, P.J.; Kirk, C.A.; Klausner, J.S. Prevalence and Risk Factors for Obesity in Adult Cats from Private US Veterinary Practices. *Int. J. Appl. Res. Vet. Med.* **2005**, *3*, 88–96.

13. Brewis, A.; SturtzSreetharan, C.; Wutich, A. Obesity stigma as a globalizing health challenge. *Glob. Health* **2018**, *14*, 20. [CrossRef]

14. Friedman, M. Mother blame, fat shame, and moral panic:"Obesity" and child welfare. *Fat Stud.* **2015**, *4*, 14–27. [CrossRef]

15. Pearl, R.L.; Wadden, T.A.; Bach, C.; Leonard, S.M.; Michel, K.E. Who's a good boy? Effects of dog and owner body weight on veterinarian perceptions and treatment recommendations. *Int. J. Obes. (Lond.)* **2020**. [CrossRef] [PubMed]

16. German, A.; Ramsey, I.; Lhermette, P. We should classify pet obesity as a disease. *Vet. Rec.* **2019**, *185*, 735. [CrossRef] [PubMed]

17. van der Klaauw, A.A.; Farooqi, I.S. The hunger genes: Pathways to obesity. *Cell* **2015**, *161*, 119–132. [CrossRef]

18. Silventoinen, K.; Magnusson, P.K.; Tynelius, P.; Kaprio, J.; Rasmussen, F. Heritability of body size and muscle strength in young adulthood: A study of one million Swedish men. *Genet. Epidemiol.* **2008**, *32*, 341–349. [CrossRef]

19. Wardle, J.; Carnell, S.; Haworth, C.M.; Plomin, R. Evidence for a strong genetic influence on childhood adiposity despite the force of the obesogenic environment. *Am. J. Clin. Nutr.* **2008**, *87*, 398–404. [CrossRef]

20. Ingalls, A.M.; Dickie, M.M.; Snell, G.D. Obese, a new mutation in the house mouse. *J. Hered.* **1950**, *41*, 317–318. [CrossRef]

21. Hummel, K.P.; Dickie, M.M.; Coleman, D.L. Diabetes, a new mutation in the mouse. *Science* **1966**, *153*, 1127–1128. [CrossRef]

22. Yen, T.T.; Stienmetz, J.; Simpson, P.J. Blood volume of obese (ob-ob) and diabetic (db-db) mice. *Proc. Soc. Exp. Biol. Med.* **1970**, *133*, 307–308. [CrossRef]

23. Coleman, D.L. Effects of parabiosis of obese with diabetes and normal mice. *Diabetologia* **1973**, *9*, 294–298. [CrossRef] [PubMed]

24. Tartaglia, L.A. The leptin receptor. *J. Biol. Chem.* **1997**, *272*, 6093–6096. [CrossRef] [PubMed]

25. Zhang, Y.; Proenca, R.; Maffei, M.; Barone, M.; Leopold, L.; Friedman, J.M. Positional cloning of the mouse obese gene and its human homologue. *Nature* **1994**, *372*, 425–432. [CrossRef] [PubMed]

26. Montague, C.T.; Farooqi, I.S.; Whitehead, J.P.; Soos, M.A.; Rau, H.; Wareham, N.J.; Sewter, C.P.; Digby, J.E.; Mohammed, S.N.; Hurst, J.A.; et al. Congenital leptin deficiency is associated with severe early-onset obesity in humans. *Nature* **1997**, *387*, 903–908. [CrossRef]

27. Wabitsch, M.; Funcke, J.B.; Lennerz, B.; Kuhnle-Krahl, U.; Lahr, G.; Debatin, K.M.; Vatter, P.; Gierschik, P.; Moepps, B.; Fischer-Posovszky, P. Biologically inactive leptin and early-onset extreme obesity. *N. Engl. J. Med.* **2015**, *372*, 48–54. [CrossRef]

28. Strobel, A.; Issad, T.; Camoin, L.; Ozata, M.; Strosberg, A.D. A leptin missense mutation associated with hypogonadism and morbid obesity. *Nat. Genet.* **1998**, *18*, 213–215. [CrossRef]

29. Zhao, Y.; Hong, N.; Liu, X.; Wu, B.; Tang, S.; Yang, J.; Hu, C.; Jia, W. A novel mutation in leptin gene is associated with severe obesity in Chinese individuals. *Biomed. Res. Int.* **2014**, *2014*, 912052. [CrossRef]

30. Clement, K.; Vaisse, C.; Lahlou, N.; Cabrol, S.; Pelloux, V.; Cassuto, D.; Gourmelen, M.; Dina, C.; Chambaz, J.; Lacorte, J.M.; et al. A mutation in the human leptin receptor gene causes obesity and pituitary dysfunction. *Nature* **1998**, *392*, 398–401. [CrossRef]

31. Farooqi, I.S.; Wangensteen, T.; Collins, S.; Kimber, W.; Matarese, G.; Keogh, J.M.; Lank, E.; Bottomley, B.; Lopez-Fernandez, J.; Ferraz-Amaro, I.; et al. Clinical and molecular genetic spectrum of congenital deficiency of the leptin receptor. *N. Engl. J. Med.* **2007**, *356*, 237–247. [CrossRef]

32. Hannema, S.E.; Wit, J.M.; Houdijk, M.E.; van Haeringen, A.; Bik, E.C.; Verkerk, A.J.; Uitterlinden, A.G.; Kant, S.G.; Oostdijk, W.; Bakker, E.; et al. Novel Leptin Receptor Mutations Identified in Two Girls with Severe Obesity Are Associated with Increased Bone Mineral Density. *Horm. Res. Paediatr.* **2016**, *85*, 412–420. [CrossRef]

33. Farr, O.M.; Gavrieli, A.; Mantzoros, C.S. Leptin applications in 2015: What have we learned about leptin and obesity? *Curr. Opin. Endocrinol. Diabetes Obes.* **2015**, *22*, 353–359. [CrossRef] [PubMed]

34. Dubern, B.; Clement, K. Leptin and leptin receptor-related monogenic obesity. *Biochimie* **2012**, *94*, 2111–2115. [CrossRef] [PubMed]

35. Nunziata, A.; Funcke, J.B.; Borck, G.; von Schnurbein, J.; Brandt, S.; Lennerz, B.; Moepps, B.; Gierschik, P.; Fischer-Posovszky, P.; Wabitsch, M. Functional and Phenotypic Characteristics of Human Leptin Receptor Mutations. *J. Endocr. Soc.* **2019**, *3*, 27–41. [CrossRef] [PubMed]

36. Farooqi, I.S.; O'Rahilly, S. 20 years of leptin: Human disorders of leptin action. *J. Endocrinol.* **2014**, *223*, T63–T70. [CrossRef]

37. Garfield, A.S.; Lam, D.D.; Marston, O.J.; Przydzial, M.J.; Heisler, L.K. Role of central melanocortin pathways in energy homeostasis. *Trends Endocrinol. Metab.* **2009**, *20*, 203–215. [CrossRef]

38. Barr, V.A.; Malide, D.; Zarnowski, M.J.; Taylor, S.I.; Cushman, S.W. Insulin stimulates both leptin secretion and production by rat white adipose tissue. *Endocrinology* **1997**, *138*, 4463–4472. [CrossRef]

39. Amitani, M.; Asakawa, A.; Amitani, H.; Inui, A. The role of leptin in the control of insulin-glucose axis. *Front. Neurosci.* **2013**, *7*, 51. [CrossRef]

40. Cummings, D.E.; Schwartz, M.W. Genetics and pathophysiology of human obesity. *Annu. Rev. Med.* **2003**, *54*, 453–471. [CrossRef]

41. Friedman, J. Leading the charge in leptin research: An interview with Jeffrey Friedman. *Dis. Model. Mech.* **2012**, *5*, 576–579.

42. Oswal, A.; Yeo, G.S. The leptin melanocortin pathway and the control of body weight: Lessons from human and murine genetics. *Obes. Rev.* **2007**, *8*, 293–306. [CrossRef]

43. Krude, H.; Biebermann, H.; Luck, W.; Horn, R.; Brabant, G.; Gruters, A. Severe early-onset obesity, adrenal insufficiency and red hair pigmentation caused by POMC mutations in humans. *Nat. Genet.* **1998**, *19*, 155–157. [CrossRef] [PubMed]

44. Krude, H.; Biebermann, H.; Schnabel, D.; Tansek, M.Z.; Theunissen, P.; Mullis, P.E.; Gruters, A. Obesity due to proopiomelanocortin deficiency: Three new cases and treatment trials with thyroid hormone and ACTH4-10. *J. Clin. Endocrinol. Metab.* **2003**, *88*, 4633–4640. [CrossRef] [PubMed]

45. Farooqi, I.S.; Drop, S.; Clements, A.; Keogh, J.M.; Biernacka, J.; Lowenbein, S.; Challis, B.G.; O'Rahilly, S. Heterozygosity for a POMC-null mutation and increased obesity risk in humans. *Diabetes* **2006**, *55*, 2549–2553. [CrossRef] [PubMed]

46. O'Rahilly, S.; Farooqi, I.S.; Yeo, G.S.; Challis, B.G. Minireview: Human obesity-lessons from monogenic disorders. *Endocrinology* **2003**, *144*, 3757–3764. [CrossRef] [PubMed]

47. Burnett, L.C.; LeDuc, C.A.; Sulsona, C.R.; Paull, D.; Rausch, R.; Eddiry, S.; Carli, J.F.; Morabito, M.V.; Skowronski, A.A.; Hubner, G.; et al. Deficiency in prohormone convertase PC1 impairs prohormone processing in Prader-Willi syndrome. *J. Clin. Investig.* **2017**, *127*, 293–305. [CrossRef] [PubMed]

48. Ramachandrappa, S.; Raimondo, A.; Cali, A.M.; Keogh, J.M.; Henning, E.; Saeed, S.; Thompson, A.; Garg, S.; Bochukova, E.G.; Brage, S.; et al. Rare variants in single-minded 1 (SIM1) are associated with severe obesity. *J. Clin. Investig.* **2013**, *123*, 3042–3050. [CrossRef] [PubMed]

49. Bonnefond, A.; Raimondo, A.; Stutzmann, F.; Ghoussaini, M.; Ramachandrappa, S.; Bersten, D.C.; Durand, E.; Vatin, V.; Balkau, B.; Lantieri, O.; et al. Loss-of-function mutations in SIM1 contribute to obesity and Prader-Willi-like features. *J. Clin. Investig.* **2013**, *123*, 3037–3041. [CrossRef]

50. Yeo, G.S.; Farooqi, I.S.; Aminian, S.; Halsall, D.J.; Stanhope, R.G.; O'Rahilly, S. A frameshift mutation in MC4R associated with dominantly inherited human obesity. *Nat. Genet.* **1998**, *20*, 111–112. [CrossRef]

51. Vaisse, C.; Clement, K.; Guy-Grand, B.; Froguel, P. A frameshift mutation in human MC4R is associated with a dominant form of obesity. *Nat. Genet.* **1998**, *20*, 113–114. [CrossRef]

52. Kobayashi, H.; Ogawa, Y.; Shintani, M.; Ebihara, K.; Shimodahira, M.; Iwakura, T.; Hino, M.; Ishihara, T.; Ikekubo, K.; Kurahachi, H.; et al. A Novel homozygous missense mutation of melanocortin-4 receptor (MC4R) in a Japanese woman with severe obesity. *Diabetes* **2002**, *51*, 243–246. [CrossRef]

53. Farooqi, I.S.; Yeo, G.S.; Keogh, J.M.; Aminian, S.; Jebb, S.A.; Butler, G.; Cheetham, T.; O'Rahilly, S. Dominant and recessive inheritance of morbid obesity associated with melanocortin 4 receptor deficiency. *J. Clin. Investig.* **2000**, *106*, 271–279. [CrossRef] [PubMed]

54. Loid, P.; Mustila, T.; Makitie, R.E.; Viljakainen, H.; Kampe, A.; Tossavainen, P.; Lipsanen-Nyman, M.; Pekkinen, M.; Makitie, O. Rare Variants in Genes Linked to Appetite Control and Hypothalamic Development in Early-Onset Severe Obesity. *Front. Endocrinol. (Lausanne)* **2020**, *11*, 81. [CrossRef] [PubMed]

55. Doulla, M.; McIntyre, A.D.; Hegele, R.A.; Gallego, P.H. A novel MC4R mutation associated with childhood-onset obesity: A case report. *Paediatr. Child Health* **2014**, *19*, 515–518. [CrossRef] [PubMed]

56. Farooqi, I.S. Monogenic human obesity. *Front. Horm. Res.* **2008**, *36*, 1–11.

57. Chami, N.; Preuss, M.; Walker, R.W.; Moscati, A.; Loos, R.J.F. The role of polygenic susceptibility to obesity among carriers of pathogenic mutations in MC4R in the UK Biobank population. *PLoS Med.* **2020**, *17*, e1003196. [CrossRef]

58. Loos, R.J.; Lindgren, C.M.; Li, S.; Wheeler, E.; Zhao, J.H.; Prokopenko, I.; Inouye, M.; Freathy, R.M.; Attwood, A.P.; Beckmann, J.S.; et al. Common variants near MC4R are associated with fat mass, weight and risk of obesity. *Nat. Genet.* **2008**, *40*, 768–775. [CrossRef]

59. Lotta, L.A.; Mokrosinski, J.; Mendes de Oliveira, E.; Li, C.; Sharp, S.J.; Luan, J.; Brouwers, B.; Ayinampudi, V.; Bowker, N.; Kerrison, N.; et al. Human Gain-of-Function MC4R Variants Show Signaling Bias and Protect against Obesity. *Cell* **2019**, *177*, 597–607.e9. [CrossRef]

60. van der Klaauw, A.A.; Croizier, S.; Mendes de Oliveira, E.; Stadler, L.K.J.; Park, S.; Kong, Y.; Banton, M.C.; Tandon, P.; Hendricks, A.E.; Keogh, J.M.; et al. Human Semaphorin 3 Variants Link Melanocortin Circuit Development and Energy Balance. *Cell* **2019**, *176*, 729–742.e18. [CrossRef]

61. Cordeira, J.; Rios, M. Weighing in the role of BDNF in the central control of eating behavior. *Mol. Neurobiol.* **2011**, *44*, 441–448. [CrossRef]

62. Pearce, L.R.; Atanassova, N.; Banton, M.C.; Bottomley, B.; van der Klaauw, A.A.; Revelli, J.P.; Hendricks, A.; Keogh, J.M.; Henning, E.; Doree, D.; et al. KSR2 mutations are associated with obesity, insulin resistance, and impaired cellular fuel oxidation. *Cell* **2013**, *155*, 765–777. [CrossRef]

63. Minster, R.L.; Hawley, N.L.; Su, C.T.; Sun, G.; Kershaw, E.E.; Cheng, H.; Buhule, O.D.; Lin, J.; Reupena, M.S.; Viali, S.; et al. A thrifty variant in CREBRF strongly influences body mass index in Samoans. *Nat. Genet.* **2016**, *48*, 1049–1054. [CrossRef] [PubMed]

64. da Fonseca, A.C.P.; Mastronardi, C.; Johar, A.; Arcos-Burgos, M.; Paz-Filho, G. Genetics of non-syndromic childhood obesity and the use of high-throughput DNA sequencing technologies. *J. Diabetes Complicat.* **2017**, *31*, 1549–1561. [CrossRef] [PubMed]

65. Yang, J.; Bakshi, A.; Zhu, Z.; Hemani, G.; Vinkhuyzen, A.A.; Lee, S.H.; Robinson, M.R.; Perry, J.R.; Nolte, I.M.; van Vliet-Ostaptchouk, J.V.; et al. Genetic variance estimation with imputed variants finds negligible missing heritability for human height and body mass index. *Nat. Genet.* **2015**, *47*, 1114–1120. [CrossRef] [PubMed]

66. Xue, A.; Wu, Y.; Zhu, Z.; Zhang, F.; Kemper, K.E.; Zheng, Z.; Yengo, L.; Lloyd-Jones, L.R.; Sidorenko, J.; Wu, Y.; et al. Genome-wide association analyses identify 143 risk variants and putative regulatory mechanisms for type 2 diabetes. *Nat. Commun.* **2018**, *9*, 2941. [CrossRef] [PubMed]

67. Locke, A.E.; Kahali, B.; Berndt, S.I.; Justice, A.E.; Pers, T.H.; Day, F.R.; Powell, C.; Vedantam, S.; Buchkovich, M.L.; Yang, J.; et al. Genetic studies of body mass index yield new insights for obesity biology. *Nature* **2015**, *518*, 197–206. [CrossRef] [PubMed]

68. Cho, Y.S.; Go, M.J.; Kim, Y.J.; Heo, J.Y.; Oh, J.H.; Ban, H.J.; Yoon, D.; Lee, M.H.; Kim, D.J.; Park, M.; et al. A large-scale genome-wide association study of Asian populations uncovers genetic factors influencing eight quantitative traits. *Nat. Genet.* **2009**, *41*, 527–534. [CrossRef]

69. Pulit, S.L.; Stoneman, C.; Morris, A.P.; Wood, A.R.; Glastonbury, C.A.; Tyrrell, J.; Yengo, L.; Ferreira, T.; Marouli, E.; Ji, Y.; et al. Meta-analysis of genome-wide association studies for body fat distribution in 694 649 individuals of European ancestry. *Hum. Mol. Genet.* **2019**, *28*, 166–174. [CrossRef]

70. Lotta, L.A.; Gulati, P.; Day, F.R.; Payne, F.; Ongen, H.; van de Bunt, M.; Gaulton, K.J.; Eicher, J.D.; Sharp, S.J.; Luan, J.; et al. Integrative genomic analysis implicates limited peripheral adipose storage capacity in the pathogenesis of human insulin resistance. *Nat. Genet.* **2017**, *49*, 17–26. [CrossRef]

71. Rask-Andersen, M.; Karlsson, T.; Ek, W.E.; Johansson, A. Genome-wide association study of body fat distribution identifies adiposity loci and sex-specific genetic effects. *Nat. Commun.* **2019**, *10*, 339. [CrossRef]

72. Hebebrand, J.; Volckmar, A.L.; Knoll, N.; Hinney, A. Chipping away the 'missing heritability': GIANT steps forward in the molecular elucidation of obesity–but still lots to go. *Obes. Facts* **2010**, *3*, 294–303. [CrossRef]

73. Llewellyn, C.H.; Trzaskowski, M.; Plomin, R.; Wardle, J. Finding the missing heritability in pediatric obesity: The contribution of genome-wide complex trait analysis. *Int. J. Obes. (Lond.)* **2013**, *37*, 1506–1509. [CrossRef] [PubMed]

74. Loos, R.J. Genetic determinants of common obesity and their value in prediction. *Best Pract. Res. Clin. Endocrinol. Metab.* **2012**, *26*, 211–226. [CrossRef] [PubMed]

75. Herrera, B.M.; Lindgren, C.M. The genetics of obesity. *Curr. Diabetes Rep.* **2010**, *10*, 498–505. [CrossRef]

76. Xia, Q.; Grant, S.F. The genetics of human obesity. *Ann. N. Y. Acad. Sci.* **2013**, *1281*, 178–190. [CrossRef] [PubMed]

77. Karlsson, E.K.; Lindblad-Toh, K. Leader of the pack: Gene mapping in dogs and other model organisms. *Nat. Rev. Genet.* **2008**, *9*, 713–725. [CrossRef]

78. Hall, A.B.; Tolonen, A.C.; Xavier, R.J. Human genetic variation and the gut microbiome in disease. *Nat. Rev. Genet.* **2017**, *18*, 690–699. [CrossRef]

79. Inouye, M.; Abraham, G.; Nelson, C.P.; Wood, A.M.; Sweeting, M.J.; Dudbridge, F.; Lai, F.Y.; Kaptoge, S.; Brozynska, M.; Wang, T.; et al. Genomic Risk Prediction of Coronary Artery Disease in 480,000 Adults: Implications for Primary Prevention. *J. Am. Coll. Cardiol.* **2018**, *72*, 1883–1893. [CrossRef]

80. Lambert, S.A.; Abraham, G.; Inouye, M. Towards clinical utility of polygenic risk scores. *Hum. Mol. Genet.* **2019**, *28*, R133–R142. [CrossRef]

81. Speakman, J.R.; Loos, R.J.F.; O'Rahilly, S.; Hirschhorn, J.N.; Allison, D.B. GWAS for BMI: A treasure trove of fundamental insights into the genetic basis of obesity. *Int. J. Obes. (Lond.)* **2018**, *42*, 1524–1531. [CrossRef]

82. Farooqi, I.S. Chapter 4: Genetics of Obesity. In *Handbook of Obesity Treatment*; Guilford Publications: New York, NY, USA, 2018; pp. 64–74.

83. Claussnitzer, M.; Dankel, S.N.; Kim, K.H.; Quon, G.; Meuleman, W.; Haugen, C.; Glunk, V.; Sousa, I.S.; Beaudry, J.L.; Puviindran, V.; et al. FTO Obesity Variant Circuitry and Adipocyte Browning in Humans. *N. Engl. J. Med.* **2015**, *373*, 895–907. [CrossRef]

84. O'Rahilly, S.; Coll, A.P.; Yeo, G.S. FTO Obesity Variant and Adipocyte Browning in Humans. *N. Engl. J. Med.* **2016**, *374*, 191. [CrossRef] [PubMed]

85. Leow, M.K. FTO Obesity Variant and Adipocyte Browning in Humans. *N. Engl. J. Med.* **2016**, *374*, 191–192. [CrossRef] [PubMed]

86. Apovian, C.M. Obesity: Definition, comorbidities, causes, and burden. *Am. J. Manag. Care* **2016**, *22*, s176–s185.

87. Kyrou, I.; Randeva, H.S.; Tsigos, C.; Kaltsas, G.; Weickert, M.O. Clinical Problems Caused by Obesity. In *Endotext [Internet]*; Feingold, K.R., Anawalt, B., Eds.; Endotext, MDText.com, Inc.: South Dartmouth, MA, USA, 2000.

88. Pi-Sunyer, X. The medical risks of obesity. *Postgrad. Med.* **2009**, *121*, 21–33. [CrossRef] [PubMed]

89. Grundy, S.M. Metabolic syndrome update. *Trends Cardiovasc. Med.* **2016**, *26*, 364–373. [CrossRef] [PubMed]

90. Han, T.S.; Lean, M.E. A clinical perspective of obesity, metabolic syndrome and cardiovascular disease. *JRSM Cardiovasc. Dis.* **2016**, *5*, 2048004016633371. [CrossRef]

91. Stefan, N.; Haring, H.U.; Hu, F.B.; Schulze, M.B. Metabolically healthy obesity: Epidemiology, mechanisms, and clinical implications. *Lancet Diabetes Endocrinol.* **2013**, *1*, 152–162. [CrossRef]

92. Eckel, R.H.; Kahn, S.E.; Ferrannini, E.; Goldfine, A.B.; Nathan, D.M.; Schwartz, M.W.; Smith, R.J.; Smith, S.R.; Endocrine, S.; American Diabetes, A.; et al. Obesity and type 2 diabetes: What can be unified and what needs to be individualized? *Diabetes Care* **2011**, *34*, 1424–1430. [CrossRef]

93. Semple, R.K. How does insulin resistance arise, and how does it cause disease? Human genetic lessons. *Eur. J. Endocrinol.* **2016**, *174*, R209–R223. [CrossRef]

94. World Health Organisation. Appropriate body-mass index for Asian populations and its implications for policy and intervention strategies. *WHO Consult. Lancet* **2004**, *363*, 157–163.

95. Goodarzi, M.O. Genetics of obesity: What genetic association studies have taught us about the biology of obesity and its complications. *Lancet Diabetes Endocrinol.* **2018**, *6*, 223–236. [CrossRef]

96. Romeo, S.; Sanyal, A.; Valenti, L. Leveraging Human Genetics to Identify Potential New Treatments for Fatty Liver Disease. *Cell Metab.* **2020**, *31*, 35–45. [CrossRef] [PubMed]

97. Rung, J.; Cauchi, S.; Albrechtsen, A.; Shen, L.; Rocheleau, G.; Cavalcanti-Proenca, C.; Bacot, F.; Balkau, B.; Belisle, A.; Borch-Johnsen, K.; et al. Genetic variant near IRS1 is associated with type 2 diabetes, insulin resistance and hyperinsulinemia. *Nat. Genet.* **2009**, *41*, 1110–1115. [CrossRef] [PubMed]

98. Robbins, A.L.; Savage, D.B. The genetics of lipid storage and human lipodystrophies. *Trends Mol. Med.* **2015**, *21*, 433–438. [CrossRef] [PubMed]

99. Sorensen, T.I.A. From fat cells through an obesity theory. *Eur. J. Clin. Nutr.* **2018**, *72*, 1329–1335. [CrossRef]

100. Virtue, S.; Vidal-Puig, A. Adipose tissue expandability, lipotoxicity and the Metabolic Syndrome—An allostatic perspective. *Biochim. Biophys. Acta* **2010**, *1801*, 338–349. [CrossRef]

101. German, A.J. The growing problem of obesity in dogs and cats. *J. Nutr.* **2006**, *136*, 1940S–1946S. [CrossRef]

102. Lucena, S.; Lamy, E.; Capela, F.; Lavrador, C.; Tvarijonaviciute, A. Human and Canine Prevalence of Obesity and Feeding Habits–a One Health Approach in Portugal. In Proceedings of the Conference Proceedings: ICAAM—Comunicações—Em Congressos Científicos Internacionais, Évora, Portugal, 15–16 October 2018. Available online: http://hdl.handle.net/10174/24279 (accessed on 9 September 2020).

103. Colliard, L.; Ancel, J.; Benet, J.J.; Paragon, B.M.; Blanchard, G. Risk Factors for Obesity in Dogs in France. *J. Nutr.* **2006**, *136*, 1951S–1954S. [CrossRef]

104. Mao, J.; Xia, Z.; Chen, J.; Yu, J. Prevalence and risk factors for canine obesity surveyed in veterinary practices in Beijing, China. *Prev. Vet. Med.* **2013**, *112*, 438–442. [CrossRef]

105. German, A.J.; Hervera, M.; Hunter, L.; Holden, S.L.; Morris, P.J.; Biourge, V.; Trayhurn, P. Improvement in insulin resistance and reduction in plasma inflammatory adipokines after weight loss in obese dogs. *Domest. Anim. Endocrinol.* **2009**, *37*, 214–226. [CrossRef]

106. Chandler, M.; Cunningham, S.; Lund, E.M.; Khanna, C.; Naramore, R.; Patel, A.; Day, M.J. Obesity and Associated Comorbidities in People and Companion Animals: A One Health Perspective. *J. Comp. Pathol.* **2017**, *156*, 296–309. [CrossRef] [PubMed]

107. Hill, R.C. Nutritional therapies to improve health: Lessons from companion animals. Conference on "Multidisciplinary approaches to nutritional problems". Symposium on "Nutrition and health". *Proc. Nutr. Soc.* **2009**, *68*, 98–102. [CrossRef] [PubMed]

108. Costa-Santos, K.; Damasceno, K.; Portela, R.D.; Santos, F.L.; Araujo, G.C.; Martins-Filho, E.F.; Silva, L.P.; Barral, T.D.; Santos, S.A.; Estrela-Lima, A. Lipid and metabolic profiles in female dogs with mammary carcinoma receiving dietary fish oil supplementation. *BMC Vet. Res.* **2019**, *15*, 401. [CrossRef] [PubMed]

109. Tvarijonaviciute, A.; Ceron, J.J.; Holden, S.L.; Cuthbertson, D.J.; Biourge, V.; Morris, P.J.; German, A.J. Obesity-related metabolic dysfunction in dogs: A comparison with human metabolic syndrome. *BMC Vet. Res.* **2012**, *8*, 147. [CrossRef]

110. Montoya-Alonso, J.A.; Bautista-Castano, I.; Pena, C.; Suarez, L.; Juste, M.C.; Tvarijonaviciute, A. Prevalence of Canine Obesity, Obesity-Related Metabolic Dysfunction, and Relationship with Owner Obesity in an Obesogenic Region of Spain. *Front. Vet. Sci.* **2017**, *4*, 59. [CrossRef] [PubMed]

111. Hoenig, M. Comparative Aspects of Diabetes Mellitus in Dogs and Cats. *Mol. Cell. Endocrinol.* **2002**, *197*, 221–229. [CrossRef]

112. Stachowiak, M.; Szczerbal, I.; Switonski, M. Genetics of Adiposity in Large Animal Models for Human Obesity-Studies on Pigs and Dogs. *Prog. Mol. Biol. Transl. Sci.* **2016**, *140*, 233–270.

113. German, A.J.; Blackwell, E.; Evans, M.; Westgarth, C. Overweight dogs are more likely to display undesirable behaviours: Results of a large online survey of dog owners in the UK. *J. Nutr. Sci.* **2017**, *6*, e14. [CrossRef]

114. Raffan, E.; Smith, S.P.; O'Rahilly, S.; Wardle, J. Development, factor structure and application of the Dog Obesity Risk and Appetite (DORA) questionnaire. *PeerJ* **2015**, *3*, e1278. [CrossRef]

115. Alegria-Moran, R.A.; Guzman-Pino, S.A.; Egana, J.I.; Munoz, C.; Figueroa, J. Food Preferences in Dogs: Effect of Dietary Composition and Intrinsic Variables on Diet Selection. *Animals (Basel)* **2019**, *9*, 372. [CrossRef]

116. Gough, A.; Thomas, A.; O'Neill, D. *Breed. Predispositions to Disease in Dogs and Cats*, 3rd ed.; Wiley: Hoboken, NJ, USA, 2018.

117. Farrell, L.L.; Schoenebeck, J.J.; Wiener, P.; Clements, D.N.; Summers, K.M. The challenges of pedigree dog health: Approaches to combating inherited disease. *Canine Genet. Epidemiol.* **2015**, *2*, 1–14. [CrossRef]

118. Wilbe, M.; Jokinen, P.; Truve, K.; Seppala, E.H.; Karlsson, E.K.; Biagi, T.; Hughes, A.; Bannasch, D.; Andersson, G.; Hansson-Hamlin, H.; et al. Genome-wide association mapping identifies multiple loci for a canine SLE-related disease complex. *Nat. Genet.* **2010**, *42*, 250–254. [CrossRef] [PubMed]

119. Switonski, M.; Mankowska, M. Dog obesity—The need for identifying predisposing genetic markers. *Res. Vet. Sci.* **2013**, *95*, 831–836. [CrossRef]

120. Mankowska, M.; Krzeminska, P.; Graczyk, M.; Switonski, M. Confirmation that a deletion in the POMC gene is associated with body weight of Labrador Retriever dogs. *Res. Vet. Sci.* **2017**, *112*, 116–118. [CrossRef]

121. Chandler, M. New thoughts about obesity. *Companion Anim.* **2018**, *23*, 686–695. [CrossRef]

122. Crane, S.W. Occurrence and Management of Obesity in Companion Animals. *J. Small Anim. Pract.* **1991**, *31*, 275–282. [CrossRef]

123. Plassais, J.; Rimbault, M.; Williams, F.J.; Davis, B.W.; Schoenebeck, J.J.; Ostrander, E.A. Analysis of large versus small dogs reveals three genes on the canine X chromosome associated with body weight, muscling and back fat thickness. *PLoS Genet.* **2017**, *13*, e1006661. [CrossRef]

124. Mawby, D.I.; Bartges, J.W.; d'Avignon, A.; Laflamme, D.P.; Moyers, T.D.; Cottrell, T. Comparison of various methods for estimating body fat in dogs. *J. Am. Anim. Hosp. Assoc.* **2004**, *40*, 109–114. [CrossRef]

125. Laflamme, D.R. Development and validation of a body condition score system for dogs.: A clinical tool. *Canine Pract.* **1997**, *22*, 10–15.

126. German, A.J.; Holden, S.L.; Moxham, G.L.; Holmes, K.L.; Hackett, R.M.; Rawlings, J.M. A simple, reliable tool for owners to assess the body condition of their dog or cat. *J. Nutr.* **2006**, *136*, 2031S–2033S. [CrossRef] [PubMed]

127. Davison, L.J.; Holder, A.; Catchpole, B.; O'Callaghan, C.A. The Canine POMC Gene, Obesity in Labrador Retrievers and Susceptibility to Diabetes Mellitus. *J. Vet. Intern. Med.* **2017**, *31*, 343–348. [CrossRef] [PubMed]

128. Lourenço, N.O.; Albuquerque, A.L.H.; Basso, R.M.; Trecenti, A.S.; Albertino, L.G.; Melchert, A.; Borges, A.S.; Oliveira-Filho, J.P. Canine POMC deletion (P187fs) allele frequency in Labrador Retrievers in Brazil. *Pesqui. Vet. Bras.* **2019**, *39*, 909–914. [CrossRef]

129. Lee, Y.S.; Challis, B.G.; Thompson, D.A.; Yeo, G.S.; Keogh, J.M.; Madonna, M.E.; Wraight, V.; Sims, M.; Vatin, V.; Meyre, D.; et al. A POMC variant implicates beta-melanocyte-stimulating hormone in the control of human energy balance. *Cell Metab.* **2006**, *3*, 135–140. [CrossRef]

130. Challis, B.G.; Pritchard, L.E.; Creemers, J.W.; Delplanque, J.; Keogh, J.M.; Luan, J.; Wareham, N.J.; Yeo, G.S.; Bhattacharyya, S.; Froguel, P.; et al. A missense mutation disrupting a dibasic prohormone processing site in pro-opiomelanocortin (POMC) increases susceptibility to early-onset obesity through a novel molecular mechanism. *Hum. Mol. Genet.* **2002**, *11*, 1997–2004. [CrossRef] [PubMed]

131. Martinelli, C.E.; Keogh, J.M.; Greenfield, J.R.; Henning, E.; van der Klaauw, A.A.; Blackwood, A.; O'Rahilly, S.; Roelfsema, F.; Camacho-Hubner, C.; Pijl, H.; et al. Obesity due to melanocortin 4 receptor (MC4R) deficiency is associated with increased linear growth and final height, fasting hyperinsulinemia, and incompletely suppressed growth hormone secretion. *J. Clin. Endocrinol. Metab.* **2011**, *96*, E181–E188. [CrossRef]

132. Yan, J.; Tao, Y.X. Pharmacological characterization of canine melancortin-4 receptor and its natural variant V213F. *Domest. Anim. Endocrinol.* **2011**, *41*, 91–97. [CrossRef]

133. Skorczyk, A.; Stachowiak, M.; Szczerbal, I.; Klukowska-Roetzler, J.; Schelling, C.; Dolf, G.; Switonski, M. Polymorphism and chromosomal location of the MC4R (melanocortin-4 receptor) gene in the dog and red fox. *Gene* **2007**, *392*, 247–252. [CrossRef]

134. van den Berg, L.; van den Berg, S.M.; Martens, E.E.; Hazewinkel, H.A.; Dijkshoorn, N.A.; Delemarre-van de Waal, H.A.; Heutink, P.; Leegwater, P.A.; Heuven, H.C. Analysis of variation in the melanocortin-4 receptor gene (mc4r) in Golden Retriever dogs. *Anim. Genet.* **2010**, *41*, 557. [CrossRef]

135. Zeng, R.; Zhang, Y.; Du, P. SNPs of melanocortin 4 receptor (MC4R) associated with body weight in Beagle dogs. *Exp. Anim.* **2014**, *63*, 73–78. [CrossRef]

136. Mankowska, M.; Nowacka-Woszuk, J.; Graczyk, A.; Ciazynska, P.; Stachowiak, M.; Switonski, M. Polymorphism and methylation of the MC4R gene in obese and non-obese dogs. *Mol. Biol. Rep.* **2017**, *44*, 333–339. [CrossRef]

137. Dubern, B.; Clement, K.; Pelloux, V.; Froguel, P.; Girardet, J.P.; Guy-Grand, B.; Tounian, P. Mutational analysis of melanocortin-4 receptor, agouti-related protein, and alpha-melanocyte-stimulating hormone genes in severely obese children. *J. Pediatr.* **2001**, *139*, 204–209. [CrossRef] [PubMed]

138. Grzes, M.; Szczerbal, I.; Fijak-Nowak, H.; Szydlowski, M.; Switonski, M. Two candidate genes (FTO and INSIG2) for fat accumulation in four canids: Chromosome mapping, gene polymorphisms and association studies of body and skin weight of red foxes. *Cytogenet. Genome Res.* **2011**, *135*, 25–32. [CrossRef] [PubMed]

139. Grzemski, A.; Stachowiak, M.; Flisikowski, K.; Mankowska, M.; Krzeminska, P.; Gogulski, M.; Aleksiewicz, R.; Szydlowski, M.; Switonski, M.; Nowacka-Woszuk, J. FTO and IRX3 genes are not promising markers for obesity in Labrador retriever dogs. *Ann. Anim. Sci.* **2019**, *19*, 343–357. [CrossRef]

140. Skorczyk, A.; Flisikowski, K.; Szydlowski, M.; Cieslak, J.; Fries, R.; Switonski, M. Association of MC3R gene polymorphisms with body weight in the red fox and comparative gene organization in four canids. *Anim. Genet.* **2011**, *42*, 104–107. [CrossRef]

141. Lee, B.; Koo, J.; Yun Jun, J.; Gavrilova, O.; Lee, Y.; Seo, A.Y.; Taylor-Douglas, D.C.; Adler-Wailes, D.C.; Chen, F.; Gardner, R.; et al. A mouse model for a partially inactive obesity-associated human MC3R variant. *Nat. Commun.* **2016**, *7*, 10522. [CrossRef]

142. Tao, Y.X. Mutations in the melanocortin-3 receptor (MC3R) gene: Impact on human obesity or adiposity. *Curr. Opin. Investig. Drugs* **2010**, *11*, 1092–1096.

143. Ghamari-Langroudi, M.; Cakir, I.; Lippert, R.N.; Sweeney, P.; Litt, M.J.; Ellacott, K.L.J.; Cone, R.D. Regulation of energy rheostasis by the melanocortin-3 receptor. *Sci. Adv.* **2018**, *4*, eaat0866. [CrossRef]

144. Girardet, C.; Begriche, K.; Ptitsyn, A.; Koza, R.A.; Butler, A.A. Unravelling the mysterious roles of melanocortin-3 receptors in metabolic homeostasis and obesity using mouse genetics. *Int. J. Obes. Suppl.* **2014**, *4*, S37–S44. [CrossRef]

145. Herbert, A.; Gerry, N.P.; McQueen, M.B.; Heid, I.M.; Pfeufer, A.; Illig, T.; Wichmann, H.E.; Meitinger, T.; Hunter, D.; Hu, F.B.; et al. A common genetic variant is associated with adult and childhood obesity. *Science* **2006**, *312*, 279–283. [CrossRef]

146. Hinney, A.; Hebebrand, J. Polygenic obesity in humans. *Obes. Facts* **2008**, *1*, 35–42. [CrossRef]

147. Hudson, B.D.; Shimpukade, B.; Mackenzie, A.E.; Butcher, A.J.; Pediani, J.D.; Christiansen, E.; Heathcote, H.; Tobin, A.B.; Ulven, T.; Milligan, G. The pharmacology of TUG-891, a potent and selective agonist of the free fatty acid receptor 4 (FFA4/GPR120), demonstrates both potential opportunity and possible challenges to therapeutic agonism. *Mol. Pharmacol.* **2013**, *84*, 710–725. [CrossRef] [PubMed]

148. Stone, V.M.; Dhayal, S.; Brocklehurst, K.J.; Lenaghan, C.; Sorhede Winzell, M.; Hammar, M.; Xu, X.; Smith, D.M.; Morgan, N.G. GPR120 (FFAR4) is preferentially expressed in pancreatic delta cells and regulates somatostatin secretion from murine islets of Langerhans. *Diabetologia* **2014**, *57*, 1182–1191. [CrossRef] [PubMed]

149. Ichimura, A.; Hirasawa, A.; Poulain-Godefroy, O.; Bonnefond, A.; Hara, T.; Yengo, L.; Kimura, I.; Leloire, A.; Liu, N.; Iida, K.; et al. Dysfunction of lipid sensor GPR120 leads to obesity in both mouse and human. *Nature* **2012**, *483*, 350–354. [CrossRef] [PubMed]

150. Miyabe, M.; Gin, A.; Onozawa, E.; Daimon, M.; Yamada, H.; Oda, H.; Mori, A.; Momota, Y.; Azakami, D.; Yamamoto, I.; et al. Genetic variants of the unsaturated fatty acid receptor GPR120 relating to obesity in dogs. *J. Vet. Med. Sci.* **2015**, *77*, 1201–1206. [CrossRef] [PubMed]

151. Barak, Y.; Kim, S. Genetic manipulations of PPARs: Effects on obesity and metabolic disease. *PPAR Res.* **2007**, *2007*, 12781. [CrossRef]

152. Vidal-Puig, A.; Jimenez-Linan, M.; Lowell, B.B.; Hamann, A.; Hu, E.; Spiegelman, B.; Flier, J.S.; Moller, D.E. Regulation of PPAR gamma gene expression by nutrition and obesity in rodents. *J. Clin. Investig.* **1996**, *97*, 2553–2561. [CrossRef]

153. Nishii, N.; Takasu, M.; Soe, O.K.; Maeda, S.; Ohba, Y.; Inoue-Murayama, M.; Kitagawa, H. Cloning, expression and investigation for polymorphisms of canine peroxisome proliferator-activated receptors. *Comp. Biochem. Physiol. B Biochem. Mol. Biol.* **2007**, *147*, 690–697. [CrossRef]

154. Mankowska, M.; Stachowiak, M.; Graczyk, A.; Ciazynska, P.; Gogulski, M.; Nizanski, W.; Switonski, M. Sequence analysis of three canine adipokine genes revealed an association between TNF polymorphisms and obesity in Labrador dogs. *Anim. Genet.* **2016**, *47*, 245–249. [CrossRef]

155. Yu, Z.; Han, S.; Cao, X.; Zhu, C.; Wang, X.; Guo, X. Genetic polymorphisms in adipokine genes and the risk of obesity: A systematic review and meta-analysis. *Obesity (Silver Spring)* **2012**, *20*, 396–406. [CrossRef]

156. Ellulu, M.S.; Patimah, I.; Khaza'ai, H.; Rahmat, A.; Abed, Y. Obesity and inflammation: The linking mechanism and the complications. *Arch. Med. Sci.* **2017**, *13*, 851–863. [CrossRef]

157. Vandendriessche, V.L.; Picavet, P.; Hesta, M. First detailed nutritional survey in a referral companion animal population. *J. Anim. Physiol. Anim. Nutr. (Berl.)* **2017**, *101* (Suppl. S1), S4–S14. [CrossRef] [PubMed]

158. Courcier, E.A.; O'Higgins, R.; Mellor, D.J.; Yam, P.S. Prevalence and risk factors for feline obesity in a first opinion practice in Glasgow, Scotland. *J. Feline Med. Surg.* **2010**, *12*, 746–753. [CrossRef] [PubMed]

159. Scarlett, J.M.; Donoghue, S.; Saidla, J.; Wills, J. Overweight cats: Prevalence and risk factors. *Int. J. Obes. Relat. Metab. Disord.* **1994**, *18* (Suppl. S1), S22–S28. [PubMed]

160. Courcier, E.A.; Mellor, D.J.; Pendlebury, E.; Evans, C.; Yam, P.S. An investigation into the epidemiology of feline obesity in Great Britain: Results of a cross-sectional study of 47 companion animal practises. *Vet. Rec.* **2012**, *171*, 560. [CrossRef] [PubMed]

161. Wall, M.; Cave, N.J.; Vallee, E. Owner and Cat-Related Risk Factors for Feline Overweight or Obesity. *Front. Vet. Sci.* **2019**, *6*, 266. [CrossRef]

162. Tarkosova, D.; Story, M.M.; Rand, J.S.; Svoboda, M. Feline obesity–prevalence, risk factors, pathogenesis, associated conditions and assessment: A review. *Vet. Med.* **2016**, *61*, 295–307. [CrossRef]

163. Scarlett, J.M.; Donoghue, S. Associations between body condition and disease in cats. *J. Am. Vet. Med. Assoc.* **1998**, *212*, 1725–1731.

164. Kocabağlı, N.; Kutay, H.C.; Dokuzeylül, B.; Süer, İ.N.E.; Apt, M. The Analysis of Computer Data regarding Obesity and Associated Diseases in Cats Examined at Private Veterinary Practices. *Acta Sci. Vet.* **2017**, *45*, 5. [CrossRef]

165. Center, S.A. Feline hepatic lipidosis. *Vet. Clin. N. Am. Small Anim. Pract.* **2005**, *35*, 225–269. [CrossRef]

166. Hoenig, M.; Thomaseth, K.; Waldron, M.; Ferguson, D.C. Insulin sensitivity, fat distribution, and adipocytokine response to different diets in lean and obese cats before and after weight loss. *Am. J. Physiol. Regul. Integr. Comp. Physiol.* **2007**, *292*, R227–R234. [CrossRef]

167. Raffan, E. The big problem: Battling companion animal obesity. *Vet. Rec.* **2013**, *173*, 287–291. [CrossRef] [PubMed]

168. Kooistra, H.S.; Galac, S.; Buijtels, J.J.; Meij, B.P. Endocrine diseases in animals. *Horm. Res.* **2009**, *71* (Suppl. S1), S144–S147. [CrossRef] [PubMed]

169. Van de Velde, H.; Janssens, G.P.; de Rooster, H.; Polis, I.; Peters, I.; Ducatelle, R.; Nguyen, P.; Buyse, J.; Rochus, K.; Xu, J.; et al. The cat as a model for human obesity: Insights into depot-specific inflammation associated with feline obesity. *Br. J. Nutr.* **2013**, *110*, 1326–1335. [CrossRef] [PubMed]

170. Jordan, E.; Kley, S.; Le, N.A.; Waldron, M.; Hoenig, M. Dyslipidemia in obese cats. *Domest. Anim. Endocrinol.* **2008**, *35*, 290–299. [CrossRef] [PubMed]

171. Hoenig, M. The cat as a model for human obesity and diabetes. *J. Diabetes Sci. Technol.* **2012**, *6*, 525–533. [CrossRef] [PubMed]

172. Rand, J.S.; Fleeman, L.M.; Farrow, H.A.; Appleton, D.J.; Lederer, R. Canine and feline diabetes mellitus: Nature or nurture? *J. Nutr.* **2004**, *134*, 2072S–2080S. [CrossRef]

173. Osto, M.; Lutz, T.A. Translational value of animal models of obesity-Focus on dogs and cats. *Eur. J. Pharmacol.* **2015**, *759*, 240–252. [CrossRef]

174. Osto, M.; Zini, E.; Reusch, C.E.; Lutz, T.A. Diabetes from humans to cats. *Gen. Comp. Endocrinol.* **2013**, *182*, 48–53. [CrossRef]

175. Zini, E.; Osto, M.; Franchini, M.; Guscetti, F.; Donath, M.Y.; Perren, A.; Heller, R.S.; Linscheid, P.; Bouwman, M.; Ackermann, M.; et al. Hyperglycaemia but not hyperlipidaemia causes beta cell dysfunction and beta cell loss in the domestic cat. *Diabetologia* **2009**, *52*, 336–346. [CrossRef]

176. Clark, M.; Hoenig, M. Metabolic Effects of Obesity and Its Interaction with Endocrine Diseases. *Vet. Clin. N. Am. Small Anim. Pract.* **2016**, *46*, 797–815. [CrossRef]

177. Häring, T.; Haase, B.; Zini, E.; Hartnack, S.; Uebelhart, D.; Gaudenz, D.; Wichert, B.A. Overweight and impaired insulin sensitivity present in growing cats. *J. Anim. Physiol. Anim. Nutr. (Berl.)* **2013**, *97*, 813–819. [CrossRef] [PubMed]

178. Center, S.A.; Crawford, M.A.; Guida, L.; Erb, H.N.; King, J. A retrospective study of 77 cats with severe hepatic lipidosis: 1975-1990. *J. Vet. Intern. Med.* **1993**, *7*, 349–359. [CrossRef] [PubMed]

179. Verbrugghe, A.; Bakovic, M. Peculiarities of one-carbon metabolism in the strict carnivorous cat and the role in feline hepatic lipidosis. *Nutrients* **2013**, *5*, 2811–2835. [CrossRef] [PubMed]

180. Corbee, R.J. Obesity in show cats. *J. Anim. Physiol. Anim. Nutr. (Berl.)* **2014**, *98*, 1075–1080. [CrossRef]

181. Ohlund, M.; Palmgren, M.; Holst, B.S. Overweight in adult cats: A cross-sectional study. *Acta Vet. Scand.* **2018**, *60*, 5. [CrossRef]

182. Colliard, L.; Paragon, B.M.; Lemuet, B.; Benet, J.J.; Blanchard, G. Prevalence and risk factors of obesity in an urban population of healthy cats. *J. Feline Med. Surg.* **2009**, *11*, 135–140. [CrossRef]

183. Alhaddad, H.; Khan, R.; Grahn, R.A.; Gandolfi, B.; Mullikin, J.C.; Cole, S.A.; Gruffydd-Jones, T.J.; Haggstrom, J.; Lohi, H.; Longeri, M.; et al. Extent of linkage disequilibrium in the domestic cat, Felis silvestris catus, and its breeds. *PLoS ONE* **2013**, *8*, e53537. [CrossRef]

184. Zhang, W.; Schoenebeck, J.J. The ninth life of the cat reference genome, Felis_catus. *PLoS Genet.* **2020**, *16*, e1009045. [CrossRef]

185. Forcada, Y.; Holder, A.; Church, D.B.; Catchpole, B. A polymorphism in the melanocortin 4 receptor gene (MC4R:c.92C>T) is associated with diabetes mellitus in overweight domestic shorthaired cats. *J. Vet. Intern. Med.* **2014**, *28*, 458–464. [CrossRef]

186. Häring, T.; Wichert, B.; Dolf, G.; Haase, B. Segregation analysis of overweight body condition in an experimental cat population. *J. Hered.* **2011**, *102* (Suppl. S1), S28–S31.

187. Wichert, B.; Trossen, J.; Uebelhart, D.; Wanner, M.; Hartnack, S. Energy requirement and food intake behaviour in young adult intact male cats with and without predisposition to overweight. *Sci. World J.* **2012**, *2012*, 509854. [CrossRef] [PubMed]

188. Speakman, J.R.; Levitsky, D.A.; Allison, D.B.; Bray, M.S.; de Castro, J.M.; Clegg, D.J.; Clapham, J.C.; Dulloo, A.G.; Gruer, L.; Haw, S.; et al. Set points, settling points and some alternative models: Theoretical options to understand how genes and environments combine to regulate body adiposity. *Dis. Model. Mech.* **2011**, *4*, 733–745. [CrossRef] [PubMed]

189. Ghielmetti, V.; Wichert, B.; Ruegg, S.; Frey, D.; Liesegang, A. Food intake and energy expenditure in growing cats with and without a predisposition to overweight. *J. Anim. Physiol. Anim. Nutr. (Berl.)* **2018**, *102*, 1401–1410. [CrossRef]

190. Keller, C.; Liesegang, A.; Frey, D.; Wichert, B. Metabolic response to three different diets in lean cats and cats predisposed to overweight. *BMC Vet. Res.* **2017**, *13*, 184. [CrossRef] [PubMed]

191. Wichert, B.; Häring, T.; Dolf, G.; Trossen, J.; Haase, B.; Szymecko, R.; Iben, C.; Burlikowska, K.; Sitkowska, B. Feline Bodyweight: Genetic Aspects of Food Intake. In Proceedings of the 16th Congress of the European Society of Veterinary and Comparative Nutrition, Bydgoszcz, Poland, 13–15 September 2012; European Society of Veterinary & Comparative Nutrition: Zürich, Switzerland, 2012; Volume 31.

192. Zobel, D.P.; Andreasen, C.H.; Grarup, N.; Eiberg, H.; Sorensen, T.I.; Sandbaek, A.; Lauritzen, T.; Borch-Johnsen, K.; Jorgensen, T.; Pedersen, O.; et al. Variants near MC4R are associated with obesity and influence obesity-related quantitative traits in a population of middle-aged people: Studies of 14,940 Danes. *Diabetes* **2009**, *58*, 757–764. [CrossRef]

193. Cauchi, S.; Stutzmann, F.; Cavalcanti-Proenca, C.; Durand, E.; Pouta, A.; Hartikainen, A.L.; Marre, M.; Vol, S.; Tammelin, T.; Laitinen, J.; et al. Combined effects of MC4R and FTO common genetic variants on obesity in European general populations. *J. Mol. Med. (Berl.)* **2009**, *87*, 537–546. [CrossRef]

194. Forcada, Y.; Boursnell, M.; Catchpole, B.; Church, D.B. A Genome-Wide Association Study Identifies Novel Candidate Genes for Susceptibility to Diabetes Mellitus in DSH Cats. In Proceedings of the Conference Proceedings: 25th ECVIM-CA Congress, Lisbon, Portugal, 10–12 September 2015.

195. Forcada, Y.; Boursnell, M.; Catchpole, B.; Church, D.B. A Genome-Wide Association Study Identifies Novel Candidate Genes for the Susceptibility to Diabetes Mellitus in DSH Cats. In Proceedings of the Conference Proceedings: ACVIM, Am College Vet Internal Med Forum, Denver, CO, USA, 9–11 June 2016.

196. Hazuchova, H.; Wallace, M.; Church, D.B.; Catchpole, B.; Forcada, Y. Analysis of GWAS Data in Domestic Shorthair and Burmese Cats Identifies Diabetes-associated Loci Near the DPP9 and Within the DPP10 Gene. In Proceedings of the Conference Proceedings: 29th ECVIM-CA Congress, European Coll Vet Int Med, Milano, Italy, 19–21 September 2019.

197. Rendle, D.; McGregor-Argo, C.; Bowen, M.; Carslake, H.; German, A.; Harris, P.; Knowles, E.; Menzies-Gow, N.; Morgan, R. Equine obesity: Current perspectives. *UK Vet. Equine* **2018**, *2*, 1–19. [CrossRef]

198. McCue, M.E.; Geor, R.J.; Schultz, N. Equine metabolic syndrome: A complex disease influenced by genetics and the environment. *J. Equine Vet. Sci.* **2015**, *35*, 367–375. [CrossRef]

199. Thatcher, C.D.; Pleasant, R.S.; Geor, R.J.; Elvinger, F. Prevalence of overconditioning in mature horses in southwest Virginia during the summer. *J. Vet. Intern. Med.* **2012**, *26*, 1413–1418. [CrossRef]

200. Stephenson, H.M.; Green, M.J.; Freeman, S.L. Prevalence of obesity in a population of horses in the UK. *Vet. Rec.* **2011**, *168*, 131. [CrossRef]

201. Johnson, P.J. The equine metabolic syndrome peripheral Cushing's syndrome. *Vet. Clin. N. Am. Equine Pract.* **2002**, *18*, 271–293. [CrossRef]

202. Durham, A.E.; Frank, N.; McGowan, C.M.; Menzies-Gow, N.J.; Roelfsema, E.; Vervuert, I.; Feige, K.; Fey, K. ECEIM consensus statement on equine metabolic syndrome. *J. Vet. Intern. Med.* **2019**, *33*, 335–349. [CrossRef] [PubMed]

203. de Laat, M.A.; McGree, J.M.; Sillence, M.N. Equine hyperinsulinemia: Investigation of the enteroinsular axis during insulin dysregulation. *Am. J. Physiol. Endocrinol. Metab.* **2016**, *310*, E61–E72. [CrossRef] [PubMed]

204. Potter, S.J.; Bamford, N.J.; Harris, P.A.; Bailey, S.R. Prevalence of obesity and owners' perceptions of body condition in pleasure horses and ponies in south-eastern Australia. *Aust. Vet. J.* **2016**, *94*, 427–432. [CrossRef] [PubMed]

205. Giles, S.L.; Rands, S.A.; Nicol, C.J.; Harris, P.A. Obesity prevalence and associated risk factors in outdoor living domestic horses and ponies. *PeerJ* **2014**, *2*, e299. [CrossRef]

206. Morrison, P.K.; Harris, P.A.; Maltin, C.A.; Grove-White, D.; Barfoot, C.F.; Argo, C.M. Perceptions of obesity and management practices in a UK population of leisure-horse owners and managers. *J. Equine Vet. Sci.* **2017**, *53*, 19–29. [CrossRef]

207. Jensen, R.B.; Danielsen, S.H.; Tauson, A.H. Body condition score, morphometric measurements and estimation of body weight in mature Icelandic horses in Denmark. *Acta Vet. Scand.* **2016**, *58*, 59. [CrossRef]

208. Harker, I.J.; Harris, P.A.; Barfoot, C.F. The body condition score of leisure horses competing at an unaffiliated championship in the UK. *J. Equine Vet. Sci.* **2011**, *5*, 253–254. [CrossRef]

209. Sánchez-Guerrero, M.J.; Ramos, J.; Valdés, M.; Valera, M. Prevalence, Environmental Risk Factors and Heritability of Body Condition in Pura Raza Español Horses. *Livest. Sci.* **2019**, *230*, 103851. [CrossRef]

210. Bamford, N.J.; Potter, S.J.; Harris, P.A.; Bailey, S.R. Breed differences in insulin sensitivity and insulinemic responses to oral glucose in horses and ponies of moderate body condition score. *Domest. Anim. Endocrinol.* **2014**, *47*, 101–107. [CrossRef]

211. Freestone, J.F.; Shoemaker, K.; Bessin, R.; Wolfsheimer, J.K. Insulin and glucose response following oral glucose administration in well-conditioned ponies. *Equine Vet. J. Suppl.* **1992**, 13–17. [CrossRef] [PubMed]

212. Jeffcott, L.B.; Field, J.R.; McLean, J.G.; O'Dea, K. Glucose tolerance and insulin sensitivity in ponies and Standardbred horses. *Equine Vet. J.* **1986**, *18*, 97–101. [CrossRef] [PubMed]

213. Robie, S.M.; Janson, C.H.; Smith, S.C.; O'Connor, J.T., Jr. Equine serum lipids: Serum lipids and glucose in Morgan and Thoroughbred horses and Shetland ponies. *Am. J. Vet. Res.* **1975**, *36*, 1705–1708. [PubMed]

214. Norton, E.M.; Schultz, N.E.; Rendahl, A.K.; Mcfarlane, D.; Geor, R.J.; Mickelson, J.R.; McCue, M.E. Heritability of Metabolic Traits Associated with Equine Metabolic Syndrome in Welsh Ponies and Morgan Horses. *Equine Vet. J.* **2019**, *51*, 475–480. [CrossRef]

215. Treiber, K.H.; Kronfeld, D.S.; Hess, T.M.; Byrd, B.M.; Splan, R.K.; Staniar, W.B. Evaluation of genetic and metabolic predispositions and nutritional risk factors for pasture-associated laminitis in ponies. *J. Am. Vet. Med. Assoc.* **2006**, *228*, 1538–1545. [CrossRef] [PubMed]

216. Lewis, S.L.; Holl, H.M.; Streeter, C.; Posbergh, C.; Schanbacher, B.J.; Place, N.J.; Mallicote, M.F.; Long, M.T.; Brooks, S.A. Genomewide association study reveals a risk locus for equine metabolic syndrome in the Arabian horse. *J. Anim. Sci.* **2017**, *95*, 1071–1079. [CrossRef] [PubMed]

217. Cash, C.M.; Fitzgerald, D.M.; Spence, R.J.; de Laat, M.A. Preliminary analysis of the FAM174A gene suggests it lacks a strong association with equine metabolic syndrome in ponies. *Domest. Anim. Endocrinol.* **2020**, *72*, 106439. [CrossRef] [PubMed]

218. Roy, M.M.; Norton, E.M.; Rendahl, A.K.; Schultz, N.E.; McFarlane, D.; Geor, R.J.; Mickelson, J.R.; McCue, M.E. Assessment of the FAM174A 11G allele as a risk allele for equine metabolic syndrome. *Anim. Genet.* **2020**, *51*, 607–610. [CrossRef]

219. Norton, E.; Schultz, N.; Geor, R.; McFarlane, D.; Mickelson, J.; McCue, M. Genome-Wide Association Analyses of Equine Metabolic Syndrome Phenotypes in Welsh Ponies and Morgan Horses. *Genes (Basel)* **2019**, *10*, 893. [CrossRef]

220. Norton, E.M.; Avila, F.; Schultz, N.E.; Mickelson, J.R.; Geor, R.J.; McCue, M.E. Evaluation of an HMGA2 variant for pleiotropic effects on height and metabolic traits in ponies. *J. Vet. Intern. Med.* **2019**, *33*, 942–952. [CrossRef]

221. Martin, A.R.; Kanai, M.; Kamatani, Y.; Okada, Y.; Neale, B.M.; Daly, M.J. Clinical use of current polygenic risk scores may exacerbate health disparities. *Nat. Genet.* **2019**, *51*, 584–591. [CrossRef] [PubMed]

222. Hayward, J.J.; Castelhano, M.G.; Oliveira, K.C.; Corey, E.; Balkman, C.; Baxter, T.L.; Casal, M.L.; Center, S.A.; Fang, M.; Garrison, S.J.; et al. Complex disease and phenotype mapping in the domestic dog. *Nat. Commun.* **2016**, *7*, 10460. [CrossRef] [PubMed]

223. Dodman, N.H.; Karlsson, E.K.; Moon-Fanelli, A.; Galdzicka, M.; Perloski, M.; Shuster, L.; Lindblad-Toh, K.; Ginns, E.I. A canine chromosome 7 locus confers compulsive disorder susceptibility. *Mol. Psychiatry* **2010**, *15*, 8–10. [CrossRef] [PubMed]

224. Hoeppner, M.P.; Lundquist, A.; Pirun, M.; Meadows, J.R.; Zamani, N.; Johnson, J.; Sundstrom, G.; Cook, A.; FitzGerald, M.G.; Swofford, R.; et al. An improved canine genome and a comprehensive catalogue of coding genes and non-coding transcripts. *PLoS ONE* **2014**, *9*, e91172. [CrossRef]

225. Halo, J.; Pendelton, A.L.; Shen, F.; Doucet, A.J.; Derrien, T.; Hitte, C.; Kirby, L.E.; Myers, B.; Sliwerska, E.; Emery, S.; et al. Preprint—Long-read assembly of a Great Dane genome highlights the contribution of GC-rich sequence and mobile elements to canine genomes. *bioRxiv* **2020**. preprints. [CrossRef]

226. Bannasch, D.; Young, A.; Myers, J.; Truve, K.; Dickinson, P.; Gregg, J.; Davis, R.; Bongcam-Rudloff, E.; Webster, M.T.; Lindblad-Toh, K.; et al. Localization of canine brachycephaly using an across breed mapping approach. *PLoS ONE* **2010**, *5*, e9632. [CrossRef]

227. Friedenberg, S.G.; Meurs, K.M. Genotype imputation in the domestic dog. *Mamm. Genome* **2016**, *27*, 485–494. [CrossRef]

228. Hayward, J.J.; White, M.E.; Boyle, M.; Shannon, L.M.; Casal, M.L.; Castelhano, M.G.; Center, S.A.; Meyers-Wallen, V.N.; Simpson, K.W.; Sutter, N.B.; et al. Imputation of canine genotype array data using 365 whole-genome sequences improves power of genome-wide association studies. *PLoS Genet.* **2019**, *15*, e1008003. [CrossRef]

229. Gandolfi, B.; Alhaddad, H.; Abdi, M.; Bach, L.H.; Creighton, E.K.; Davis, B.W.; Decker, J.E.; Dodman, N.H.; Ginns, E.I.; Grahn, J.C.; et al. Applications and efficiencies of the first cat 63K DNA array. *Sci. Rep.* **2018**, *8*, 7024. [CrossRef]

230. Kalbfleisch, T.S.; Rice, E.S.; DePriest, M.S.; Walenz, B.P.; Hestand, M.S.; Vermeesch, J.R.; O'Connell, B.L.; Fiddes, I.T.; Vershinina, A.O.; Petersen, J.L.; et al. Preprint—EquCab3, an updated reference genome for the domestic horse. *bioRxiv* **2018**, 306928. [CrossRef]

231. McCue, M.E.; Bannasch, D.L.; Petersen, J.L.; Gurr, J.; Bailey, E.; Binns, M.M.; Distl, O.; Guerin, G.; Hasegawa, T.; Hill, E.W.; et al. A high density SNP array for the domestic horse and extant Perissodactyla: Utility for association mapping, genetic diversity, and phylogeny studies. *PLoS Genet.* **2012**, *8*, e1002451. [CrossRef]

232. Schaefer, R.J.; Schubert, M.; Bailey, E.; Bannasch, D.L.; Barrey, E.; Bar-Gal, G.K.; Brem, G.; Brooks, S.A.; Distl, O.; Fries, R.; et al. Developing a 670k genotyping array to tag ~2M SNPs across 24 horse breeds. *BMC Genom.* **2017**, *18*, 565. [CrossRef] [PubMed]

233. Schaefer, R.J.; McCue, M.E. Equine Genotyping Arrays. *Vet. Clin. N. Am. Equine Pract.* **2020**, *36*, 183–193. [CrossRef]

234. Chassier, M.; Barrey, E.; Robert, C.; Duluard, A.; Danvy, S.; Ricard, A. Genotype imputation accuracy in multiple equine breeds from medium- to high-density genotypes. *J. Anim. Breed. Genet.* **2018**, *135*, 420–431. [CrossRef] [PubMed]

235. Samaha, G.; Beatty, J.; Wade, C.M.; Haase, B. The Burmese cat as a genetic model of type 2 diabetes in humans. *Anim. Genet.* **2019**, *50*, 319–325. [CrossRef] [PubMed]

236. Brito-Casillas, Y.; Melian, C.; Wagner, A.M. Study of the pathogenesis and treatment of diabetes mellitus through animal models. *Endocrinol. Nutr.* **2016**, *63*, 345–353. [CrossRef]

237. Srinivasan, K.; Ramarao, P. Animal models in type 2 diabetes research: An overview. *Indian J. Med. Res.* **2007**, *125*, 451–472.

238. Rimbault, M.; Ostrander, E.A. So many doggone traits: Mapping genetics of multiple phenotypes in the domestic dog. *Hum. Mol. Genet.* **2012**, *21*, R52–R57. [CrossRef]

239. Shearin, A.L.; Ostrander, E.A. Leading the way: Canine models of genomics and disease. *Dis. Model. Mech.* **2010**, *3*, 27–34. [CrossRef]

240. Switonski, M. Dog as a model in studies on human hereditary diseases and their gene therapy. *Reprod. Biol.* **2014**, *14*, 44–50. [CrossRef]

241. Momozawa, Y.; Merveille, A.C.; Battaille, G.; Wiberg, M.; Koch, J.; Willesen, J.L.; Proschowsky, H.F.; Gouni, V.; Chetboul, V.; Tiret, L.; et al. Genome wide association study of 40 clinical measurements in eight dog breeds. *Sci. Rep.* **2020**, *10*, 6520. [CrossRef]

242. Sutter, N.B.; Eberle, M.A.; Parker, H.G.; Pullar, B.J.; Kirkness, E.F.; Kruglyak, L.; Ostrander, E.A. Extensive and breed-specific linkage disequilibrium in Canis familiaris. *Genome Res.* **2004**, *14*, 2388–2396. [CrossRef]

243. Marsden, C.D.; Ortega-Del Vecchyo, D.; O'Brien, D.P.; Taylor, J.F.; Ramirez, O.; Vila, C.; Marques-Bonet, T.; Schnabel, R.D.; Wayne, R.K.; Lohmueller, K.E. Bottlenecks and selective sweeps during domestication have increased deleterious genetic variation in dogs. *Proc. Natl. Acad. Sci. USA* **2016**, *113*, 152–157. [CrossRef] [PubMed]

244. Gurda, B.L.; Bradbury, A.M.; Vite, C.H. Canine and Feline Models of Human Genetic Diseases and Their Contributions to Advancing Clinical Therapies. *Yale J. Biol. Med.* **2017**, *90*, 417–431. [PubMed]

245. Oh, A.; Pearce, J.W.; Gandolfi, B.; Ceighton, E.K.; Suedmeyer, W.K.; Selig, M.; Bosiack, A.P.; Castaner, L.J.; Whiting, R.E.; Belknap, E.B.; et al. Early-Onset Progressive Retinal Atrophy Associated with an IQCB1 Variant in African Black-Footed Cats (Felis nigripes). *Sci. Rep.* **2017**, *7*, 43918. [CrossRef] [PubMed]

246. Lonker, N.S.; Fechner, K.; Wahed, A.A.E. Horses as a Crucial Part of One Health. *Vet. Sci.* **2020**, *7*, 28. [CrossRef]

17

A Missense Variant in *ALDH5A1* Associated with Canine Succinic Semialdehyde Dehydrogenase Deficiency (SSADHD) in the Saluki Dog

Karen M. Vernau [1,*], Eduard Struys [2], Anna Letko [3], Kevin D. Woolard [4], Miriam Aguilar [5], Emily A. Brown [5], Derek D. Cissell [1], Peter J. Dickinson [1], G. Diane Shelton [6], Michael R. Broome [7], K. Michael Gibson [8], Phillip L. Pearl [9], Florian König [10], Thomas J. Van Winkle [11], Dennis O'Brien [12], B. Roos [2], Kaspar Matiasek [13], Vidhya Jagannathan [3], Cord Drögemüller [3], Tamer A. Mansour [5,14], C. Titus Brown [5] and Danika L. Bannasch [5,*]

[1] Department of Surgical and Radiological Sciences, University of California Davis, Davis, CA 95616, USA; ddcissell@ucdavis.edu (D.D.C.); pjdickinson@ucdavis.edu (P.J.D.)

[2] Department of Clinical Chemistry, VU University Medical Center, 1081 HV Amsterdam, The Netherlands; E.Struys@vumc.nl (E.S.); b.roos@amsterdamumc.nl (B.R.)

[3] Institute of Genetics, Vetsuisse Faculty, University of Bern, 3001 Bern, Switzerland; anna.letko@vetsuisse.unibe.ch (A.L.); vidhya.jagannathan@vetsuisse.unibe.ch (V.J.); cord.droegemueller@vetsuisse.unibe.ch (C.D.)

[4] Department of Pathology, Microbiology and Immunology, University of California Davis, Davis, CA 95616, USA; kdwoolard@ucdavis.edu

[5] Department of Population Health and Reproduction, University of California Davis, Davis, CA 95616, USA; miraguilar@ucdavis.edu (M.A.); eabrown@ucdavis.edu (E.A.B.); drtamermansour@gmail.com (T.A.M.); ctbrown@ucdavis.edu (C.T.B.)

[6] Department of Pathology, University of California San Diego, La Jolla, CA 92093, USA; gshelton@health.ucsd.edu

[7] Advanced Veterinary Medical Imaging, Tustin, CA 92780, USA; mbroome@avmi.net

[8] College of Pharmacy and Pharmaceutical Sciences, Washington State University, Spokane, WA 99202, USA; mike.gibson@wsu.edu

[9] Harvard Medical School, Boston, MA 02115, USA; Phillip.Pearl@childrens.harvard.edu

[10] Fachtierarzt fur Kleintiere, Am Berggewann 13, 65199 Wiesbaden, Germany; fk@neurovet.de

[11] Department of Pathobiology, School of Veterinary Medicine, University of Pennsylvania, Philadelphia, PA 19104, USA; tomvw@vet.upenn.edu

[12] College of Veterinary Medicine, University of Missouri, Columbia, MO 65211, USA; ObrienD@missouri.edu

[13] Clinical and Comparative Neuropathology, Ludwig-Maximilians-Universitaet München, 80539 Munchen, Germany; kaspar.matiasek@neuropathologie.de

[14] Department of Clinical Pathology, School of Medicine, Mansoura University, Mansoura 35516, Egypt

*   Correspondence: kmvernau@ucdavis.edu (K.M.V.); dlbannasch@ucdavis.edu (D.L.B.)

Abstract: Dogs provide highly valuable models of human disease due to the similarity in phenotype presentation and the ease of genetic analysis. Seven Saluki puppies were investigated for neurological abnormalities including seizures and altered behavior. Magnetic resonance imaging showed a diffuse, marked reduction in cerebral cortical thickness, and symmetrical T2 hyperintensity in specific brain regions. Cerebral cortical atrophy with vacuolation (status spongiosus) was noted on necropsy. Genome-wide association study of 7 affected and 28 normal Salukis revealed a genome-wide significantly associated region on CFA 35. Whole-genome sequencing of three confirmed cases from three different litters revealed a homozygous missense variant within the aldehyde dehydrogenase 5 family member A1 (*ALDH5A1*) gene (XM_014110599.2: c.866G>A; XP_013966074.2: p.(Gly288Asp)). *ALDH5A1* encodes a succinic semialdehyde dehydrogenase (SSADH) enzyme critical in the gamma-aminobutyric acid neurotransmitter (GABA) metabolic pathway. Metabolic screening of affected dogs showed markedly elevated gamma-hydroxybutyric acid in serum, cerebrospinal fluid

(CSF) and brain, and elevated succinate semialdehyde in urine, CSF and brain. SSADH activity in the brain of affected dogs was low. Affected Saluki dogs had striking similarities to SSADH deficiency in humans although hydroxybutyric aciduria was absent in affected dogs. *ALDH5A1*-related SSADH deficiency in Salukis provides a unique translational large animal model for the development of novel therapeutic strategies.

Keywords: inborn error of metabolism; encephalopathy; SSADHD; *ALDH5A1*; GABA; 4-hydroxybutyric acid; succinic semialdehyde; encephalopathy; whole-genome sequencing; precision medicine; GWAS; inherited

1. Introduction

Inborn errors of metabolism (IEMs) are a group of diseases caused by an enzymatic deficiency in a metabolic pathway, most commonly caused by a genetic mutation. While individually these diseases are rare, as a group they are relatively common, with more than 500 IEM diseases reported in people [1]; in animals, they are becoming increasingly recognized [2–6]. In diseases caused by an IEM, clinical signs are due to the reduced or lack of production of a biochemical product, or accumulation of an abnormal amount of substrate or substrates produced by alternative metabolic pathways, secondary to the enzymatic deficiency. The diagnosis of an IEM may be a challenging, as clinical signs can be vague and non-specific, and targeted diagnostic testing is required [7]. IEMs are often recognized in young people and animals, and many have neurological manifestations [8,9].

Seizures are a common neurological sign in dogs [10]. Disorders causing seizures arise either extracranially (reactive seizures), or intracranially [11] Epilepsy is a brain disease characterized by a lasting predisposition to generate seizures, which is classified in dogs as structural epilepsy or idiopathic epilepsy (OMIA 000344-9615) [11]. Causes of structural epilepsy include inflammation (e.g., granulomatous meningoencephalitis), neoplasia, nutritional alterations (e.g., thiamine deficiency), infection, anomalous entities (e.g., hydrocephalus), inborn errors of metabolism and trauma [11]. Dogs with idiopathic epilepsy (IE) are typically 6 months to 6 years of age and usually have normal physical and neurological examinations between seizures [12]. Dogs younger than 6 months or older than 6 years of age usually have reactive seizures or structural epilepsy, rather than idiopathic epilepsy [12].

A seizure disorder reported in Salukis is called central nervous system status spongiosus in Saluki dogs (SSSD). There are only brief reports of this disease in the literature [13,14]. One affected 8-month-old male puppy from a litter of 9 was reported with a 5 month history of seizures and behavioral changes. The sire and dam were full siblings. All nine puppies and the sire were euthanized; pathological changes were noted in the affected puppy and in two clinically normal littermates, and the rest of the puppies and the sire were pathologically normal. Pathological changes in the clinically affected puppy included widespread bilaterally symmetrical status spongiosis of the cerebrum, brainstem and cerebellum at the grey–white matter junction, which extended into both the grey and white matter. There were also lesions in the thalamus, optic nerve and internal capsule but no lesions were noted in the spinal cord [13].

Recognized causes of early-onset symmetrical brain lesions include metabolic, nutritional and toxin-induced diseases [15]. In Saluki dogs with SSSD, the clinical signs and lesions on MRI and pathology appear to be breed specific, identical in distribution and type, and diagnosed in multiple dogs over a long period of time (1987 [13] to 2020). Clinical signs developed while puppies were still with the breeders, making toxicity a less likely cause; pathology differed from previously reported nutritional [16] or toxic [17–19] central nervous system problems, and thus a genetic cause was considered most likely. Although a metabolic disorder was not identified by routine diagnostic testing in affected Salukis, an underlying genetic abnormality causing a metabolic problem was most likely based on the age of onset of clinical signs.

The purpose of this study was to define the phenotype of Salukis with SSSD and to determine the underlying genetic cause in this breed. Comprehensive evaluations including MRI and necropsy, as well as metabolic and enzyme activity testing, were performed on urine, serum, cerebrospinal fluid and brain tissue from four affected puppies from two litters from the USA and a litter with three affected puppies from Germany. All seven affected dogs were used for a genome-wide association study (GWAS) followed by whole-genome sequence analysis of three affected puppies, which identified a private homozygous missense variant in the canine *ALDH5A1* gene.

2. Materials and Methods

2.1. Affected Dogs

From 2005 to 2015, seven Saluki dogs affected with SSSD from the USA (4) and Germany (3) had DNA collected. Four dogs were examined—three dogs at the William R. Pritchard Veterinary Medical Teaching Hospital at the University of California Davis (UCD) and one dog was evaluated at Fachtierarzt fur Kleintiere, in Wiesbaden, Germany. All 4 dogs were presented by their breeders for examination. A fifth Saluki dog affected with SSSD from the USA had a necropsy completed at UCD Two additional German dogs were not evaluated clinically beyond the breeder's description of the clinical signs.

2.2. Control Dogs

2.2.1. MRI Evaluation

Four unaffected Saluki dogs related to the affected USA Saluki dogs were examined and had magnetic resonance imaging of their brain and completed at Advanced Veterinary Medicine Imaging in Los Angeles, California.

2.2.2. Targeted Metabolic Testing

Archived urine = 4, serum = 4, cerebrospinal fluid (3) and brain tissue (4) from 15 different non-Saluki dogs unaffected by SSSD were utilized as control samples.

2.3. Affected Saluki Dogs

Blood work (complete blood count, and serum biochemical profile) was performed by the referring veterinarians in two dogs (dogs 3 and 4). Cerebrospinal fluid sample (CSF) was collected in two dogs (dogs 1 and 5). One CSF sample was routinely analyzed in Germany and the other sample was collected at UCD and frozen at −80 degrees for further analysis. Two dogs had quantitative urine organic acid testing completed at the University of California San Diego Biochemical Genetics Laboratory (dogs 1 and 2). Urine was shipped to the lab by the breeder and was analyzed by the lab 18 days later. Four dogs had complete necropsies completed at UCD, and one had a necropsy at Ludwig Maximilians Universität München in Germany. The owners consented to the necropsy and processing of postmortem samples. Following necropsy, the brain was immediately immersed in 10% neutral buffered formalin followed by standard paraffin embedding. Selected regions were sectioned at 5 μm slice thickness and stained with hematoxylin-eosin and luxol fast blue-cresyl violet.

MRI and Histopathology

Six Saluki dogs underwent MRI of the brain—two affected Saluki dogs underwent magnetic resonance imaging (MRI) of the brain at UC Davis, and four unaffected Saluki dogs had imaging of the brain at Advanced Veterinary Medicine Imaging in Los Angeles, California. Both locations used a 1.5 T MRI system (GE Signa, GE Healthcare, Waukesha, WI, USA), with paired 5″ general purpose radiofrequency coils. Sagittal T1-weighted (T1W) and T2-weighted (T2W) images, transverse T1W, T2W, fluid attenuating inversion recovery (FLAIR), and T2*-weighted (T2*W) images, and dorsal T2W images were acquired of the brain. Sagittal, transverse, and dorsal T1W images were repeated after intravenous administration of 0.1 mmol/kg gadopentetate dimeglumine (Magnevist, Bayer, Whippany, NJ, USA).

2.4. Sample Collection and DNA Extraction

Blood samples, pedigree, and phenotype information were collected from 7 affected dogs and 18 close relatives of affected dogs including 4 parents (Figure 1). Additional samples were collected from 48 healthy Saluki dogs. Healthy dogs of other breeds (n = 228) were used that were part of a DNA repository at UC Davis. DNA was extracted from EDTA whole blood samples using Gentra Puregene DNA purification extraction kit (Qiagen, Valencia, CA, USA). Collection of canine samples was approved by the University of California, Davis Animal Care and Use Committee (protocol #18561) and the Cantonal Committee for Animal Experiments (Canton of Bern; permit 75/16).

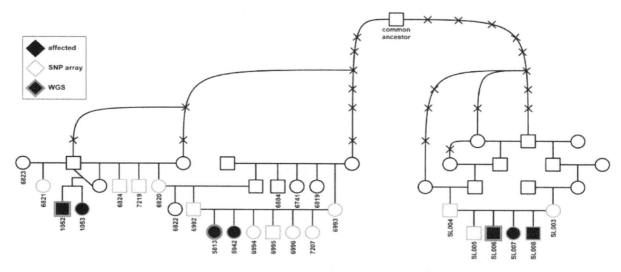

Figure 1. Pedigree of seven succinic semialdehyde dehydrogenase deficiency (SSADHD)-affected Saluki dogs. Females are depicted by circles and males by squares. Black fill indicates affected puppies. Numbers indicate 25 dogs from which samples were available. The blue contour indicates animals that were genotyped on SNP array, and the red contour the three affected dogs selected for the WGS. Note that the two litters on the left were seen in the USA and the third litter on the right in Germany. A common male ancestor illustrates the genealogical relatedness.

2.5. Genome-Wide Association Scan

SNP genotyping was performed using the Illumina Canine HD 174,000 SNP array (Illumina, San Diego, CA, USA) for 7 affected cases and 28 neurologically normal adult Saluki controls. Genome-wide association analysis was performed using Plink [20]. SNPs were pruned from analysis if the minor allele frequency was <5% and the call rate <90%. Chi-square association analysis, Bonferroni adjustments, and genomic inflation calculations were performed in Plink. Figure 5 was made in R using ggplot2 [21,22].

2.6. Whole-Genome Sequence

Whole-genome sequencing (WGS) was performed on the two affected Salukis from the USA and compared to 98 controls dogs from various breeds as reported, and coverage was 6.4× for 1052 and 5.3× for 5813 SRA: SRR5311685 and SRR5311664 (study: PRJNA377155) [23]. Segregation of variants was performed using 2 cases compared to 98 controls within the homozygous interval identified by visual inspection of genotype calls from the array data. Variant Effect Predictor (VEP), as employed in Ensembl using Refseq annotation and additional EST/CCDs, was used to predict the effect of segregating variants [24]. Polyphen2 [25] and SIFT [26] were used to evaluate the severity of the missense variants.

In one German Saluki (dog 5), whole-genome sequencing using genomic DNA isolated from the blood sample of the affected dog was performed as described previously [27]. Data corresponding to approximately 15× coverage of the genome was collected on an Illumina HiSeq2000 instrument (2 × 100 bp). Read mapping and variant calling were carried out as previously described [28], with respect to the CanFam3.1 genome reference assembly and the NCBI annotation release 105. Variant filtering was performed against 581 dog and 8 wolf genomes which were publicly available [28]. WGS data of the affected dog was made available under study accession PRJEB16012 at the European Nucleotide Archive.

Annotations within the canine *ALDH5A1* gene refer to the NCBI mRNA accession no. XM_014110599.2 and the protein accession no. XP_013966074.2. Annotations within the *GPLD1* gene refer to the NCBI mRNA accession no. XM_005640079.3 and the protein accession number XP_005640136.1. Annotations for the putative *PTCHD3* gene refer to the mRNA accession no. ENSCAFT00000039442.3 and the protein accession no. ENSCAFP00000035301.

2.7. Genotyping

The variant in *ALDH5A1* disrupted a Sau96I restriction enzyme site, allowing rapid genotyping by PCR-RFLP analysis. PCR primers were designed using primer 3 [29] to amplify an 872 bp product, which upon digestion with Sau96I produced 700 and 150 bp fragments for the variant allele and 550 and 150 bp fragments for the wild-type allele. All PCR was carried out using Qiagen HotStart DNA polymerase kit (Qiagen, Valencia, CA, USA) at an annealing temperature of 58 degrees using the following PCR primers: F_TCCCGAGTTAGGGGTTCTTT, R_TCACGTTTTCCTGATTTCACC. The same primers were used to verify the mutation by Sanger sequencing on an Applied Biosystems 3500 Genetic Analyzer using the Big Dye Terminator Sequencing Kit (Life Technologies, Burlington, ON, Canada).

2.8. RT-PCR

RT-PCR was performed for liver cDNA from a case and control. *RPS5* was included as a housekeeping gene control [27]. Primers were designed using Primer3 (SAL_2F: TTGTATTTGACAGC GCCAAC, SAL_2R: CAAGGCCAGATTGCTTCAC) except for RPS5, in which the primers were as recommended [30]. Each reaction included 13.9 μL of water, 2 μL of 10× buffer with MgCl$_2$, 1 μL of dNTP, 1 μL of each forward and reverse primers (20 μM), 1 μL of HotStarTaq DNA Polymerase (Qiagen, Valenica, CA, USA), and 1 μL of cDNA made from 1000 ng of RNA. Amplified products were visualized on a 2% agarose gel.

2.9. Targeted Metabolic Testing

Gamma-hydroxybutyrate (GHB) and succinate semialdehyde (SSA):
GHB and SSA in fluids and brain tissue were quantified by isotope dilution mass spectrometric methodology, as previously described [31,32].
The 4,5-dihydroxyhexanoic acid (DHHA):
Analysis of DHHA in fluids and brain was comparable to that for GHB as previously described [31], with some modifications. ^{2}H$_3$-DHHA was used as the internal standard and the samples were extracted a single time with ethylacetate. For quantitation, positive chemical ionization was employed.
Succinic semialdehyde dehydrogenase (SSADH) activity:
SSADH activity was quantified fluorometrically in brain tissue samples using the NADH/NAD couple and SSA as substrate, as previously described [33].

3. Results

3.1. Affected Dogs

Four dogs from two litters from the USA were closely related, and the third litter from Germany was distantly related to the other two litters. There were four females and three males affected (Figure 1).

3.2. Clinical Phenotype

The breeders of affected Saluki puppies noted that puppies were first abnormal between six and ten weeks of age. Historical clinical signs included seizures, abnormal behavior such as episodes of vocalization (Video S1, Supplementary Materials), and difficulty being aroused from sleep. Four puppies (dogs 1 and 3–5) were evaluated by a board-certified veterinary neurologist (Table 1). No abnormalities were noted on physical examination. On neurological examination, puppies had mild generalized ataxia with thoracic limb hypermetria (two puppies) (Video S2, Supplementary Materials), absent menace reflex in both eyes and delayed proprioceptive positioning in all four limbs, consistent with a multifocal disease process. Two dogs (dogs 3 and 4) had a normal CBC and serum biochemical profile completed by their referring veterinarian, and two dogs had normal quantitative urine organic acid analysis (Biochemical Genetics Laboratory, University of California San Diego, San Diego, CA, USA). One dog (dog 5) had a normal cisternal cerebrospinal fluid analysis. Five dogs were treated for seizures with oral phenobarbital or levetiracetam. Although clinical signs did not progress, all affected dogs were euthanized as puppies at the request of the breeders when they were still in their care. Puppies were euthanized between three and nine months of age for quality of life concerns, primarily due to the recurrent episodes of vocalization. Five dogs (dogs 1–5) had necropsies completed.

3.3. MRI and Histopathology

Two affected dogs (dogs 1 and 2) and four other related but unaffected dogs had an MRI of the brain. All four unaffected dogs had unremarkable MR images. Both affected dogs exhibited prominent sulci (Figure 2A,C–E) compared to normal dogs (Figure 2F), consistent with diffuse cortical atrophy. Bilateral, symmetrical, T2 and FLAIR hyperintensity was present in the diencephalon, deep cerebellar nuclei (Figure 2A–C), midbrain (Figure 2D), and multiple basal nuclei (Figure 2E). Multifocal, symmetrical T2 and FLAIR hyperintensity was also present in the deep cortical laminae of the grey matter throughout the cerebral cortex (Figure 2A–F).

No hypointense lesions or signal voids were observed associated within the brain parenchyma on T2*W images.

Histopathologically, there was severe bilaterally symmetric spongiform change, worse within the mesencephalon (Figure 3), brainstem, and deep cerebellar nuclei, but also severe in the thalamic nuclei and deep cortical grey matter. The corpus striatum was less affected but exhibited similar lesions most notably in the entopeduncular nuclei and putamen. Neurons exhibited single to multiple, clear, well-demarcated vacuoles that compressed and displaced the nucleus (Figure 4). There was marked proliferation of enlarged astrocytes associated with the spongiform change, and both neurons and astrocytes appear affected. The grey matter was more severely affected, particularly at the grey–white matter junction. The spinal cord was not affected.

Table 1. Clinical information for seven SSADHD-affected Saluki dogs. (OU = oculus uterque (both eyes)).

Dog No.	Sample ID	Country	Sex	Age of Onset	Clinical Signs	Neurological Examination	Outcome
1	5813	USA	F	10 weeks	Generalized epileptic seizures, episodes of vocalization, abnormal behavior, generalized ataxia with thoracic limb hypermetria	Mild generalized ataxia with thoracic limb hypermetria. Delayed proprioceptive positioning present in all 4 limbs	Treated with anticonvulsants (phenobarbital), euthanized at 32 weeks of age
2	4942	USA	F	10 weeks	Generalized epileptic seizures, episodes of vocalization, abnormal behavior, generalized ataxia with thoracic limb hypermetria	Not done	Treated with anticonvulsants (phenobarbital), euthanized at 39 weeks of age
3	1053	USA	F	6 weeks	Focal epileptic seizures, episodes of vocalization, normal between episodes. Unable to arouse when sleeping	Absent menace response OU	Treated with anticonvulsants (phenobarbital), euthanized at 17 weeks of age
4	1052	USA	M	6 weeks	Generalized and focal epileptic seizures, episodes of vocalization, normal between episodes. Unable to arouse when sleeping	Absent menace response OU	Treated with anticonvulsants (phenobarbital), euthanized at 17 weeks of age
5	SL006	Germany	M	9 weeks	Focal epileptic seizures, deep sleep	Thoracic limb hypermetria, mild ataxia, reduced proprioceptive positioning, absent menace	Treated with levetiracetam, euthanized at 4 months of age
6	SL008	Germany	M	9 weeks	Focal epileptic seizures, episodes of vocalization	Not done	Euthanized at unknown age
7	SL007	Germany	F	9 weeks	Focal epileptic seizures	Not done	Euthanized at unknown age

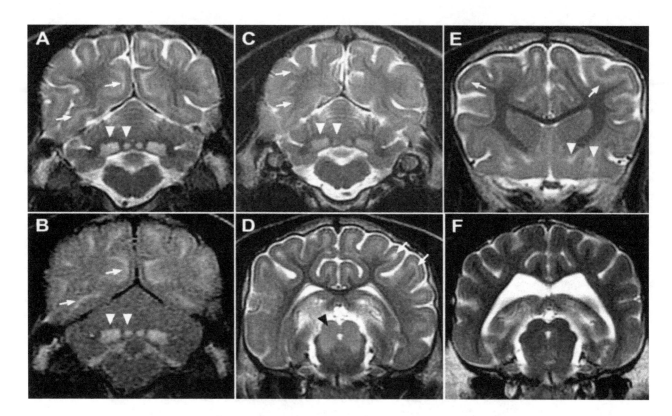

Figure 2. MRI abnormalities in SSADHD-affected Saluki Dogs. Transverse T2-weighted (**A,C–F**) and FLAIR (**B**) MR images at the level of the cerebellum (**A–C**), midbrain (**D,F**) and corpus striatum (**E**) demonstrating symmetrical involvement of predominantly grey matter structures. Images from dog 1 (**A,B,D,E**), dog 2 (**C**) and an unaffected littermate (**F**). Consistent bilateral symmetrical T2 hyperintensity of the deep cerebellar nuclei ((**A–C**); white arrowheads) is the most prominent finding. Similar bilaterally symmetrical hyperintensity is seen involving the tectum and dorsal tegmentum ((**D**); black arrowhead) and endopeduncular (medial) and lentiform nuclei ((**E**); white arrowheads) but not present in unaffected dog images (**F**). Sulci are prominent (**D**) compared to an unaffected age matched control (**F**), consistent with atrophy of cortical grey matter. Hyperintensity of deep cortical grey mater laminae is evident on T2-weighted and FLAIR images at all levels (white arrows) is not present on unaffected dog MR images (**F**).

3.4. Genetic Analysis

Both sexes are affected and in-depth pedigree analysis revealed the presence of a common male ancestor connecting the American and European families (Figure 1). As all parents of affected offspring show no clinical signs, it could be speculated that the observed disease phenotype follows autosomal monogenic recessive inheritance. Genome-wide association was performed using DNA samples from the seven affected dogs (Figure 1) and 28 phenotypically normal Saluki controls. After quality control, there were 108579 SNPs available for association. A single genome-wide significant association signal based on a $p_{Bonferroni}$ (0.006) on CFA 35 (chr35: g23,654,869; p_{raw} 5.27 × 10^{-8}) was identified (Figure 5). Furthermore, a 2.683 Mb region of homozygosity was identified in the seven affected dogs on CFA 35: 21,925,974–24,608,949 bp (CanFam3.1).

In order to identify a causative variant, initially paired-end whole-genome sequences of 2 affected puppies from two American litters (1052, 5813: Figure 1) and 98 unaffected controls from various breeds were investigated in the associated interval. There were 35,982 single-nucleotide variants (SNVs) and 16,832 insertion/deletion (indel) variants identified within the critical interval defined by homozygosity: CFA 35: 21,925,974–24,608,949 bp (CanFam3.1). There were 259 SNVs and 41 indels that segregated with the phenotype in the 100 animals. There were three coding variants identified: a synonymous variant (g.22,506,956G>A) in the *GPLD1* gene, and two protein-changing missense variants, g.22,572,768G>A in the *ALDH5A1* gene, and g.23,908,560T>C in the putative *PTCHD3* gene. The synonymous variant in *GPLD1* was not investigated further.

The two missense variants in *ALDH5A1* (XM_014110599.2: c.866G>A; XP_013966074.2: p.(Gly288Asp)) and *PTCHD3* (ENSCAFT00000039442.3: c.1247T>C; ENSCAFP00000035301: p.(Iso416Thr)) were evaluated to identify whether the substitutions were potentially deleterious. There is a gap in the canine genome assembly that likely contains at least one additional exon of the *ALDH5A1* gene. Aligning the predicted canine ALDH5A1 protein sequence with the human protein sequence places the canine missense variant at amino acid 381 in human (NP_001071.1). Both PolyPhen2 [25] (probably damaging—1.0) and SIFT [26] (deleterious—0.0) predicted this amino acid substitution to be deleterious. It occurs in a well -conserved portion of the protein (Figure 6B). The missense variant in *PTCHD3* is not predicted to affect the protein based on PolyPhen2 [25] (benign-0.436) and SIFT [26] (tolerated-0.05). In addition, based on the known functions of these two proteins and the independent findings presented below, the *ALDH5A1* variant was the only one pursued further.

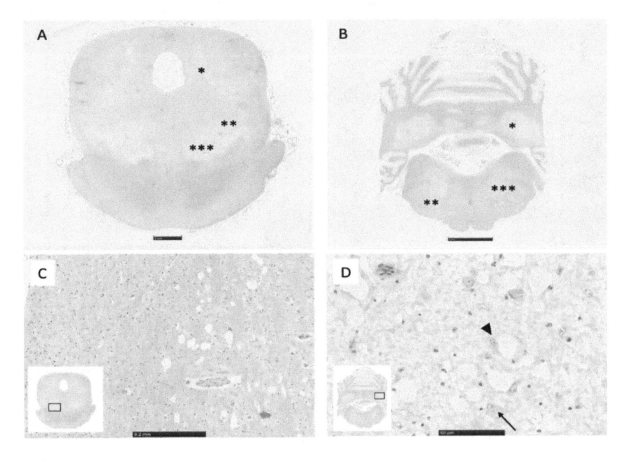

Figure 3. Histopathology of mesencephalon and brainstem from dog 1. (**A**) Bilaterally, the mesencephalic nuclei of cranial nerve V (*), the red nuclei (**), and the substantia nigra (***) exhibit decreased staining intensity (H&E). (**B**) Bilaterally, the deep cerebellar nuclei (*), the dorsal nuclei of the trapezoid body (**), and the reticular formations (***) exhibit decreased staining intensity (H&E). (**C**) Higher magnification of (**A**), inset. The substantia nigra shows prominent vacuolation of affected neurons. (**D**) Higher magnification of (**B**), inset. The interpositial nucleus shows reactive astrocytes (arrow), some of which also contain prominent cytoplasmic vacuolation (arrowhead).

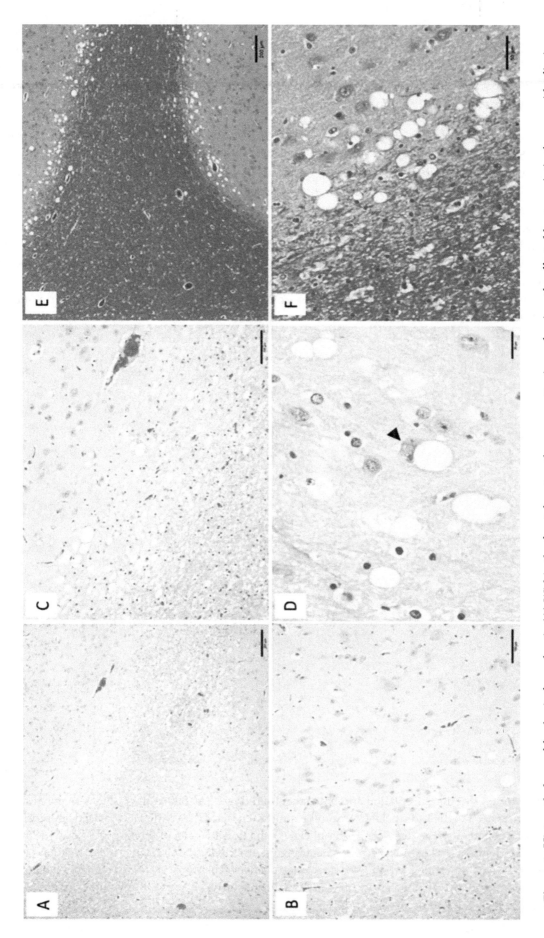

Figure 4. Histopathology of forebrain from dog 1. (**A**) Within the frontal cortex, the grey matter is predominantly affected by spongiotic change, with gliosis. (**B**) The spongiosis within the forebrain is most severe in the deep laminar cortex. (**C**) The caudate nucleus is also affected at the grey–white matter junction. (**D**) Affected neurons are characterized by enlarged, vacuolated cytoplasm with a peripheralized nucleus (arrowhead). Luxol fast blue (LFB) staining highlights the deep cortical nature of the vacuolation (**E**) within the cerebrum. (**F**) Vacuolation is discrete and often displaces cellular nuclei LFB staining.

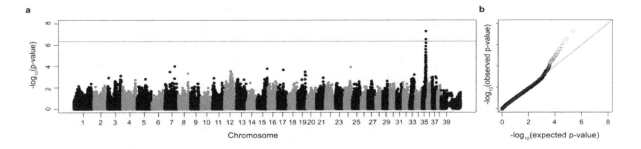

Figure 5. GWAS for SSADHD-affected Saluki dogs. (**a**) Manhattan plot showing −log10 of the raw p-values for each genotyped SNP by chromosome (*x*-axis). Genomic inflation was 1.25. Line denotes genome-wide significance based on Bonferroni-corrected p-values. (**b**) Q–Q plot of samples used in GWAS showing the −log10 of the expected versus the observed p-values. The SNPs on CFA35 are shown in light grey.

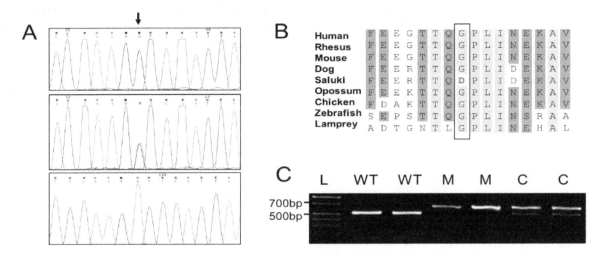

Figure 6. SSADHD-associated *ALDH5A1* missense variant in Saluki dogs. (**A**) The electropherograms from a normal dog (top panel), a heterozygous dog (middle panel) and a dog homozygous for the variant in *ALDH5A1* indicated by an arrow. (**B**) The amino acid alignment around the missense variant in ALDH5A1 (XP_013966074.2: p.(Gly288Asp)). Yellow boxes indicate 100% conservation across the species listed to the left and blue boxes indicate 75% conservation. The variant amino acid residue is boxed and the variant allele detected in affected Salukis is shown in red. (**C**) The PCR-RFLP genotyping assay for the *ALDH5A1* missense variant is shown. After PCR amplification, the products were digested with Sau96I. L is the DNA ladder, WT stands for wild type (542 bp), C for carrier and M for mutant (702 bp).

Independently, the genome of an affected puppy (dog 5) from the German litter was sequenced. No private variants were found in the *GPLD1* and *PTCHD3* genes. Furthermore, only one protein-changing missense variant (*ALDH5A1*: XM_014110599.2: c.866G>A) remained after filtering for homozygous private variants in the region of interest on chromosome 35 against the 589 control genomes from the Dog Biomedical Variant Database Consortium (DBVDC) variant catalog [27].

The *ALDH5A1* variant was confirmed by Sanger sequencing of genomic DNA (Figure 6A). In order to genotype the *ALDH5A1* missense variant, a PCR-RFLP genotyping assay was used (Figure 6C).

Genotyping of the *ALDH5A1* missense variant was performed in the seven affected dogs used for the GWAS, and the four available parents (Figure 1). The variant was homozygous in all cases and heterozygous in the parents. Siblings and other relatives, as well as unrelated Saluki dogs, were genotyped; 13 were heterozygous carriers and 48 were homozygous wild type. The segregation of the *ALDH5A* variant fits perfectly with the assumed monogenic recessive Mendelian inheritance within the studied family. In-depth pedigree analysis revealed the presence of a common male ancestor connecting the American and European families (Figure 1). To experimentally determine whether the *ALDH5A* variant was a common canine variant, 228 dogs from various other breeds were genotyped and all were found to have the wild-type allele, which was also confirmed by the absence of the variant in 581 dogs from 125 breeds and eight wolves of the DBVDC cohort [27].

The presence of the variant in cDNA of an affected dog was verified by Sanger sequencing of RT-PCR product from liver of an affected Saluki compared to a control unaffected dog. There was no obvious difference in expression level between the case and the control. Quantitative evaluation was not possible since only one affected dog sample was available.

3.5. Targeted Metabolic Testing

Targeted quantitative organic acids were analyzed on urine, serum, CSF, and brain tissue (Table 2) in affected ($n = 1$ to 4) and control dogs ($n = 2$ to 4). Compared to control dogs, there were marked elevations in urine succinate semialdehyde (SSA) and urine 4,5-dihydroxyhexanoic acid (DHHA) but levels of gamma hydroxybutyrate (GHB) in the urine were normal. Serum GHB and serum DHHA from affected dogs were markedly elevated compared to controls. Serum SSA could not be measured in either affected or control dogs. In cisternal cerebrospinal fluid (CSF) and brain, SSA, GHB and DHHA were markedly elevated in the affected dog compared to controls, with the CSF GHB having the highest elevation (by a factor of at least 4800). Activity of succinate semialdehyde dehydrogenase (SSADH) was absent or markedly reduced to 0.18% of normal in the affected dogs compared to control dogs.

Table 2. Specific quantitative organic acids in urine, serum, CSF, and brain tissue in affected and control dogs (nd = not done).

Dog Number	Urine SSA, mmol/mol Creatinine	Urine GHB, mmol/mol Creatinine	Urine DHHA mmol/mol Creatinine	Serum GHB, µmol/L	Serum DHHA, µmol/L	CSF SSA, µmol/L	CSF GHB, µmol/L	CSF DHHA, µmol/L	Brain GHB, nmol/mg Brain	Brain DHHA, nmol/mg Brain	Brain SSA, nmol/mg Brain	Brain SSA Activity, pmol/min/mg Protein
1	9.23	1.06	5.85	6.59	0.45	69	>1500	43.3	2.43	0.22	0.23	10
2	nd	nd	nd	nd	nd	nd	nd	nd	2.93	0.28	0.18	0
5	38.7	nd	11.8	nd	0.41	nd	nd	nd	nd	nd	nd	nd
6	30.9	0.67	10.4	nd	0.61	nd	nd	nd	nd	nd	nd	nd
7	nd	nd	nd	nd	0.56	nd	nd	nd	nd	nd	nd	nd
Number of affected dogs	3	2	3	1	4	1	1	1	2	2	2	2
Number of control dogs	4	4	4	4	4	2	3	3	4	nd	nd	5
median affected	30.9	0.87	10.4	n/a	0.51	n/a	n/a	n/a	2.68	0.25	0.21	5
range affected	9.23–38.7	0.67–1.06	5.85–11.8	n/a	0.41–0.61	n/a	n/a	n/a	2.43–2.93	0.22–0.28	0.18–0.23	0–10
median control	0.86	0.82	0.29	0.38	0.08	0.24	0.31	0.11	0.03	0	0.11	5587
range control	0.64–0.9	0.29–2.04	0.18–0.65	0.28–0.59	0.07–0.1	0.02–0.46	0.23–0.8	0.1–0.2	0–0.05	0–0	0.06–0.14	4214–5942

4. Discussion

A pathogenic variant in the canine *ALDH5A1* gene associated with recessive SSADH deficiency, formerly known as status spongiosus in Saluki dogs (SSSD) [13]. Seven Saluki puppies from two continents had an onset of multifocal cranial neurological signs at 10 weeks of age or younger. Blood work was normal. On MRI of the brain, lesions were similar in all dogs, with bilateral and symmetrical lesions of the cerebrum, brainstem and cerebellum, predominantly affecting grey matter structures. Because this disorder occurred in purebred Saluki puppies from different environments with a consistent clinical phenotype and a normal extracranial work up, structural epilepsy from an inborn error of metabolism was considered the most likely etiology. Using genome-wide association, followed by whole-genome sequencing, a missense mutation in the *ALDH5A1* gene was identified as the presumed cause of status spongiosus in Saluki dogs, previously reported in Saluki puppies [13]. The mutation segregated completely in family members as an apparently fully penetrant monogenic recessive disorder.

The *ALDH5A1* gene encodes the mitochondrial enzyme succinic semialdehyde dehydrogenase (NAD+) (SSADH), which is involved in the catabolism of the inhibitory neurotransmitter gamma-aminobutyric acid (GABA) (Figure 7). GABA is the major inhibitory neurotransmitter in the central nervous system(CNS), where it is utilized in up to 30% of cerebral synapses [34]; it is also found in non-nervous-system tissue. GABA is synthesized from L-glutamate via glutamate decarboxylase (GAD). The first step in GABA metabolism is by GABA-transaminase (GABA-T) to form succinic semialdehyde (SSA). SSA is then oxidized by the mitochondrial protein succinic semialdehyde dehydrogenase (NAD+) (SSADH) to succinic acid, which then enters the tricarboxylic acid (TCA) cycle for energy generation (Figure 7). In people, recognized disorders of GABA synthesis are GAD deficiency, and recognized disorders of GABA degradation are GABA transaminase deficiency and succinic semialdehyde dehydrogenase (NAD+) (SSADH) deficiency.

The SSADH protein is expressed in the mammalian brain, as well as liver, pituitary, heart, ovary and kidney [35]. In people, the *ALDH5A1* gene is located on chromosome 6p22, and is 10 exons long extending over 38 kb [36]. Succinic semialdehyde dehydrogenase (NAD+) is an enzyme which is member of the aldehyde dehydrogenase family of proteins. In people with SSADH enzyme deficiency, SSA is not catabolized to succinic acid, and thus excess levels of SSA build up in tissues and fluids (Figure 7). Excess succinic semialdehyde is converted to 4-hydroxybutyric acid (GHB) by succinic semialdehyde reductase. Excess SSA may also interact with an intermediate in the pyruvate dehydrogenase complex to form 4,5-dihydroxyhexanoic acid (DHHA). People with a deficiency of SSADH have elevations of SSA, DHHA, and GHB in body fluids [35]. The activity of SSADH is reduced in people, and thus levels of SSA rise, with associated high levels of GHB and DHHA (Figure 7) [37]. The hallmark of SSADH deficiency in people is persistent and elevated levels of the GHB in urine, plasma and CSF [37]. The diagnosis is confirmed by molecular genetics by sequencing the *ALDH5A1* gene for pathogenic variants. There is no effective therapy [37].

In Saluki dogs with SSADH deficiency, levels of SSA and DHHA are elevated in urine, serum, CSF and brain, and GHB is elevated in serum, CSF and brain. Unlike in people, where GHB is elevated in urine, the level of GHB in urine in Saluki dogs with SSADH deficiency is normal. Since the activity of succinate semialdehyde dehydrogenase (NAD+) (SSADH) was absent or markedly reduced, along with elevated levels of SSA, DHHA and GHB, we believe that the previously described central nervous system status spongiosus in Saluki dogs should be more appropriately termed succinic semialdehyde dehydrogenase deficiency (SSADHD).

In people, SSADH deficiency is a rare autosomal recessive neurological disorder caused by a mutation in the *ALDH5A1* gene, reported in 1981 (OMIM 271980) [38]. There are 44 unique mutations in the *ALDH5A1* gene, which occur in exons 1–10; there are no other mutations in genes other than *ALDH5A1* associated with SSADH deficiency in people [36]. The clinical features in people include developmental delay, hypotonia, intellectual disability, ataxia, seizures, hyperkinetic behavior, aggression and sleep disturbances. Approximately 50% of patients have seizures, 45% have neuropsychiatric problems such as sleep disturbances, and many patients also have behavioral abnormalities [34], which all worsen with age [39]. The encephalopathy is considered non-progressive and has wide phenotypic heterogeneity from mild to severe. Symptoms are first noted at a mean of 11 months (range 0–44 months of age), with a mean age at diagnosis of 6.6 years (range of 0 to 25 years) [40]. On MR imaging in people with SSADHD, MR images may be normal, or there may be hyperintensities on T2-weighted imaging in the globus pallidus, cerebellar dentate nuclei and brainstem [41]. A small percentage of people are reported with cerebral white matter hyperintensity on MR imaging as well [41]. There is one single case report of the pathology of SSADH deficiency in a young adult, where there was discoloration of the globus pallidi, congestion of the leptomeninges and scar tissue in the cerebral cortex [42].

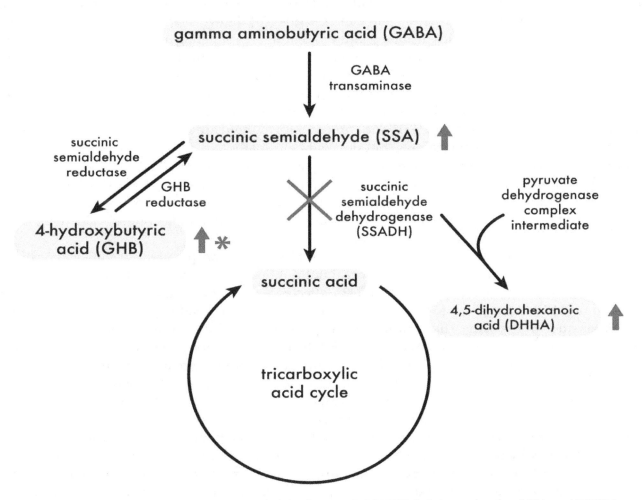

Figure 7. GABA catabolism pathway. In Saluki dogs with SSADH deficiency, levels of SSA and DHHA are elevated in urine, serum, CSF and brain, and GHB is elevated in serum, CSF and brain (red arrows) as in people with SSADH deficiency. Unlike in people, where GHB is elevated in urine (red arrow), the level of GHB in urine (red *) in Saluki dogs with SSADH deficiency is normal.

The pathophysiology of SSADH deficiency in people is complex. The disease is thought to be caused primarily by the elevation of GHB in the brain, particularly during neurodevelopment or due to the imbalance of neurotransmitters [43] but also potentially from oxidative stress in the brain [44]. GHB is a neuromodulator with a wide array of pharmacological effects [45]. It was initially produced as an injectable anesthetic agent but is now longer utilized for this purpose due to adverse effects but is prescribed to treat cataplexy in narcolepsy/cataplexy, opiate dependency and alcoholism, and is a drug of abuse, where its street names include Grievous Bodily Harm, Liquid Ecstasy and Soap [46]. GHB may cause anxiolytic, hypnotic and euphoric effects as well as short-term memory loss and CNS depression, causing sedation [44,47]; intoxication may cause bradycardia, myoclonus and seizures, hypoventilation, coma and death from respiratory depression [33]. GHB is a monocarboxylate that is primarily cleared from the plasma via metabolism in a dose-dependent fashion through the Kreb's cycle. Renal clearance of GHB is minor and non-linear, due to the carrier-mediated saturable renal reabsorption of GHB through the proximal tubules via sodium-dependent and pH-dependent monocarboxylate transporters. Methods to increase the renal excretion of GHB have been investigated in animals as part of a treatment plan for people with GHB intoxication, such as with the intravenous administration of L-Lactate which increases the renal excretion of GHB [48,49].

As there are no effective specific treatments for SSADH deficiency in people, treatment is currently aimed at managing the clinical signs of seizures and neurobehavioral disturbances [34]. Broad-spectrum anticonvulsants are generally utilized, avoiding valproate which inhibits SSADH which may worsen GHB accumulation and clinical signs [50]. However, there are many therapeutic options under investigation which include pharmacological (e.g., targeting neurotransmitter receptors), enzyme-replacement therapy, gene therapy and treatment with pharmacological chaperones [51,52].

In animals, SSADH has been produced in knockout mice; clinical signs are progressive ataxia, failure to thrive, seizure and death at a young age [53,54], and thus they are utilized as a model for the severe and poor survival phenotype in humans. There are no reports of the MR imaging features of SSADH-knockout mice [51] and, on pathology, there are no reported abnormalities on routine hematoxylin and eosin staining, but detailed neuropathological examinations have not been performed [55]. There is a single case report of a dog with suspected SSADH deficiency, which had a progressive encephalopathy with profound and persistent lactic acidosis, elevated urine GHB and a 30% reduced activity of SSADH measured in cultured lymphoblasts compared to normal dogs. Intracranial MR imaging of the brain was not performed; on histopathology of the brain, there was a spongiform change in the cerebral cortex [56].

Saluki dogs have a more severe phenotype of SSADHD than people, but with very similar clinical signs of seizures, abnormal behavior, abnormalities of sleep and multifocal brain disease on neurological examination. Like people [42], affected Salukis have multifocal abnormalities in the brain on MR imaging, where affected dogs have identical bilaterally symmetrical T2-weighted hyperintensities in the same anatomical areas as people such as the basal nuclei, deep cerebellar nuclei, and brain stem. In people with SSADH deficiency, these abnormalities have considerable consistency, and are almost universal. However, in some people, there are reports of non-specific hyperintensities in subcortical white matter and the substantia nigra in the brainstem, as well as cerebellar atrophy [57,58]. These abnormalities are not considered specific for SSADHD, but considered to be imaging characteristics of cytotoxic edema, secondary to oxidative stress from the underlying SSADHD [43]. Differently to what is noted in people, dogs have hyperintensity of the deep cortical laminae of the grey matter of the cerebral cortex and atrophy of the cerebral cortex. On histopathology in dogs with SSADH deficiency, there is bilaterally symmetric multifocal spongiform change in the brainstem, deep cerebellar nuclei, but also severe in the thalamic nuclei and deep cortical grey matter. The brain lesions in affected Salukis on MRI (two dogs) and pathology (three dogs (same two dogs that had MRI plus one other) were identical. There is only one case report of the pathology of SSADHD in a person where the histopathology was not described and thus the comparative pathology between dogs and people is not possible [42].

Unlike in people with SSADHD, where GHB is elevated in the urine and therefore is an excellent biomarker, GHB is not elevated in the urine of affected dogs. GHB is, however, elevated in the serum, CSF and brain tissue of affected dogs. Since GHB is extensively reabsorbed from the proximal tubules in the kidney [59], it is possible that species differences in handling GHB resulted in extensive reabsorption of GHB and in a normal level of GHB in the affected dog's urine. It is also plausible that since urine GHB was evaluated in only two affected dogs, that evaluation of additional SSADHD-affected dogs may have yielded elevated levels of urine GHB. There may also have been loss of GHB in the samples during shipping to the lab or storage, as GHB is a volatile compound [40] and a reduction in GHB levels is reported with storage, which varied between 10% loss at just 3 days and in excess of 20% after

4 weeks of storage [60]. If the activity of the D-2-hydroxyglutarate dehydrogenase in liver (non-cofactor enzyme converting GHB to SSA and ketoglutarate to D-2-hydroxyglutarate) was very active in the liver of Salukis, this could be a plausible explanation for why GHB was not elevated in the urine; however, D-2-HG was not measured in affected or control dogs. Otherwise, aside from serum SSA that we were not able to measure in dogs with SSADHD, dogs are similar to human patients in regards to elevated body fluid levels of SSA, DHHA and GHB, and zero to low levels of brain SSA activity.

5. Conclusions

Saluki dogs with SSADHD have a disease phenotype resembling SSADHD in people, although it appears to be more severe clinically. On the other hand, it appears to be less severe than the phenotype described in in knockout mice, which is lethal [58]. Furthermore, GHB may not be an acceptable biomarker for the disease in dogs; alternatively, urine SSA or GHB in serum may be more appropriate biomarkers. Compared to mice models of human disease, dog models have naturally occurring disease, are more similar to humans in regards to size, and have more longevity than mice. Dogs are proven and valuable models of human disease, particularly in the field of lysosomal storage diseases [6]. This first *ALDH5A1*-related large animal model for SSADHD may provide an opportunity for evaluation of potential therapeutics for this rare orphan disease in people. Dogs may be a more appropriate disease model than the murine SSADH model, as dogs appear to have a more similar disease phenotype and similar MR imaging features to people. The identification of the pathogenic *ALDH5A1* variant will allow the screening of carriers to avoid producing further affected puppies and thereby contribute to maintaining breed health.

Author Contributions: Conceptualization, K.M.V., D.L.B., E.S., P.L.P., K.M.G., and C.D.; methodology, D.L.B. and E.S.; software, D.L.B.; validation, D.L.B., E.S., and Z.Z.; formal analysis, D.L.B., E.S., B.R., and A.L.; investigation, K.M.V., D.L.B., D.D.C., E.A.B., M.A., K.D.W., G.D.S., F.G., M.R.B., K.M., T.A.M., M.R.B., A.L., V.J., D.L.B., T.J.V.W., and F.K.; resources, D.L.B., E.S., and C.D.; data curation, D.L.B. and E.S.; writing—original draft preparation, K.M.V. and D.L.B.; writing—review and editing, D.L.B., P.J.D., C.D., K.D.W., E.S., P.L.P., K.M.G., G.D.S., F.K.,T.A.M., D.O., and A.L.; visualization, K.M.V., D.L.B., and A.L; supervision, D.L.B., C.T.B., and C.D.; project administration, K.M.V.; funding acquisition, D.L.B. and K.M.V. All authors have read and agreed to the published version of the manuscript.

Acknowledgments: The authors acknowledge the support of Sharron Kinney, Lorrie Boldrick, Ember, Encore, Khrome, Kara, Yamal, Yari, Yanam and Kelly Kohen for this study. We acknowledge the Next-Generation Sequencing Platform and the Interfaculty Bioinformatics Unit of the University of Bern for performing the whole-genome sequencing experiments and for providing the computational infrastructure.

References

1. El-Hattab, A.W. Inborn errors of metabolism. *Clin. Perinatol.* **2015**, *42*, 413–439. [CrossRef]

2. Seijo-Martinez, M.; Navarro, C.; Castro del Rio, M.; Vila, O.; Puig, M.; Ribes, A.; Butron, M. L-2-hydroxyglutaric aciduria: Clinical, neuroimaging, and neuropathological findings. *Arch. Neurol.* **2005**, *62*, 666–670. [CrossRef] [PubMed]

3. Jolly, R.D.; Walkley, S.U. Lysosomal storage diseases of animals: An essay in comparative pathology. *Vet. Pathol.* **1997**, *34*, 527–548. [CrossRef]

4. Mansour, T.A.; Woolard, K.D.; Vernau, K.L.; Ancona, D.M.; Thomasy, S.M.; Sebbag, L.; Moore, B.A.; Knipe, M.F.; Seada, H.A.; Cowan, T.M.; et al. Whole genome sequencing for mutation discovery in a single case of lysosomal storage disease (MPS type 1) in the dog. *Sci. Rep.* **2020**, *10*, 6558. [CrossRef] [PubMed]

5. Lucot, K.L.; Dickinson, P.J.; Finno, C.J.; Mansour, T.A.; Letko, A.; Minor, K.M.; Mickelson, J.R.; Drogemuller, C.; Brown, C.T.; Bannasch, D.L. A Missense Mutation in the Vacuolar Protein Sorting 11 (VPS11) Gene Is Associated with Neuroaxonal Dystrophy in Rottweiler Dogs. *G3 Genes Genomes Genet.* **2018**, *8*, 2773–2780. [CrossRef]

6. Haskins, M.E.; Giger, U.; Patterson, D.F. Animal models of lysosomal storage diseases: Their development and clinical relevance. In *Fabry Disease: Perspectives from 5 Years of FOS*; Mehta, A., Beck, M., Sunder-Plassmann, G., Eds.; Oxford PharmaGenesis: Oxford, UK, 2006.

7. Kamboj, M. Clinical approach to the diagnoses of inborn errors of metabolism. *Pediatr. Clin. N. Am.* **2008**, *55*, 1113–1127. [CrossRef]

8. Saudubray, J.M.; Garcia-Cazorla, A. An overview of inborn errors of metabolism affecting the brain: From neurodevelopment to neurodegenerative disorders. *Dialogues Clin. Neurosci.* **2018**, *20*, 301–325. [CrossRef]

9. Sewell, A.C.; Haskins, M.E.; Giger, U. Inherited metabolic disease in companion animals: Searching for nature's mistakes. *Vet. J.* **2007**, *174*, 252–259. [CrossRef]

10. Lavely, J.A. Pediatric seizure disorders in dogs and cats. *Vet. Clin. N. Am. Small Anim. Pract.* **2014**, *44*, 275–301. [CrossRef]

11. Berendt, M.; Farquhar, R.G.; Mandigers, P.J.; Pakozdy, A.; Bhatti, S.F.; De Risio, L.; Fischer, A.; Long, S.; Matiasek, K.; Munana, K.; et al. International veterinary epilepsy task force consensus report on epilepsy definition, classification and terminology in companion animals. *BMC Vet. Res.* **2015**, *11*, 182. [CrossRef]

12. De Risio, L.; Bhatti, S.; Munana, K.; Penderis, J.; Stein, V.; Tipold, A.; Berendt, M.; Farqhuar, R.; Fischer, A.; Long, S.; et al. International veterinary epilepsy task force consensus proposal: Diagnostic approach to epilepsy in dogs. *BMC Vet. Res.* **2015**, *11*, 148. [CrossRef]

13. Luttgen, P.; Storts, R. Central Nervous system spongiosus of Saluki Dogs. In Proceedings of the American College of Veterinary Internal Medicine Forum, San Diego, CA, USA, 21–24 May 1987.

14. Summers, B.; Cummings, J.F.; de Lahunta, A. *Veterinary Neuropathology*; Mosby: St. Louis, MO, USA, 2005.

15. Kanekar, S.; Gustas, C. Metabolic disorders of the brain: Part I. *Semin Ultrasound CT MR* **2011**, *32*, 590–614. [CrossRef]

16. Markovich, J.E.; Heinze, C.R.; Freeman, L.M. Thiamine deficiency in dogs and cats. *J. Am. Vet. Med. Assoc.* **2013**, *243*, 649–656. [CrossRef]

17. Brauer, C.; Jambroszyk, M.; Tipold, A. Metabolic and toxic causes of canine seizure disorders: A retrospective study of 96 cases. *Vet. J.* **2011**, *187*, 272–275. [CrossRef]

18. Peterson, M.E. Bromethalin. *Top Companion Anim. Med.* **2013**, *28*, 21–23. [CrossRef]

19. Tauro, A.; Beltran, E.; Cherubini, G.B.; Coelho, A.T.; Wessmann, A.; Driver, C.J.; Rusbridge, C.J. Metronidazole-induced neurotoxicity in 26 dogs. *Aust. Vet. J.* **2018**, *96*, 495–501. [CrossRef]

20. Purcell, S.; Neale, B.; Todd-Brown, K.; Thomas, L.; Ferreira, M.A.; Bender, D.; Maller, J.; Sklar, P.; de Bakker, P.I.; Daly, M.J.; et al. PLINK(1.7): A tool set for whole-genome association and population-based linkage analyses. *Am. J. Hum. Genet.* **2007**, *81*, 559–575. [CrossRef]

21. Kierczak, M.; Jablonska, J.; Forsberg, S.K.; Bianchi, M.; Tengvall, K.; Pettersson, M.; Scholz, V.; Meadows, J.R.; Jern, P.; Carlborg, O.; et al. Cgmisc: Enhanced genome-wide association analyses and visualization. *Bioinformatics* **2015**, *31*, 3830–3831. [CrossRef]

22. Wickham. *Elegant Graphics for Data Analysis*, 1st ed.; Springer: Berlin/Heidelberg, Germany, 2009.

23. Mansour, T.A.; Lucot, K.; Konopelski, S.E.; Dickinson, P.J.; Sturges, B.K.; Vernau, K.L.; Choi, S.; Stern, J.A.; Thomasy, S.M.; Doring, S.; et al. Whole genome variant association across 100 dogs identifies a frame shift mutation in DISHEVELLED 2 which contributes to Robinow-like syndrome in Bulldogs and related screw tail dog breeds. *PLoS Genet.* **2018**, *14*, e1007850. [CrossRef]

24. McLaren, W.; Gil, L.; Hunt, S.E.; Riat, H.S.; Ritchie, G.R.; Thormann, A.; Flicek, P.; Cunningham, F. The Ensembl Variant Effect Predictor. *Genome Biol.* **2016**, *17*, 122. [CrossRef]

25. Adzhubei, I.A.; Schmidt, S.; Peshkin, L.; Ramensky, V.E.; Gerasimova, A.; Bork, P.; Kondrashov, A.S.; Sunyaev, S.R. A method and server for predicting damaging missense mutations. *Nat. Methods* **2010**, *7*, 248–249. [CrossRef]

26. Choi, Y.; Chan, A.P. PROVEAN web server: A tool to predict the functional effect of amino acid substitutions and indels. *Bioinformatics* **2015**, *31*, 2745–2747. [CrossRef]

27. Jagannathan, V.; Drögemüller, C.; Leeb, T.; Aguirre, G.; André, C.; Bannasch, D.; Becker, D.; Davis, B.; Ekenstedt, K.; Faller, K.; et al. A comprehensive biomedical variant catalogue based on whole genome sequences of 582 dogs and eight wolves. *Anim. Genet.* **2019**, *50*, 695–704. [CrossRef]

28. Minor, K.M.; Letko, A.; Becker, D.; Drogemuller, M.; Mandigers, P.J.J.; Bellekom, S.R.; Leegwater, P.A.J.; Stassen, Q.E.M.; Putschbach, K.; Fischer, A.; et al. Canine NAPEPLD-associated models of human myelin disorders. *Sci. Rep.* **2018**, *8*, 5818. [CrossRef]

29. Rozen, S.; Skaletsky, H. *Methods in Molecular Biology: Bioinformatics Methods and Protocols*; Primer3 on the WWW for general users and for biologist programmers; Humana Press: Totowa, NJ, USA, 2000; Volume 132.

30. Brinkhof, B.; Spee, B.; Rothuizen, J.; Penning, L.C. Development and evaluation of canine reference genes for accurate quantification of gene expression. *Anal. Biochem.* **2006**, *356*, 36–43. [CrossRef]

31. Gibson, K.M.; Aramaki, S.; Sweetman, L.; Nyhan, W.L.; DeVivo, D.C.; Hodson, A.K.; Jakobs, C. Stable isotope dilution analysis of 4-hydroxybutyric acid: An accurate method for quantification in physiological fluids and the prenatal diagnosis of 4-hydroxybutyric aciduria. *BioMed. Environ. Mass Spectrom.* **1990**, *19*, 89–93. [CrossRef]

32. Struys, E.A.; Jansen, E.E.; Gibson, K.M.; Jakobs, C. Determination of the GABA analogue succinic semialdehyde in urine and cerebrospinal fluid by dinitrophenylhydrazine derivatization and liquid chromatography-tandem mass spectrometry: Application to SSADH deficiency. *J. Inherit. Metab. Dis.* **2005**, *28*, 913–920. [CrossRef]

33. Gibson, K.M.; Lee, C.F.; Chambliss, K.L.; Kamali, V.; Francois, B.; Jaeken, J.; Jakobs, C. 4-Hydroxybutyric aciduria: Application of a fluorometric assay to the determination of succinic semialdehyde dehydrogenase activity in extracts of cultured human lymphoblasts. *Clin. Chim. Acta* **1991**, *196*, 219–221. [CrossRef]

34. Pearl, P.L.; Parviz, M.; Vogel, K.; Schreiber, J.; Theodore, W.H.; Gibson, K.M. Inherited disorders of gamma-aminobutyric acid metabolism and advances in ALDH5A1 mutation identification. *Dev. Med. Child Neurol.* **2015**, *57*, 611–617. [CrossRef]

35. Kim, K.J.; Pearl, P.L.; Jensen, K.; Snead, O.C.; Malaspina, P.; Jakobs, C.; Gibson, K.M. Succinic semialdehyde dehydrogenase: Biochemical-molecular-clinical disease mechanisms, redox regulation, and functional significance. *Antioxid. Redox Signal.* **2011**, *15*, 691–718. [CrossRef]

36. Liu, N.; Kong, X.D.; Kan, Q.C.; Shi, H.R.; Wu, Q.H.; Zhuo, Z.H.; Bai, Q.L.; Jiang, M. Mutation analysis and prenatal diagnosis in a Chinese family with succinic semialdehyde dehydrogenase and a systematic review of the literature of reported ALDH5A1 mutations. *J. Perinat. Med.* **2016**, *44*, 441–451. [CrossRef]

37. Parviz, M.; Vogel, K.; Gibson, K.M.; Pearl, P.L. Disorders of GABA metabolism: SSADH and GABA-transaminase deficiencies. *J. Pediatr. Epilepsy* **2014**, *3*, 217–227. [CrossRef]

38. Jakobs, C.; Bojasch, M.; Mönch, E.; Rating, D.; Siemes, H.; Hanefeld, F. Urinary excretion of gamma-hydroxybutyric acid in a patient with neurological abnormalities. The probability of a new inborn error of metabolism. *Clin. Chim. Acta* **1981**, *111*, 169–178. [CrossRef]

39. DiBacco, M.L.; Roullet, J.B.; Kapur, K.; Brown, M.N.; Walters, D.C.; Gibson, K.M.; Pearl, P.L. Age-related phenotype and biomarker changes in SSADH deficiency. *Ann. Clin. Transl. Neurol.* **2019**, *6*, 114–120. [CrossRef]

40. Pearl, P.L.; Gibson, K.M.; Acosta, M.T.; Vezina, L.G.; Theodore, W.H.; Rogawski, M.A.; Novotny, E.J.; Gropman, A.; Conry, J.A.; Berry, G.T.; et al. Clinical spectrum of succinic semialdehyde dehydrogenase deficiency. *Neurology* **2003**, *60*, 1413–1417. [CrossRef]

41. Gibson, K.M.; Christensen, E.; Jakobs, C.; Fowler, B.; Clarke, M.A.; Hammersen, G.; Raab, K.; Kobori, J.; Moosa, A.; Vollmer, B.; et al. The clinical phenotype of succinic semialdehyde dehydrogenase deficiency (4-hydroxybutyric aciduria): Case reports of 23 new patients. *Pediatrics* **1997**, *99*, 567–574. [CrossRef]

42. Knerr, I.; Gibson, K.M.; Murdoch, G.; Salomons, G.S.; Jakobs, C.; Combs, S.; Pearl, P.L. Neuropathology in succinic semialdehyde dehydrogenase deficiency. *Pediatr. Neurol.* **2010**, *42*, 255–258. [CrossRef]

43. Malaspina, P.; Roullet, J.B.; Pearl, P.L.; Ainslie, G.R.; Vogel, K.R.; Gibson, K.M. Succinic semialdehyde dehydrogenase deficiency (SSADHD): Pathophysiological complexity and multifactorial trait associations in a rare monogenic disorder of GABA metabolism. *Neurochem. Int.* **2016**, *99*, 72–84. [CrossRef]

44. Sgaravatti, A.M.; Sgarbi, M.B.; Testa, C.G.; Durigon, K.; Pederzolli, C.D.; Prestes, C.C.; Wyse, A.T.; Wannmacher, C.M.; Wajner, M.; Dutra-Filho, C.S. Gamma-hydroxybutyric acid induces oxidative stress in cerebral cortex of young rats. *Neurochem. Int.* **2007**, *50*, 564–570. [CrossRef]

45. Struys, E.A.; Verhoeven, N.M.; Jansen, E.E.; Ten Brink, H.J.; Gupta, M.; Burlingame, T.G.; Quang, L.S.; Maher, T.; Rinaldo, P.; Snead, O.C.; et al. Metabolism of gamma-hydroxybutyrate to d-2-hydroxyglutarate in mammals: Further evidence for d-2-hydroxyglutarate transhydrogenase. *Metabolism* **2006**, *55*, 353–358. [CrossRef]

46. Teter, C.J.; Guthrie, S.K. A comprehensive review of MDMA and GHB: Two common club drugs. *Pharmacotherapy* **2001**, *21*, 1486–1513. [CrossRef]

47. Kamal, R.M.; van Noorden, M.S.; Franzek, E.; Dijkstra, B.A.; Loonen, A.J.; De Jong, C.A. The Neurobiological Mechanisms of Gamma-Hydroxybutyrate Dependence and Withdrawal and Their Clinical Relevance: A Review. *Neuropsychobiology* **2016**, *73*, 65–80. [CrossRef]

48. Morris, M.E.; Hu, K.; Wang, Q. Renal clearance of gamma-hydroxybutyric acid in rats: Increasing renal elimination as a detoxification strategy. *J. Pharmacol. Exp. Ther.* **2005**, *313*, 1194–1202. [CrossRef]

49. Felmlee, M.A.; Wang, Q.; Cui, D.; Roiko, S.A.; Morris, M.E. Mechanistic toxicokinetic model for gamma-hydroxybutyric acid: Inhibition of active renal reabsorption as a potential therapeutic strategy. *AAPS J.* **2010**, *12*, 407–416. [CrossRef]

50. Shinka, T.; Ohfu, M.; Hirose, S.; Kuhara, T. Effect of valproic acid on the urinary metabolic profile of a patient with succinic semialdehyde dehydrogenase deficiency. *J. Chromatogr. B Anal. Technol. Biomed. Life Sci.* **2003**, *792*, 99–106. [CrossRef]

51. Didiasova, M.; Banning, A.; Brennenstuhl, H.; Jung-Klawitter, S.; Cinquemani, C.; Opladen, T.; Tikkanen, R. Succinic Semialdehyde Dehydrogenase Deficiency: An Update. *Cells* **2020**, *9*, 477. [CrossRef]

52. Vogel, K.R.; Ainslie, G.R.; Walters, D.C.; McConnell, A.; Dhamne, S.C.; Rotenberg, A.; Roullet, J.B.; Gibson, K.M. Succinic semialdehyde dehydrogenase deficiency, a disorder of GABA metabolism: An update on pharmacological and enzyme-replacement therapeutic strategies. *J. Inherit. Metab. Dis.* **2018**, *41*, 699–708. [CrossRef] [PubMed]

53. Drasbek, K.R.; Vardya, I.; Delenclos, M.; Gibson, K.M.; Jensen, K. SSADH deficiency leads to elevated extracellular GABA levels and increased GABAergic neurotransmission in the mouse cerebral cortex. *J. Inherit. Metab. Dis.* **2008**, *31*, 662–668. [CrossRef]

54. Gibson, K.M.; Jakobs, C.; Pearl, P.L.; Snead, O.C. Murine succinate semialdehyde dehydrogenase (SSADH) deficiency, a heritable disorder of GABA metabolism with epileptic phenotype. *IUBMB Life* **2005**, *57*, 639–644. [CrossRef]

55. Gupta, M.; Hogema, B.M.; Grompe, M.; Bottiglieri, T.G.; Concas, A.; Biggio, G.; Sogliano, C.; Rigamonti, A.E.; Pearl, P.L.; Snead, O.C., 3rd; et al. Murine succinate semialdehyde dehydrogenase deficiency. *Ann. Neurol.* **2003**, *54* (Suppl. 6), S81–S90. [CrossRef]

56. Kelmer, E.; Gibson, K.M.; Jakobs, C.; Struys, E.; Shelton, G.D.; Aroch, I.; O'Brien, D.P. Severe Lactic Acidosis Associated with a Suspected Succinic Semialdehyde Dehydrogenas (SSADH) Deficiency in a Young Chihuahua Dog. *Isr. J. Vet. Med.* **2018**, *73*, 43–48.

57. Pearl, P.L.; Wiwattanadittakul, N.; Roullet, J.B.; Gibson, K.M. Succinic Semialdehyde Dehydrogenase Deficiency. In *GeneReviews (R)*; Adam, M.P., Ardinger, H.H., Pagon, R.A., Wallace, S.E., Bean, L.J.H., Stephens, K., Amemiya, A., Eds.; University of Washington: Seattle, WA, USA, 1993.

58. Pearl, P.L.; Gibson, K.M.; Cortez, M.A.; Wu, Y.; Carter Snead, O., 3rd; Knerr, I.; Forester, K.; Pettiford, J.M.; Jakobs, C.; Theodore, W.H. Succinic semialdehyde dehydrogenase deficiency: Lessons from mice and men. *J. Inherit. Metab. Dis.* **2009**, *32*, 343–352. [CrossRef] [PubMed]

59. Wang, Q.; Lu, Y.; Morris, M.E. Monocarboxylate transporter (MCT) mediates the transport of gamma-hydroxybutyrate in human kidney HK-2 cells. *Pharm. Res.* **2007**, *24*, 1067–1078. [CrossRef]

60. Busardo, F.P.; Zaami, S.; Baglio, G.; Indorato, F.; Montana, A.; Giarratana, N.; Kyriakou, C.; Marinelli, E.; Romano, G. Assessment of the stability of exogenous gamma hydroxybutyric acid (GHB) in stored blood and urine specimens. *Eur. Rev. Med. Pharmacol. Sci.* **2015**, *19*, 4187–4194.

X-Linked Duchenne-Type Muscular Dystrophy in Jack Russell Terrier Associated with a Partial Deletion of the Canine *DMD* Gene

Barbara Brunetti [1,*]**, Luisa V. Muscatello** [1]**, Anna Letko** [2]**, Valentina Papa** [3]**, Giovanna Cenacchi** [3]**, Marco Grillini** [4]**, Leonardo Murgiano** [2,5]**, Vidhya Jagannathan** [2] **and Cord Drögemüller** [2]

[1]   Department of Veterinary Medical Sciences, University of Bologna, 40064 Bologna, Italy; luisaver.muscatello2@unibo.it
[2]   Institute of Genetics, Vetsuisse Faculty, University of Bern, 3001 Bern, Switzerland; anna.letko@vetsuisse.unibe.ch (A.L.); leomur@vet.upenn.edu (L.M.); vidhya.jagannathan@vetsuisse.unibe.ch (V.J.); cord.droegemueller@vetsuisse.unibe.ch (C.D.)
[3]   Department of Biomedical and Neuromotor Sciences, University of Bologna, 40138 Bologna, Italy; valentina.papa2@unibo.it (V.P.); giovanna.cenacchi@unibo.it (G.C.)
[4]   Pathology Unit, S Orsola Malpighi Hospital, University of Bologna, 40138 Bologna, Italy; marco.grillini@aosp.bo.it
[5]   Department of Clinical Sciences & Advanced Medicine, School of Veterinary Medicine, University of Pennsylvania, Philadelphia, PA 19104, USA
*   Correspondence: b.brunetti@unibo.it;

Abstract: A 9-month old male Jack Russell Terrier started showing paraparesis of the hindlimbs after a walk. Hospitalized, the dog went into cardiac arrest, and later died. Necroscopic examination revealed a severe thickness of the diaphragm, esophagus, and base of the tongue, leading to the diagnosis of muscular dystrophy. The histology confirmed the marked size variation, regeneration, and fibrosis replacement of the skeletal muscle fibers. Immunohistochemistry demonstrated the absence of dystrophin confirming the diagnosis. Transmission electron microscopy showed disarrangement of skeletal muscle fibers. Finally, whole-genome sequencing identified a ~368kb deletion spanning 19 exons of the canine dystrophin (*DMD*) gene. This pathogenic loss-of-function variant most likely explains the observed disease phenotype. The X-chromosomal variant was absent in seven controls of the same breed. Most likely, this partial deletion of the *DMD* gene was either transmitted on the maternal path within the family of the affected dog or arose de novo. This study revealed a spontaneous partial deletion in *DMD* gene in a Jack Russell Terrier showing a Duchenne-type muscular dystrophy due to non-functional dystrophin.

Keywords: canine; dystrophinopathy; Duchenne; immunohistochemistry; precision medicine

1. Introduction

Duchenne and Becker muscular dystrophies are X-linked recessive disorders, therefore these forms occur predominantly in males. They are caused by genetic variants in the dystrophin gene (*DMD*), the largest gene in the human genome, and as such are called dystrophinopathies [1]. The *DMD* gene spanning 2.4 Mb on the X chromosome encodes 79 exons for a 427-kD protein, called dystrophin, a rod-shaped protein located on the inner face of the plasma membrane of all types of myofibers and anchors cytoskeletal F-actin to the extracellular matrix protein laminin [2,3]. Dystrophin protein has four main functional domains. The N-terminus is the cysteine-rich actin-binding domain, while the carboxy-terminal domain interacts with β-dystroglycan as well as with dystrobrevin and syntrophin. The central rod domain comprises the majority of the mass of the dystrophin molecule, forming a flexible, rod-shaped structure [4]. In humans, a causative genetic variant in *DMD* was found in 96% of Duchenne muscular dystrophy (DMD) cases and 82% of Becker muscular dystrophy (BMD) cases. Around one third of pathogenic variants in *DMD* are spontaneously occurring de novo mutations in the affected male patients [1]. The most common genetic variants within *DMD* are large deletions (approximately 70%) or duplications (10–14%) often encompassing numerous exons of the gene [1].

Mutations may occur throughout the 79 exons of the *DMD* gene but concentrate in major (exons 45–53) and minor (exons 2–20) hotspot areas. According to Leiden's database, ~40% of *DMD* gene variants are deletions of a mean length of 6.5 exons, with exon 47 being most commonly affected [5]. These deletions tend to predominate in one of two hotspots, namely, the central rod domain around exons 44–53 (~80%) and, to a lesser extent (~20%), at the 5′-end of the gene [6,7]. Duplications occur most frequently in the region of exon 20 [5]. Dystrophin is important for the maintenance of the structural integrity of muscle fibers during contraction. Both Duchenne- and Becker-types of muscular dystrophies have similar signs and symptoms and are due to different mutations in the same gene. In human Duchenne muscular dystrophy, variants affecting the *DMD* gene result in a severely truncated, non-functional dystrophin, while in Becker muscular dystrophy, the mutations result in a truncated semi-functional dystrophin protein [8]. The two conditions differ in their severity, age of onset, and rate of progression. The signs of BMD are usually milder and more variable [9].

The diagnostic evaluation of muscular dystrophy often includes a muscle biopsy to demonstrate fibrosis, muscle fiber size variation, internalization of muscle nuclei, and more importantly, the abnormal expression of dystrophin by immunostaining or Western blot analysis. Fibro-fatty replacement, inflammation, and degenerative fibers are commonly described histological features [10]. Similar muscular dystrophies, homologous to human DMD and BMD, also occur in dogs (OMIA 001081-9615), cats (OMIA 001081-9685), pigs (OMIA 001081-9823), and mice [9]. Thus far, 12 different causative *DMD* variants for DMD have been described in several dog breeds (OMIA 001081-9615). For instance, the Golden Retriever muscular dystrophy model is widely used as a useful animal model, because these severely affected dogs show a phenotype strongly resembling human DMD on a clinical and histopathological level [10].

2. Materials and Methods

2.1. Ethics Statement

The dog in this study was privately owned, and samples were collected during the necropsy requested from the owner because the dog died unexpectedly.

2.2. Clinical History and Necropsy Request

A 9-month old male Jack Russell Terrier started showing paraparesis of the hindlimbs after a walk, but he was still able to stand and walk; during the next day, dyspnea developed and the dog was immediately taken to the veterinarian. At arrival in the practice, he went into cardiac arrest, and although resuscitation was tried, he finally died. The owner reported that the dog was originally imported from Poland, and he confirmed that the dog had always been healthy and regularly vaccinated. As a result of the sudden and unexpected death of the subject, the owner requested a necropsy to identify the causes of death.

2.3. Histopathology

During necropsy, tissue samples for histological evaluation were fixed in 10% buffered formalin. Particular attention was paid to sampling the various muscles both affected by the pathology and those that were apparently normal. Diaphragm, esophagus, tongue, thigh (quadriceps femoral), and heart muscles were sampled. The quadriceps femoris muscle macroscopically looked normal.

Tissue was fixed in 10% formalin for 24 h at room temperature, then it was embedded in paraffin and cut at a thickness of 4 microns. The sections were stained with hematoxylin and eosin (H&E) and Masson's trichrome stain.

2.4. Immunohistochemistry

Immunohistochemistry was performed using three antibodies against-dystrophin: C-terminus simultaneously specific for anti-human, -dog, and -mouse (corresponding to the 3′ end of the dystrophin gene); anti-human rod domain and anti-human N-terminus (corresponding to the 5′ end of the dystrophin gene). See specific technical data in Table S1 of supplementary material.

2.5. Transmission Electron Microscopy

Samples were fixed in 1% OsO4 in cacodylate buffer, dehydrated in graded ethanol, and embedded in Araldite. Thin sections, stained with uranyl acetate and lead citrate, were examined using a Philips TEM CM100 Transmission Electron Microscope.

2.6. Whole-Genome Sequencing (WGS)

In order to investigate the underlying molecular basis, whole-genome sequencing (WGS), using genomic DNA isolated from the blood sample of the affected dog, was performed as described before [11]. Data corresponding to roughly 29× coverage of the genome were collected on an Illumina NovaSeq6000 instrument (2 × 150 bp). Read mapping, re-alignment, and variant calling were carried out as previously described [11] with respect to the CanFam3.1 genome reference assembly and the NCBI annotation release 105. The *DMD* gene representing the functional candidate was visually inspected for structural variants using Integrative Genomics Viewer [12]. WGS of the affected dog is available at the European Nucleotide Archive [13] sample accession SAMEA6249497. Numbering within the canine *DMD* gene as reported in the paper refers to the mRNA accession no. NM_001003343.1 and the protein accession no. NP_001003343.1.

3. Results

3.1. Necropsy Examination

During necropsy, on external examination, the muscle conformation was normal without signs of muscle hypotrophy or hypertrophy and in a good state of nutrition. Interestingly, the diaphragm muscles were diffusely severely thickened, contracted with severe fibrosis, and the thickness of the muscle was about 1 cm (Figure 1A). In addition, the muscle of the base of the tongue and the distal part of esophagus were severely thickened (Figure 1B). The heart was increased in volume (cardiomegaly). As seen in the section, the right ventricular lumen was markedly dilated (dilated cardiomyopathy). The left and right atrioventricular valves were moderately swollen and edematous (valvular endocardiosis). Some sero-hemorrhagic fluid (around 10 mL) was found in the thoracic cavity with a severe acute pulmonary edema; the lungs showed multifocal petechiae and hemorrhages; whitish foam was found in the trachea and large bronchi. The sero-hemorrhagic fluid and the lung's petechiae and hemorrhages could be due to resuscitation procedures.

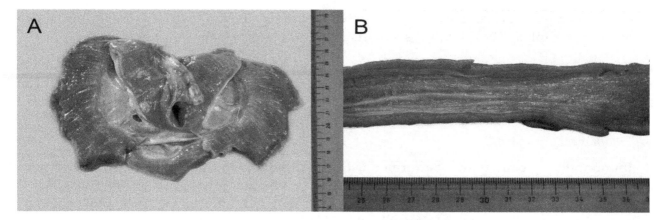

Figure 1. (**A**) Macroscopic image of diaphragm: it was severely thickened until 1 cm in section as well as the distal part of esophagus (4–5 mm thick) (**B**).

3.2. Histopathology

All the muscles examined (diaphragm, esophagus, tongue, heart, thigh muscle) showed marked alterations. In the longitudinal sections, hematoxylin-eosin (H&E) rows of central nuclei in the fibers (regeneration) and fiber splitting (Figure 2A) were evident, and a moderate fibrosis was appreciated and confirmed with Masson's trichrome stain. Cross-sections revealed marked variations in the fibers' diameter with atrophy in some and hypertrophy in others (Figure 2B). Multifocal myofibers were fragmented and hypereosinophilic with a lack of a transversal band (coagulative necrosis) and internal nuclei and were multifocally infiltrated by lymphocytes and macrophages. There was also mild to moderate adipose tissue replacement, and fiber mineralization was rare. In the myocardium, there was slight fibrosis, whereas the lymphocytic and macrophage interstitial infiltrate was multifocal and moderate. A large focal area of coagulative necrosis was present.

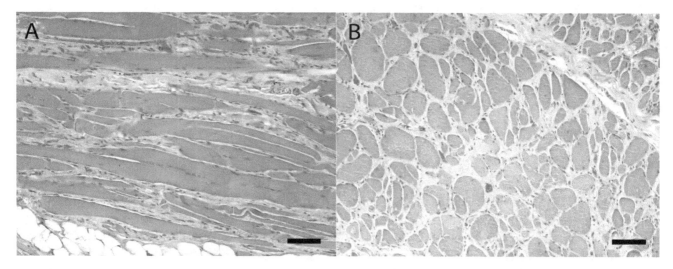

Figure 2. Longitudinal section of diaphragm stained with hematoxylin-eosin (H&E) (**A**), showing the rows of nuclei in the fibers (regeneration) and fiber splitting. (**B**). Cross-section of diaphragm stained with H&E showing marked atrophy in some muscle fibers and hypertrophy in others, and fiber splitting. A diffuse and mild fibrosis was also present. Bar = 100 micron.

3.3. Immunohistochemistry

All three antibodies tested for dystrophin gave a strong positivity and membrane positivity on the diaphragmatic muscle of a dog of the same breed used as a positive control (Figure 3A–C). On the contrary, all examined sections of the diaphragm, esophagus, tongue, and thigh muscle of the affected dog did not show anti-C-terminal (Figure 3D) and N-terminal (Figure 3F) antibody positivity, with the exception of some multifocal revertant fibers. There was weak and multifocal positivity to the anti-Rod antibody (Figure 3E).

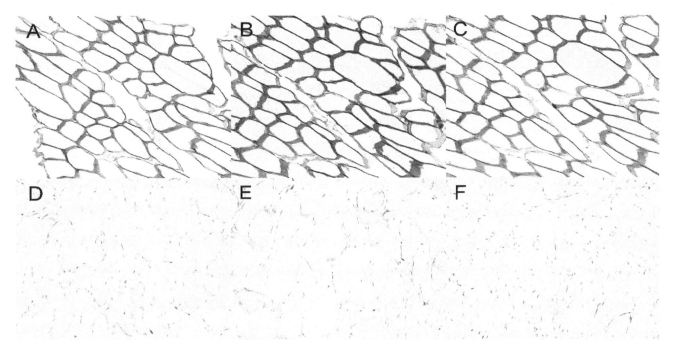

Figure 3. Control dog. Immunostains for the C-terminus (**A**), rod domain (**B**), and N-terminus (**C**) of the dystrophin in the diaphragm of a normal dog showing diffuse and strong sarcolemmal staining (positive control, transverse sections, objective 20×). In the affected dog, there was a total loss of positivity using both the anti-C-terminal (**D**) and N-terminal antibodies (**F**), and a very mild and multifocal signal with the anti-Rod antibody (**E**) (transverse sections, objective 20×).

3.4. Transmission Electron Microscopy

Transmission electron microscopy (TEM) analysis performed on the diaphragm and tongue muscle showed mild myopathic changes as Z-band streaming (Figure 4A) and myofibrillar disarray (Figure 4B) with mitochondria hyperplasia (Figure 4C).

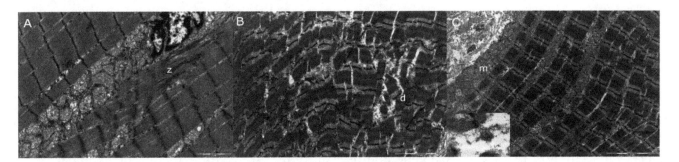

Figure 4. Electron microscopy of diaphragm muscle (**A,B**) and tongue (**C**): mild myopathic changes were seen as Z-line streaming (z), myofibrillar disarray (d), and mitochondrial hyperplasia (m): mitochondria seemed to be increased in size compared to the control (insert). 10,500×.

3.5. Whole-Genome Sequencing

In the region of the *DMD* gene, a large hemizygous structural variant was detected in the genome of the affected dog (Figure 5). The variant encompasses a 367,633 bp region upstream of exon 3, up to part of intron 21. The deletion truncates the coding sequence of 19 of the 79 *DMD* exons annotated in the canine reference genome (exon 3 to exon 21). The formal variant designation is CFAX g.[27,615,280_27,982,912del]. No further single nucleotide variants affecting the coding regions of this gene were detected. Furthermore, the variant was absent from seven (five males, two females) publicly available WGS of Jack Russell Terriers as well as 576 dogs of 125 breeds and eight wolves [11].

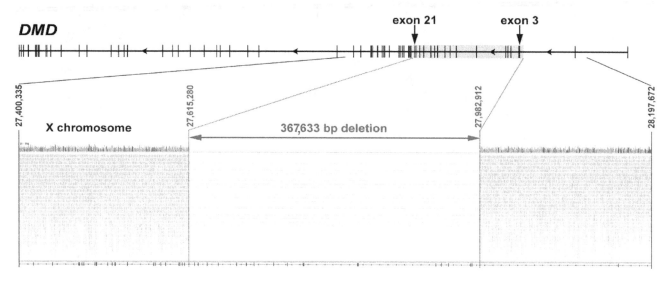

Figure 5. Large hemizygous partial deletion (CFAX g.[27,615,280_27,982,912del]) of the canine *DMD* gene in the Duchenne muscular dystrophy (DMD)-affected dog. The deletion spans exons 3–21 (highlighted by red box) and part of the flanking introns. The lower part shows an integrative genomics viewer screenshot of the region of interest from the whole-genome sequence data. Note the absence of mapped reads (shown in grey) within the region of 19 coding exons (red arrow). The light grey lines indicate read pairs, mapping across the breakpoints.

4. Discussion

This report details a dystrophin-deficient 9-month-old Jack Russell Terrier with an abrupt onset of clinical signs that resulted in death the next day. The Polish owner reported that the affected dog had never shown any health problems before, and apart from the known Polish geographical origin, there was no pedigree information available. The juvenile age of death of this subject was in line with other cases of canine DMD reported previously, with a range from a few weeks to a few months of life [5,14,15]. The great majority of Golden Retriever Muscular Dystrophy (GRMD) dogs do not survive beyond age two [16]. Only some rare cases of similarly affected dogs of up to 5.6 years of age were reported before [17]. The clinical signs probably were not observed by the owner, but in any case, considering the conditions of the diaphragm, esophagus, tongue, and heart, we may suppose that it took place. It is obviously speculative, but we can assume the occurrence of heart failure, respiratory failure, and dysphagia.

It is reported that dystrophin deficiency results in progressive gross muscle atrophy in most breeds of dogs, but it causes a marked muscular hypertrophy in the mice, cats, and in dogs such as the Rat Terrier. Muscle fiber hypertrophy occurs, especially in early stages of the disorders, but extensive fiber necrosis in most cases leads to a general muscle atrophy. At this time, there is no explanation for this phenomenon, although it would appear that muscle hypertrophy is more apparent in animals of small stature [9].

Immunostaining in dystrophinopathies routinely involves the use of three antibodies targeting the different region of dystrophin, namely, the C- and N-terminus, as well as the central rod domain. In these cases, we tested all the three antibodies on formalin-fixed paraffin-embedded (FFPE) tissue of the case and one control dog. The results obtained in the affected dog were very similar to those observed in DMD-affected human patients [18], with total loss of positivity using both the anti-C-terminal and N-terminal antibodies, and a very mild and multifocal signal with the anti-Rod antibody. These results based on the use of these antibodies working on FFPE tissue are important in veterinary medicine, as it is not always possible to obtain fresh muscle biopsies and to then freeze them to send to suitable laboratories. Furthermore, the use of these antibodies allows the diagnosis of muscular dystrophy to be verified on the sample available to the pathologist. It is also possible to work retrospectively on archived samples. The key tests performed on the biopsy sample for muscular dystrophies were immunohistochemistry and immunoblotting for dystrophin, and therefore, the presented immunohistochemistry findings in the studied Jack Russell Terrier are highly suggestive of the presence of a Duchenne-type disease phenotype.

The first identified case of canine muscular dystrophy was in a Golden Retriever in 1958. Since then, various muscular dystrophy phenotypes have been reported in at least 15 other breeds [19]. Therefore, the obtained genetic results confirmed the previous clinical and pathological suspicion of a Duchenne-type muscular dystrophy in the affected Jack Russell Terrier. Different but similar gross deletions have been reported before in the Duchenne type of muscular dystrophy in dogs encompassing the entire *DMD* gene (OMIA 001081-9615) [2,15]; or, similarly to the findings in the herein presented dog, affecting a significant number of the coding exons, as in an affected Tibetan Terrier showing a deletion encompassing *DMD* exons 8 to 29 [20]. Other previously reported *DMD*-associated loss-of-function variants causing canine Duchenne-like muscular dystrophies include structural variants such as smaller sized deletions or gross insertions, as well as variants affecting single or smaller numbers of nucleotides such as splicing variants, inversions, or nonsense (stop-gain) variants (OMIA 001081-9615).

5. Conclusions

The herein reported partial deletion of approximately a fifth of the canine *DMD* gene leads to a true null allele of the *DMD* gene, with the lack of protein expression being experimentally confirmed. The identified deletion variant might have occurred de novo during meiosis of the maternal germ cells and subsequently passed to the offspring as a consequence of low-level mosaicism in the mother, or it may have been transmitted as an X-linked recessive variant on the maternal path within the family of the affected dog. No evidence for further cases was obtained; we can, therefore, speculate that the mutation might also have occurred post-zygotically during early embryonic development of the affected dog explaining this single case. Taken together, this is the first report of a *DMD*-associated Duchenne-like muscular dystrophy in the Jack Russell Terrier breed. This study provides an example of a pathogenic disease-causing variant underlying a sporadic syndrome observed in dogs. Precision medicine using WGS has been proven to be suitable in recent years to help diagnose rare diseases in routine diagnoses in veterinary medicine: to both confirm genetic etiology and to obtain an insight into the molecular mechanisms involved. Nonetheless, the Golden Retriever muscular dystrophy continues to be the best-documented of the canine dystrophinopathies [21]. Thus far, there have been reports of 12 different canine breed-specific DMD-associated variants in the *DMD* gene (OMIA 001081-9615). The herein described phenotype of the affected Jack Russell terrier was most likely caused by the identified large genomic ~368kb deletion, spanning 19 coding exons of the *DMD* gene. This partial deletion truncates 18% of the coding sequence from exon 3 to 21 from the 79 exons annotated in the canine reference genome.

Author Contributions: Conceptualization, B.B. and L.V.M.; methodology, B.B, L.V.M., A.L., V.P, G.C., and M.G. ; software, V.J. and L.M.; validation, V.P., G.C., and M.G.; data curation, B.B.; writing—original draft preparation, B.B.; writing—review and editing, B.B., L.V.M., A.L., and C.D.; visualization, B.B., L.V.M., A.L., and V.P.; supervision, C.D.; All authors have read and agreed to the published version of the manuscript.

Acknowledgments: The Next Generation Sequencing Platform of the University of Bern is acknowledged for performing the whole-genome re-sequencing experiments and the Interfaculty Bioinformatics Unit of the University of Bern for providing high performance computing infrastructure.

References

1.   Jones, H.F.; Bryen, S.J.; Waddell, L.B.; Bournazos, A.; Davis, M.; Farrar, M.A.; Mclean, C.A.; Mowat, D.R.; Sampaio, H.; Woodcock, I.R.; et al. Importance of muscle biopsy to establish pathogenicity of DMD missense and splice variants. *Neuromuscul. Disord.* **2019**, *29*, 913–919. [CrossRef] [PubMed]

2.   Sánchez, L.; Beltrán, E.; De Stefani, A.; Guo, L.T.; Shea, A.; Shelton, G.D.; De Risio, L.; Burmeister, L.M. Clinical and genetic characterisation of dystrophin-deficient muscular dystrophy in a family of Miniature Poodle dogs. *PLoS ONE* **2018**, *13*, 1–18. [CrossRef] [PubMed]

3.   Freund, A.A.; Scola, R.H.; Arndt, R.C.; Lorenzoni, P.J.; Kay, C.K.; Werneck, L.C. Duchenne and Becker muscular dystrophy: A molecular and immunohistochemical approach. *Arq. Neuropsiquiatr.* **2007**, *65*, 73–76. [CrossRef] [PubMed]

4.   Deisch, J.K. *Muscle and Nerve Development in Health and Disease*, 6th ed.; Elsevier Inc.: Amsterdam, The Netherlands, 2017; Volume 4.

5.   Mata López, S.; Hammond, J.J.; Rigsby, M.B.; Balog-Alvarez, C.J.; Kornegay, J.N.; Nghiem, P.P. A novel canine model for Duchenne muscular dystrophy (DMD): Single nucleotide deletion in DMD gene exon 20. *Skelet. Muscle* **2018**, *8*, 18–23. [CrossRef]

6.   Elhawary, N.A.; Jiffri, E.H.; Jambi, S.; Mufti, A.H.; Dannoun, A.; Kordi, H.; Khogeer, A.; Jiffri, O.H.; Elhawary, A.N.; Tayeb, M.T. Molecular characterization of exonic rearrangements and frame shifts in the dystrophin gene in Duchenne muscular dystrophy patients in a Saudi community. *Hum. Genom.* **2018**, *12*, 1–11. [CrossRef] [PubMed]

7.   Duchenne and Becker Muscular Dystrophy. Available online: https://ghr.nlm.nih.gov/condition/duchenne-and-becker-muscular-dystrophy#sourcesforpage (accessed on 7 October 2020).

8.   Shieh, P.B. Muscular Dystrophies and Other Genetic Myopathies. *Neurol. Clin.* **2013**, *31*, 1009–1029. [CrossRef] [PubMed]

9.   Cooper, B.J.; Valentine, B. Muscle and Tendon. In *Jubb, Kennedy, and Palmer's Pathology of Domestic Animals*; Elsevier: St. Louis, MO, USA, 2016; ISBN 0702053228.

10. Walmsley, G.L.; Arechavala-Gomeza, V.; Fernandez-Fuente, M.; Burke, M.M.; Nagel, N.; Holder, A.; Stanley, R.; Chandler, K.; Marks, S.L.; Muntoni, F.; et al. A duchenne muscular dystrophy gene hot spot mutation in dystrophin-deficient Cavalier King Charles Spaniels is amenable to exon 51 skipping. *PLoS ONE* **2010**, *5*. [CrossRef] [PubMed]

11. Jagannathan, V.; Drögemüller, C.; Leeb, T.; Aguirre, G.; André, C.; Bannasch, D.; Becker, D.; Davis, B.; Ekenstedt, K.; Faller, K.; et al. A comprehensive biomedical variant catalogue based on whole genome sequences of 582 dogs and eight wolves. *Anim. Genet.* **2019**, *50*, 695–704. [CrossRef] [PubMed]

12. Thorvaldsdóttir, H.; Robinson, J.T.; Mesirov, J.P. Integrative Genomics Viewer (IGV): High-performance genomics data visualization and exploration. *Brief. Bioinform.* **2013**, *14*, 178–192. [CrossRef] [PubMed]

13. European Nucleotide Archive (ENA). Available online: www.ebi.ac.uk/ena (accessed on 7 October 2020).

14. Nguyen, F.; Cherel, Y.; Guigand, L.; Goubault-Leroux, I.; Wyers, M. Muscle lesions associated with dystrophin deficiency in neonatal golden retriever puppies. *J. Comp. Pathol.* **2002**, *126*, 100–108. [CrossRef] [PubMed]

15. Schatzberg, S.J.; Anderson, L.V.B.; Wilton, S.D.; Kornegay, J.N.; Mann, C.J.; Solomon, G.G.; Sharp, N.J.H. Alternative dystrophin gene transcripts in golden retriever muscular dystrophy. *Muscle Nerve* **1998**, *21*, 991–998. [CrossRef]

16. Vieira, N.M.; Elvers, I.; Alexander, M.S.; Moreira, Y.B.; Eran, A.; Gomes, J.P.; Marshall, J.L.; Karlsson, E.K.; Verjovski-Almeida, S.; Lindblad-Toh, K.; et al. Jagged 1 Rescues the Duchenne Muscular Dystrophy Phenotype. *Cell* **2015**, *163*, 1204–1213. [CrossRef] [PubMed]

17. Nghiem, P.P.; Bello, L.; Balog, C.; Sara, A.; López, M.; Bettis, A.; Barnett, H.; Hernandez, B.; Schatzberg, S.J.; Piercy, R.J.; et al. Whole genome sequencing reveals a 7 base-pair deletion in DMD exon 42 in a dog with muscular dystrophy. *Mamm. Genome* **2017**, *28*, 106–113. [CrossRef] [PubMed]

18. Vogel, H.; Zamecnik, J. Diagnostic immunohistology of muscle diseases. *J. Neuropathol. Exp. Neurol.* **2005**, *64*, 181–193. [CrossRef] [PubMed]

19. McGreevy, J.W.; Hakim, C.H.; McIntosh, M.A.; Duan, D. Animal models of Duchenne muscular dystrophy: From basic mechanisms to gene therapy. *Dis. Model. Mech.* **2015**, *8*, 195–213. [CrossRef] [PubMed]

20. Kornegay, J.N.; Bogan, J.R.; Bogan, D.J.; Childers, M.K.; Li, J.; Nghiem, P.; Detwiler, D.A.; Larsen, C.A.; Grange, R.W.; Bhavaraju-Sanka, R.K.; et al. Canine models of Duchenne muscular dystrophy and their use in therapeutic strategies. *Mamm. Genome* **2012**, *23*, 85–108. [CrossRef] [PubMed]

21. Shrader, S.M.; Jung, S.; Denney, T.S.; Smith, B.F. Characterization of Australian Labradoodle dystrophinopathy. *Neuromuscul. Disord.* **2018**, *28*, 927–937. [CrossRef] [PubMed]

PERMISSIONS

LIST OF CONTRIBUTORS

Doris Pereira Halfen, Douglas Segalla Caragelasco, Vivian Pedrinelli, Bruna Ruberti, Marcia Mery Kogika and Marcio Antonio Brunetto
School of Veterinary Medicine and Animal Science, University of São Paulo, Av. Prof. Dr. Orlando Marques de Paiva, 87, Cidade Universitária, São Paulo, SP 05508-270, Brazil

Juliana Paschoalin de Souza Nogueira and Patrícia Massae Oba
Animal Sciences Department, College of Agricultural, Consumer & Environmental Sciences, University of Illinois at Urbana-Champaign, Champaign, IL 217-333-3131, USA

Juliana Toloi Jeremias and Cristiana Fonseca Ferreira Pontieri
Nutrition Development Center, Grand Food Industria e Comercio Ltda (Premier Pet), Dourado, SP 13590-000, Brazil

Alexandra J Malbon
Institute of Veterinary Pathology, Vetsuisse Faculty, University of Zurich, 8057 Zurich, Switzerland
Center for Clinical Studies, Vetsuisse Faculty, University of Zurich, 8057 Zurich, Switzerland

Sonja Fonfara
Department of Clinical Studies, Ontario Veterinary College, University of Guelph, Guelph, ON N1G 2W1, Canada
Small Animal Hospital, Faculty of Veterinary Medicine, University of Helsinki, 00014 Helsinki, Finland
Department of Basic Veterinary Sciences, Faculty of Veterinary Medicine, University of Helsinki, 00014 Helsinki, Finland

Anja Kipar
Institute of Veterinary Pathology, Vetsuisse Faculty, University of Zurich, 8057 Zurich, Switzerland
Center for Clinical Studies, Vetsuisse Faculty, University of Zurich, 8057 Zurich, Switzerland
Department of Basic Veterinary Sciences, Faculty of Veterinary Medicine, University of Helsinki, 00014 Helsinki, Finland

Shelley Hahn
Department of Basic Veterinary Sciences, Faculty of Veterinary Medicine, University of Helsinki, 00014 Helsinki, Finland

Marina L Meli
Center for Clinical Studies, Vetsuisse Faculty, University of Zurich, 8057 Zurich, Switzerland
Clinical Laboratory, Vetsuisse Faculty, University of Zurich, 8057 Zurich, Switzerland

Herman Egberink
Virology Division, Department of Infectious Diseases and Immunology, Faculty of Veterinary Medicine, Utrecht University, 3584 CL Utrecht, The Netherlands

Raíssa O. Leite, Júlia F. Ferreira, César E. T. Araújo, Regina K. Takahira, Alexandre S. Borges and Jose P. Oliveira-Filho
São Paulo State University (Unesp), School of Veterinary Medicine and Animal Science, Department of Veterinary Clinical Science, 18618-681 Botucatu, Brazil

Diego J. Z. Delfiol
School of Veterinary Medicine, Universidade Federal de Uberlândia, 38405-320 Uberlândia, Brazil

Irene M. Häfliger and Julia M. Paris
Institute of Genetics, Vetsuisse Faculty, University of Bern, 3012 Bern, Switzerland

Cord Drögemüller
Institute of Genetics, Vetsuisse Faculty, University of Bern, 3012 Bern, Switzerland
Institute of Genetics, Vetsuisse Faculty, University of Bern, 3001 Bern, Switzerland

Anna Letko
Institute of Genetics, Vetsuisse Faculty, University of Bern, 3012 Bern, Switzerland
Institute of Genetics, Vetsuisse Faculty, University of Bern, 3001 Bern, Switzerland
Dermfocus, University of Bern, 3001 Bern, Switzerland

Reinie Dijkman
Royal GD, Postbus 9, 7400 AA Deventer, The Netherlands

Ben Strugnell
Farm Post Mortems Ltd., Hamsterley, Bishop Auckland, County Durham DL13 3QF, UK

Katrina Henderson, Tim Geraghty, Hannah Orr and Sandra Scholes
SRUC Consulting Veterinary Services, Pentlands Science Park, Bush Estate Loan, Penicuik, Midlothian EH26 0PZ, UK

Erica K. Creighton, Reuben M. Buckley and Leslie A. Lyons
Department of Veterinary Medicine and Surgery, College of Veterinary Medicine, University of Missouri, Columbia, MO 65211, USA

Yoshihiko Yu
Department of Veterinary Medicine and Surgery, College of Veterinary Medicine, University of Missouri, Columbia, MO 65211, USA
Laboratory of Veterinary Radiology, Nippon Veterinary and Life Science University, Musashino, Tokyo 180-8602, Japan

Aurore Laprais
The Ottawa Animal Emergency and Specialty Hospital, Ottawa, ON K1K 4C1, Canada

Thierry Olivry
Department of Clinical Sciences, College of Veterinary Medicine, North Carolina State University, Raleigh, NC 27607, USA

Matthias Christen
Institute of Genetics, Vetsuisse Faculty, University of Bern, 3001 Bern, Switzerland
Dermfocus, University of Bern, 3001 Bern, Switzerland

Tosso Leeb
Institute of Genetics, Vetsuisse Faculty, University of Bern, 3001 Bern, Switzerland
Dermfocus, University of Bern, 3001 Bern, Switzerland
Institute of Genetics, Vetsuisse Faculty, University of Bern, 3012 Bern, Switzerland

Michaela Austel and Frane Banovic
Department of Small Animal Medicine and Surgery, College of Veterinary Medicine, University of Georgia, Athens, GA 30602, USA

Vidhya Jagannathan
Institute of Genetics, Vetsuisse Faculty, University of Bern, 3001 Bern, Switzerland
Dermfocus, University of Bern, 3001 Bern, Switzerland
Institute of Genetics, Vetsuisse Faculty, University of Bern, 3012 Bern, Switzerland

Katie M. Minor and James R. Mickelson
Department of Veterinary and Biomedical Sciences, College of Veterinary Medicine, University of Minnesota, Saint Paul, MN 55108, USA
Department of Veterinary and Biomedical Sciences, University of Minnesota, Saint Paul, 55108, USA

Steven G. Friedenberg
Department of Veterinary Clinical Sciences, College of Veterinary Medicine, University of Minnesota, Saint Paul, MN 55108, USA

Jill Pesayco Salvador
Department of Pathology, School of Medicine, University of California San Diego, La Jolla, CA 92093-0709, USA

Paul J. J. Mandigers and Peter A. J. Leegwater
Department of Clinical Sciences, Utrecht University, 3584 CM Utrecht, The Netherlands
Department of Clinical Sciences, Faculty of Veterinary Medicine, Utrecht University, 3584 CM Utrecht, The Netherlands

Paige A.Winkler, Simon M. Petersen-Jones and Bryden J. Stanley
Department of Small Animal Clinical Sciences, College of Veterinary Medicine, Michigan State University, East Lansing, MI 48824, USA

Kari J. Ekenstedt
Department of Basic Medical Sciences, College of Veterinary Medicine, Purdue University, West Lafayette, IN 47907, USA

Gary S. Johnson and Liz Hansen
Department of Veterinary Pathobiology, University of Missouri, Columbia, MO 65211, USA

Sarah Kiener
Institute of Genetics, Vetsuisse Faculty, University of Bern, 3001 Bern, Switzerland
Dermfocus, University of Bern, 3001 Bern, Switzerland

Petra Roosje
Dermfocus, University of Bern, 3001 Bern, Switzerland
Division of Clinical Dermatology, Department of Clinical Veterinary Medicine, Vetsuisse Faculty, University of Bern, 3001 Bern, Switzerland

Monika M. Welle
Dermfocus, University of Bern, 3001 Bern, Switzerland
Institute of Animal Pathology, Vetsuisse Faculty, University of Bern, 3001 Bern, Switzerland

Katherine L. Gailbreath
ZNLabs Veterinary Diagnostics, Garden City, ID 83714, USA

Andrea Cannon
Westvet, Garden City, ID 83714, USA

Stephen D. White
Department of Medicine and Epidemiology, School of Veterinary Medicine, University of California Davis, Davis, CA 95616, USA

Kevin Batcher
Department of Population Health and Reproduction, School of Veterinary Medicine, University o California, Davis, CA 95616, USA

Marjo K. Hytönen and Hannes Lohi
Department of Veterinary Biosciences, University of Helsinki, 00014 Helsinki, Finland
Department of Medical and Clinical Genetics, University of Helsinki, 00014 Helsinki, Finland
Folkhälsan Research Center, 00290 Helsinki, Finland

Elizabeth A. Mauldin and Margret L. Casal
School of Veterinary Medicine, University of Pennsylvania, Philadelphia, PA 19104, USA

Suvi Mäkeläinen, Anna Darlene van der Heiden, Göran Andersson and Tomas F. Bergström
Department of Animal Breeding and Genetics, Swedish University of Agricultural Sciences (SLU), Box 7023, SE-750 07 Uppsala, Sweden

Minas Hellsand and Finn Hallböök
Department of Neuroscience, Uppsala University, SE-751 24 Uppsala, Sweden

Elina Andersson and Elina Thorsson
Section of Pathology, Department of Biomedical Sciences and Veterinary Public Health, Faculty of Veterinary Medicine and Animal Science, Swedish University of Agricultural Sciences (SLU), SE-750 07 Uppsala, Sweden

Bodil S. Holst, Jens Häggström, Ingrid Ljungvall and Björn Ekesten
Department of Clinical Sciences, Swedish University of Agricultural Sciences, Box 7054, SE-750 07 Uppsala, Sweden

Cathryn Mellersh
Canine Genetics Research Group, Kennel Club Genetics Centre, Animal Health Trust, Lanwades Park, Kentford, Newmarket, CB8 7UU Suffolk, UK

Grant Morahan
Centre for Diabetes Research, Harry Perkins Institute for Medical Research, University of Western Australia, Nedlands 6009, Australia

Lois Balmer
Centre for Diabetes Research, Harry Perkins Institute for Medical Research, University of Western Australia, Nedlands 6009, Australia
School of Medical and Health Sciences, Edith Cowan University, Joondalup, Perth 6027, Australia

Caroline Ann O'Leary, Mia Reeves-Johnson, Susan Gottlieb and Dianne Vankan
School of Veterinary Science, the University of Queensland, Gottan 4343, Australia

Marilyn Menotti-Raymond
Laboratory of Genomic Diversity, Center for Cancer Research (FNLCR), Frederick, MD 21702, USA

Victor David
Laboratory of Basic Research, Center for Cancer Research (FNLCR), National Cancer Institute, Frederick, MD 21702, USA

Stephen O'Brien
Laboratory of Genomics Diversity, Center for Computer Technologies, ITMO University, 197101 St. Petersburg, Russia
Guy Harvey Oceanographic Center, Halmos College of Arts and Sciences, Nova Southeastern University, Ft Lauderdale, FL 33004, USA

Belinda Penglis
IDEXX Laboratories, East Brisbane 4169, Australia

Sher Hendrickson
Department of Biology, Shepherd University, Shepherdstown, WV 25443, USA

Linda Fleeman
Animal Diabetes Australia, Melbourne 3155, Australia

Jacquie Rand
School of Veterinary Science, the University of Queensland, Gottan 4343, Australia
American College of Veterinary Internal Medicine, University of Zurich, 8006 Zurich, Switzerland

Fabienne Leuthard
Institute of Genetics, Vetsuisse Faculty, University of Bern, 3012 Bern, Switzerland
Institute of Genetics, Vetsuisse Faculty, University of Bern, 3001 Bern, Switzerland
Dermfocus, University of Bern, 3001 Bern, Switzerland

Daniele Corlazzoli
Clinica Veterinaria Roma Sud, 00173 Roma, Italy
Neurology & Neurosurgery Unit, Policlinico Veterinario Roma Sud, 00173 Roma, Italy

Daniela Schweizer
Division of Clinical Radiology, Vetsuisse Faculty, University of Bern, 3012 Bern, Switzerland

Jasmin Nessler and Andrea Tipold
Department of Small Animal Medicine and Surgery, University of Veterinary Medicine Hannover Foundation, 30559 Hannover, Germany

Petra Hug
Institute of Genetics, Vetsuisse Faculty, University of Bern, 3001 Bern, Switzerland

Anibh M. Das
Department of Pediatrics, Hannover Medical School, 30625 Hannover, Germany

Marco Rosati
Section of Clinical and Comparative Neuropathology, Institute of Veterinary Pathology at the Centre for Clinical Veterinary Medicine, Ludwig-Maximilians-Universität, 80539 Munich, Germany
Section of Clinical & Comparative Neuropathology, Centre for Clinical Veterinary Medicine, Ludwig Maximilians Universität Munich, 80539 Munich, Germany

Adrian C. Sewell
Biocontrol, Labor für Veterinärmedizinische Diagnostik, 55218 Ingelheim, Germany

Marion Kornberg
AniCura Tierklinik Trier GbR, 54294 Trier, Germany

Marina Hoffmann
Tierklinik Stommeln, 50259 Puhlheim, Germany

Petra Wolf
Nutritional Physiology and Animal Nutrition, University of Rostock, 18059 Rostock, Germany

Andrea Fischer
Section of Neurology, Clinic of Small Animal Medicine, Ludwig-Maximilians-Universität, 80539 Munich, Germany
Section of Neurology, Centre for Clinical Veterinary Medicine, Ludwig-Maximilians-Universität, 80539 Munich, Germany

Michaela Drögemüller
Institute of Genetics, Vetsuisse Faculty, University of Bern, 3012 Bern, Switzerland

Konrad Jurina
Small Animal Hospital, Tierklinik Haar, 85540 Haar, Germany

Susanne Medl
Small Animal Hospital, Anicura Kleintierklinik Babenhausen, 87727 Babenhausen, Germany

Thomas Gödde
Small Animal Referral Practice, Veterinary Health Centre, 83451 Piding, Germany

Stefan Rupp
Small Animal Hospital, Tierklinik Hofheim, 65719 Hofheim, Germany

Alejandro Luján Feliu-Pascual
Aúna Especialidades Veterinarias, 46980 Valencia, Spain

Monika Linek and Maren Doelle
AniCura Tierärztliche Spezialisten, 22043 Hamburg, Germany

Anina Bauer and Jan Henkel
Institute of Genetics, Vetsuisse Faculty, University of Bern, 3001 Bern, Switzerland
Dermfocus, University of Bern, 3001 Bern, Switzerland

Danika Bannasch
Institute of Genetics, Vetsuisse Faculty, University of Bern, 3001 Bern, Switzerland
Department of Population Health and Reproduction, School of Veterinary Medicine, University of California, Davis, CA 95616, USA

Monika M. Welle
Dermfocus, University of Bern, 3001 Bern, Switzerland
Institute of Animal Pathology, Vetsuisse Faculty, University of Bern, 3001 Bern, Switzerland

Natalie Wallis and Eleanor Raffan
Anatomy Building, Department of Physiology, Development and Neuroscience, University of Cambridge, Downing Street, Cambridge CB2 3DY, UK

Karen M. Vernau, Derek D. Cissell and Peter J. Dickinson
Department of Surgical and Radiological Sciences, University of California Davis, Davis, CA 95616, USA

Eduard Struys and B. Roos
Department of Clinical Chemistry, VU University Medical Center, 1081 HV Amsterdam, The Netherlands

Kevin D. Woolard
Department of Pathology, Microbiology and Immunology, University of California Davis, Davis, CA 95616, USA

Miriam Aguilar, Emily A. Brown, C. Titus Brown and Danika L. Bannasch
Department of Population Health and Reproduction, University of California Davis, Davis, CA 95616, USA

G. Diane Shelton
Department of Pathology, University of California San Diego, La Jolla, CA 92093, USA
Department of Pathology, School of Medicine, University of California San Diego, La Jolla, CA 92093-0709, USA

Michael R. Broome
Advanced Veterinary Medical Imaging, Tustin, CA 92780, USA

K. Michael Gibson
College of Pharmacy and Pharmaceutical Sciences, Washington State University, Spokane, WA 99202, USA

Phillip L. Pearl
Harvard Medical School, Boston, MA 02115, USA

Florian König
Fachtierarzt fur Kleintiere, Am Berggewann 13, 65199 Wiesbaden, Germany

Thomas J. VanWinkle
Department of Pathobiology, School of Veterinary Medicine, University of Pennsylvania, Philadelphia, PA 19104, USA

Dennis O'Brien
College of Veterinary Medicine, University of Missouri, Columbia, MO 65211, USA

Kaspar Matiasek
Clinical and Comparative Neuropathology, Ludwig-Maximilians-Universitaet München, 80539 Munchen, Germany
Section of Clinical and Comparative Neuropathology, Institute of Veterinary Pathology at the Centre for Clinical Veterinary Medicine, Ludwig-Maximilians-Universität, 80539 Munich, Germany
Section of Clinical & Comparative Neuropathology, Centre for Clinical Veterinary Medicine, Ludwig Maximilians Universität Munich, 80539 Munich, Germany

Tamer A. Mansour
Department of Clinical Pathology, School of Medicine, Mansoura University, Mansoura 35516, Egypt

Barbara Brunetti and Luisa V. Muscatello
Department of Veterinary Medical Sciences, University of Bologna, 40064 Bologna, Italy

Valentina Papa and Giovanna Cenacchi
Department of Biomedical and Neuromotor Sciences, University of Bologna, 40138 Bologna, Italy

Marco Grillini
Pathology Unit, S Orsola Malpighi Hospital, University of Bologna, 40138 Bologna, Italy

Leonardo Murgiano
Institute of Genetics, Vetsuisse Faculty, University of Bern, 3001 Bern, Switzerland
Department of Clinical Sciences & Advanced Medicine, School of Veterinary Medicine, University of Pennsylvania, Philadelphia, PA 19104, USA

Index

A

Allele, 29-31, 37-38, 43, 45, 47, 49, 56, 61, 66, 71, 74, 77-78, 82, 84-85, 91-94, 99-100, 103, 128-130, 134, 141-142, 147, 155-156, 161, 163, 165-166, 175-176, 184-185, 188, 192, 194, 202, 206, 212-213, 219-220, 235

Allelic Imbalance, 71, 169, 177

Amino Acid, 9, 17, 36-38, 40, 47, 50, 59, 62, 81-82, 87, 93-94, 117-118, 131, 134, 140-141, 143, 146, 155, 157, 165, 189, 217, 219, 226

Antioxidant Capacity, 1-2, 4, 8

Autoimmune Disease, 89, 94

B

Basement Membrane, 56-57, 60, 62, 64

Brain Malformation, 41, 43, 49

C

Canine Darier Disease, 169-170, 173, 176

Cardiomyocytes, 12-13, 16, 21-23

Causative Variant, 33, 56, 63-64, 66, 71-72, 78, 80, 88, 90, 92, 94, 136, 144, 163-164, 174, 178, 196, 216

Cholesterol Biosynthesis, 66-67, 71-72

Chromogen, 17-18

Closest Gene, 185, 193

Codon, 29, 50, 66, 99, 110-111, 118, 122, 143, 164, 175-177

Cohort, 52, 61, 76-80, 82, 95, 120, 122, 125-128, 130-131, 138, 140, 144, 163, 166, 188-194, 220

Comedones, 173, 177

Coronavirus, 12, 14, 24-26

Creatine Kinase, 147, 151

Crystalline Nephropathy, 35, 38

Cytokines, 2, 4-7, 9-10, 12-13, 16-19, 21-23, 25-27

D

Demarcation, 35, 68

Disease Phenotype, 131, 144, 165, 216, 225, 229, 235

Dystrophin, 229-236

E

Energy Expenditure, 183-184, 186, 192, 205

Epidermis, 56, 58, 68, 169-170, 173-174, 177-178

F

Feline, 8-9, 11-14, 16-18, 21, 24-27, 39, 41-47, 49-50, 52-54, 57, 71, 127-128, 131-135, 159, 191-192, 196, 204-205, 208

Feline Infectious Peritonitis, 12-14, 24-27

Felis Catus, 41, 50, 52-53, 134

Fibrosis, 108-109, 229-232

G

Gene Encoding, 31-32, 75, 89, 147-148, 154, 170, 186, 190

Genetic Disease, 28, 30

Genetic Test, 32, 39, 41, 50, 85, 166, 194-195

Genomics, 34, 40-41, 44, 54, 71, 73, 78, 87, 101, 119-122, 125, 133-134, 138, 141, 146, 163, 167, 179-180, 207, 231, 234, 236

Genotyping, 38, 43, 45, 47, 49, 76-80, 82, 90-91, 128, 130, 134, 161, 163, 165-166, 174, 181, 192, 195, 207, 212-213, 219

H

Haplotype, 44, 46-47, 50, 53, 74, 76, 80, 82, 85-86, 91, 94, 130, 132

Hepatic Transcription, 18, 22

Hepatocytes, 12-13, 18-23, 25-26

Heterozygous Carriers, 38, 166, 219

Homeostasis, 8, 116, 143, 159, 166, 176, 180-184, 186, 188, 198, 203

Homozygosity Analysis, 44, 47, 163

Hyperostotic Disorder, 136-137, 144

Hyperoxaluria, 32-33, 35, 37-40

I

Immunohistochemistry, 229, 231-232, 235

Immunohistology, 17-19, 236

Imputation, 77, 86, 195-196, 207

Inflammation, 1-2, 5, 8-12, 19, 22, 39, 60, 90, 94, 97, 137, 186, 191, 194, 204, 210, 230

Inflammatory Cell, 17

Inflammatory Cytokines, 2, 6, 10, 12-13, 18-19, 23, 27

Infundibular Cysts, 169-170, 174, 177

Interventricular Septum, 16, 18

L

Laminin, 56-58, 61-65, 81-82, 229

Laminitis, 193-195, 206

Laryngeal Paralysis, 74-77, 83-86

Lesional Skin, 66, 70-71, 172, 177

Lesions, 12-15, 17, 19, 21-24, 33, 38, 59, 61, 63, 66-73, 87-90, 108, 143, 162, 170-174, 176-177, 210, 214, 222, 224, 236

M

Metabolic Disease, 32-33, 39, 156, 180, 193, 196, 203, 226

Mineral Metabolism, 1-2

Muscle Fibers, 229-230, 232

Mutant Allele, 56, 61, 66, 71, 82, 93-94, 142, 147, 155, 161, 165, 175-176

N

Necropsy, 43, 50, 68, 70, 99, 108, 209, 211, 230-231

Neurodevelopment, 41, 223, 226

Neutrophils, 10, 19, 68, 172

Nucleic Acids, 26, 68, 94, 96, 122, 146, 179

O

Oxalate Nephropathy, 32-34, 39

Oxidative Stress, 1-2, 5, 8-11, 223-224, 227

P

Pathogenesis, 2, 12, 21-25, 39, 66, 73, 95, 143, 162, 185, 200, 204, 207

Pathophysiology, 26, 179-180, 184, 186, 191, 198, 223

Phenotypes, 42, 49-50, 56, 62, 65-67, 76, 84, 117, 120, 123-124, 143, 148, 155, 167, 170, 180, 188-190, 193-195, 206-207, 235

Precision Medicine, 32, 38, 54, 56, 64, 66, 136-137, 144, 146, 148, 161, 169, 210, 229, 235

Protein Accession, 213, 231

S

Sanger Sequencing, 34, 38, 41, 45, 49-50, 59, 61, 66, 68, 70-71, 78, 82, 91, 93, 117, 147, 151, 154-155, 163-166, 171, 213, 219-220

Skin Biopsy, 69, 71, 150

Skin Lesion, 170

Skin Phenotype, 66, 71

Small Clefts, 173-174

Stratification, 44, 50, 190-191, 194

Superficial Dermis, 68-69

V

Variant Calling, 47, 59, 91, 144, 151, 171, 213, 231

Vocal Cord Palsy, 74, 81

W

Whole-genome Sequencing, 32-33, 54, 74-75, 78, 136-137, 143, 146, 161-163, 166, 209-210, 212-213, 222, 225, 229, 231, 233

Printed in the USA
CPSIA information can be obtained
at www.ICGtesting.com
JSHW060040230124
55870JS00006B/46

9 781647 403751